Real-time Ultrasound Imaging
in the Abdomen

Real-time Ultrasound Imaging in the Abdomen

M. Leon Skolnick, M.D.

Associate Professor of Radiology
University of Pittsburgh
School of Medicine

Director of Ultrasound Laboratories
Presbyterian-University Hospital
Pittsburgh, Pennsylvania

With 386 Illustrations

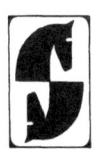

Springer-Verlag
New York   Heidelberg   Berlin

M. Leon Skolnick, M.D.
Associate Professor of Radiology
University of Pittsburgh
School of Medicine
Pittsburgh, Pennsylvania 15261 U.S.A.

Sponsoring Editor: Larry W. Carter
Production and Design: Berta Steiner

Library of Congress Cataloging in Publication Data
Skolnick, M. Leon.
    Real-time ultrasound imaging in the abdomen.
    Bibliography: p.
    Includes index.
    1. Abdomen—Radiography.   2. Diagnosis,
Ultrasonic.   I. Title.   [DNLM: 1. Ultra-
sonics—Diagnostic use.   2. Abdomen.
WI 900 S628r]
RC944.S56   617′.5507543   81-5740
                            AACR2

9 8 7 6 5 4 3 2 1

ISBN-13: 978-1-4612-5921-3   e-ISBN-13: 978-1-4612-5919-0
DOI: 10.1007/978-1-4612-5919-0

Dedications

To the memory of my father, Samuel, who inspired me to write this book, and to my family—Irene, David, Karen, and Eric—who encouraged and supported me through these endeavors

Contents

Preface

Diagnostic ultrasound is changing dramatically because of the development of a variety of high resolution real-time scanning instruments. Until recently the standard instrument was the articulated arm contact scanner. Real-time scanners were viewed as adjunct instruments for specific and limited purposes. The roles are reversing with real-time instruments more frequently accepted as the primary diagnostic tool and the contact scanner becoming the ancillary instrument for use mainly for viewing a large field that cannot be scanned with real-time instruments.

Two recent editorials stated that real-time instruments were used as the sole diagnostic instrument for between 80% [Cooperberg (2)] and 98% [Bartrum and Crow (1)] of their abdominal examinations.

This book introduces the reader to the field of real-time scanning in the abdomen. It presupposes an understanding of basic physical concepts of ultrasound, the appearance of both normal and pathologic conditions as produced by static articulated arm contact scanning, and a familiarity with the techniques of contact scanning. It is designed to acquaint the reader with the spectrum of real-time instrumentation, provide a basic understanding of the physics of ultrasound as related to these instruments, emphasize the special skills required in the use of this equipment, and describe applications of real-time scanning for various parts of the abdomen. While numerous illustrations of both normal and pathologic anatomy are shown, the book is an all-inclusive study of abdominal pathology as demonstrated by real-time imaging.

Obstetrics and gynecology were intentionally omitted from this work. I believe that these subjects are sufficiently broad that adequate coverage would require publication in a separate book. The adrenal gland was excluded because our experience with real-time studies of this organ was quite limited.

Unless otherwise noted, all of the ultrasound images in this book are printed so that: 1) on transverse scans, the right side (R) of the subject is on the viewer's left; and (2) on sagittal scans, the direction of the subject's head (H) is on the viewer's left.

REFERENCES

1. Bartrum RJ, Crow HC: Real-time ultrasound: Its role in abdominal examinations. Radiology 133:823–824, 1979
2. Cooperberg P: Real-time ultrasound of the abdomen: Clinical usefulness and limitations. Appl Radiology, p. 130, November–December, 1980

Acknowledgments

The writing and producing of a book involves many people in addition to the author. Several persons who have been especially vital to the success of this project and whom I wish to individually acknowledge and thank for their efforts are: Janice French, my devoted secretary, for typing and organizing the manuscript; Denise Basara, Abbe Greenberg, and Lois Galentine, our excellent technologists who worked with me in performing the ultrasound examinations; Jon Coulter and Ron Filer, for the artwork; Norman Rabinovitz and his staff for photographic support; and Larry Carter, Berta Steiner, and Ute Bujard of Springer-Verlag for producing this volume.

M. Leon Skolnick, M.D.
Pittsburgh, Pennsylvania

1
Advantages of Real-time Imaging

1. STATIC VERSUS REAL-TIME IMAGING

There are two basic types of ultrasound imaging instrumentation: those producing static images and those producing images in motion (real-time or dynamic imaging).

The articulated arm contact scanner is the main type of instrument used to produce static images. Such images are formed as the operator manually moves a transducer attached to a multijointed (articulated) arm over the patient's skin. The plane through which the image is obtained depends upon the orientation of the arm and can only be changed by varying the arm position (Fig. 1.1). Images produced by contact scanners cover a larger field of view and usually are of higher resolution than those produced by real-time instruments. Image quality produced by contact scanning greatly depends upon the skill of the operator since the transducer must be manually moved over the patient to form an image. Thus, image quality can vary from scan to scan. In addition, since each image takes several seconds to form, highest resolution images are obtained during suspended respiration. Improper scanning techniques, especially during compound scanning, can introduce artifacts into the images, which if not appreciated by the physician or technologist may lead to incorrect interpretation of the images (Fig. 1.2).

In real-time systems, image formation is automatic, and new images are continuously produced many times per second. The transducer assembly can be freely moved over the patient to produce images in any axis, and images can be produced as the transducer is being moved (Fig. 1.3). Organs can be displayed in motion and patients need not suspend respiration during the scanning procedure. Since the equipment automatically produces each new image in the same way as the previous one, image quality is consistent from image to image and is not dependent upon operator skill (Table 1.1).

It is much easier to train a person to op-

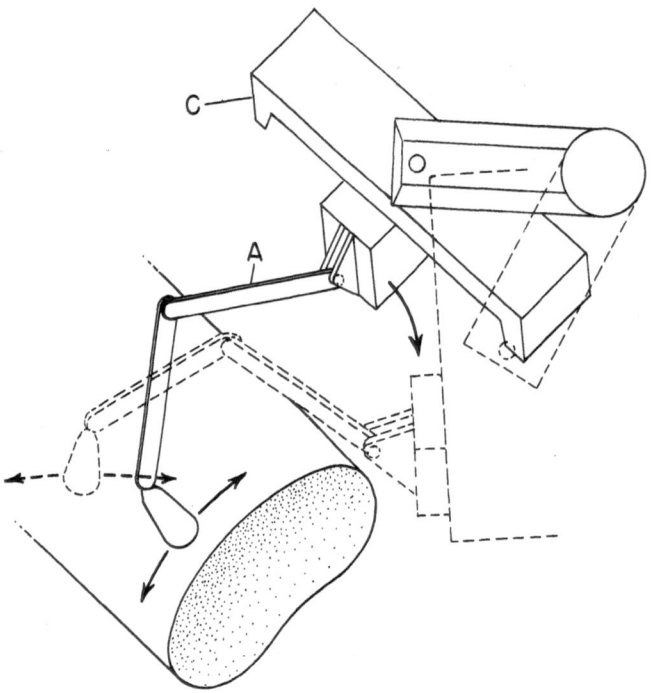

Fig. 1.1. To change the plane of the scan (*solid* or *dotted arrows*) in the articulated arm contact scanner, the entire arm assembly (*A*) and support carriage (*C*) must be rotated.

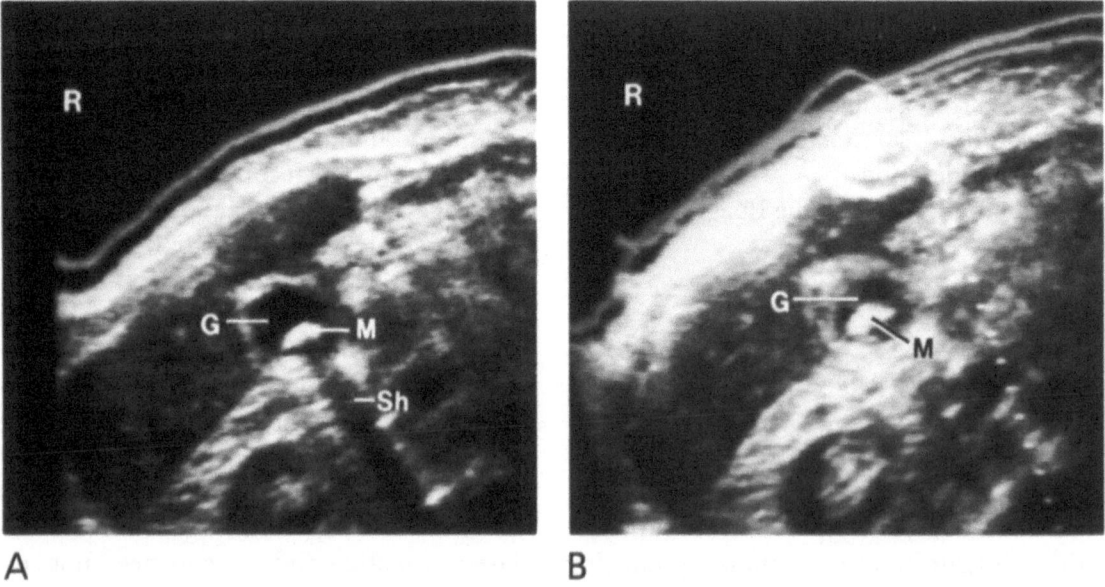

Fig. 1.2. Artifacts introduced by improper scanning techniques. Transverse scans through right upper abdomen showing a mass (*M*) in gallbladder (*G*). *R*, right side of patient. **A** Single sweep scan. Mass identified as gallstone because of acoustic shadow (*Sh*) cast by mass. **B** Compound scan. Acoustic shadow not seen because compounding movements of transducer allow ultrasound beam to reach tissues behind gallbladder without being shadowed by mass. Mass can be mistaken for polyp in gallbladder.

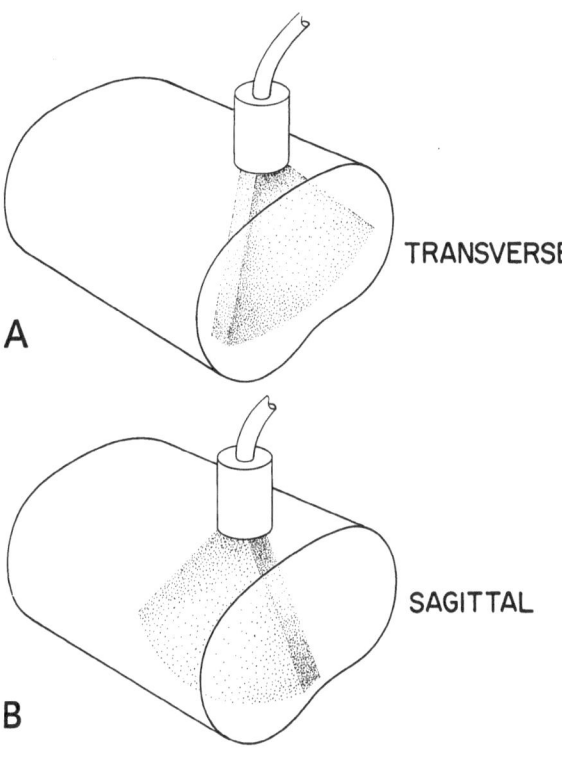

TRANSVERSE

A

SAGITTAL

B

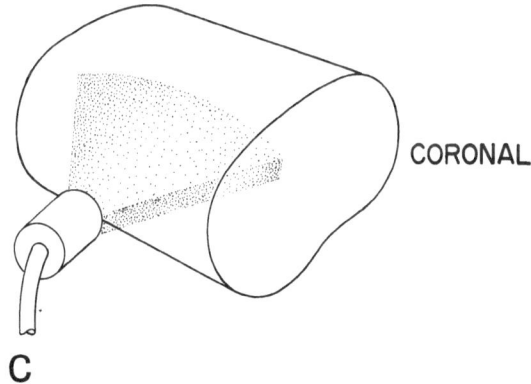

CORONAL

C

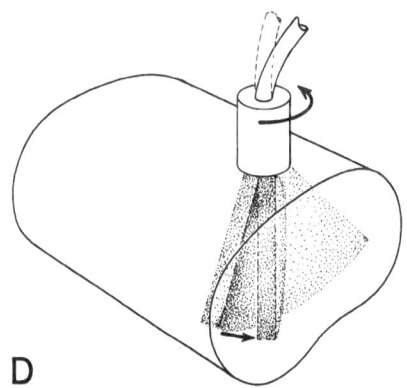

D

Fig. 1.3. Real-time transducer readily allows imaging in a variety of planes (**A–C**) and during rotation from one plane to another (**D**).

erate a real-time scanner than a contact scanner because image quality is unrelated to operator skill. However, a greater knowledge of abdominal anatomy is required of an operator using a real-time rather than a contact scanning instrument because the real-time scanner produces a smaller field of view which makes anatomic orientation more difficult.

The above remarks are not meant to intimidate the reader or to scare him away from the field of real-time scanning. We feel that real-time ultrasound imaging is the most exciting, stimulating, and challenging form of abdominal imaging because of the physiologic and anatomic data that can be obtained without injury to the patient. We only wish to caution the reader that the skills required for the mastery of real-time scanning differ somewhat from those required for contact scanning. Such mastery can only in part be gained from reading texts such as this one.

Table 1.1. Respective qualities of contact scanners and real-time scanners.

Contact Scanner	Real-time Scanner
Large field of view; full cross section of abdomen	Small field of view; rectangular, sector, or trapezoid shape depending upon specific instrument
Image manually produced	Image formation automatic
Image quality depends upon and varies with operator skill	Image quality constant and unrelated to operator manual skill
Each image takes several seconds to form	Many images per second are produced
Images are static display of internal anatomy	Organs are displayed in actual motion
Because transducer is attached to articulated arm assembly, changing image plane is a relatively slow process	Image plane can be rapidly changed *during* scanning because transducer is hand held and freely maneuverable
Large physical size of equipment; not portable	Many units are portable on cart; some are compact enough to be hand carried

Much depends upon actual clinical experience with real-time scanners.

The main thrust of this book involves the operation and application of real-time scanners with hand-held, compact, and freely maneuverable transducer assemblies. Such instruments possess two crucial characteristics: (1) the frame rate is faster than the flicker fusion rate of the eye (greater than 16 frames/s) so that images are continuously displayed in motion; and (2) the transducer assembly can be freely moved over the abdomen to produce images in any plane and with the patient in any position that the operator desires.

Real-time instrumentation comes in different sizes and shapes and produces different fields of view ranging from the rectangular to the sector. For particular applications, a given instrument size or field of view can be much more useful than for other applications. Therefore, it is important for the reader to bear in mind that certain applications of real-time scanning may be most successful with a particular design of the instrument.

There are also several instruments that produce what we call quasi–real-time imaging because images are displayed at a rate of 4 to 12 frames/s which is below the flicker fusion rate of the eye. In these instruments each frame is displayed until it is updated by the next frame. The transducer assemblies are mounted on a supporting arm because they are too bulky and heavy to be held by hand. Although these assemblies possess a considerable freedom of movement over the abdomen, they do not have as much freedom as the truly hand-held instruments. Therefore, their applications are more limited. Specific descriptions of various types of instrumentation will be presented in the next chapter.

One can compare contact scanning to radiography since both modalities produce large-field static images, one using ultrasound and the other x rays. Real-time imaging is akin to fluoroscopy in that both of these modalities produce images in motion and view small fields, but allow the operator to examine a large region by moving the instrument from area to area.

2. WHY IS REAL-TIME IMAGING IMPORTANT?

A. Demonstration of Organs in Motion

Observing motion is important for two reasons: (1) certain types of normal and abnormal anatomy can only be appreciated by seeing organs in motion, and (2) the need to suspend respiration is eliminated. Therefore, patients who cannot suspend respiration can be satisfactorily examined with real-time imaging, whereas during the contact ultrasound examination indistinct images or distortions of organ size and contour may occur because of organ motion during the scan (Fig. 1.4).

Types of motion identifiable by real-time imaging are:

1) Respiratory motion. Typical examples are the changes of diaphragm position between inspiration and expiration or the sliding of one organ over the other, such as the movement of the liver over the kidneys. Absence of organ motion during respiration often implies a disease process. Lack of diaphragm motion may indicate phrenic nerve injury or an inflammatory process in the lung base or subdiaphragmatic region. Failure of the liver or kidney to move with respiration suggests either an inflammatory or neoplastic process that binds that organ to its surrounding structures.

2) Vascular motion. While it is frequently easy to distinguish arteries, veins, and bile ducts by their anatomic positions within the abdomen, this distinction is not always possible by position alone. Intrinsic motion is a helpful supplement. The rhythmic pulsatile movement of arteries can be distinguished from the respiration-induced changing contours of vein from the nonchanging caliber of bile ducts.

3) Bowel motion—peristalsis. This motion is important for distinguishing fluid-filled loops of bowel from extraluminal

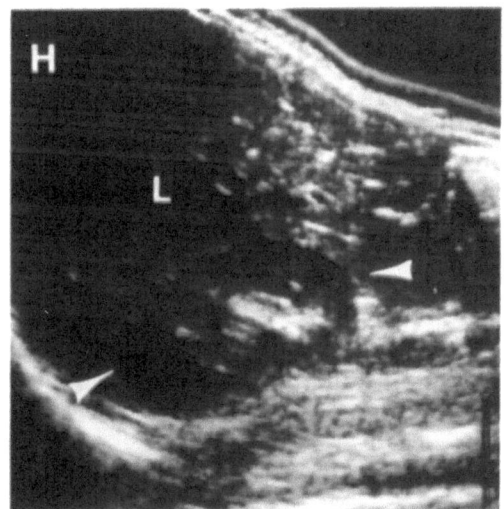

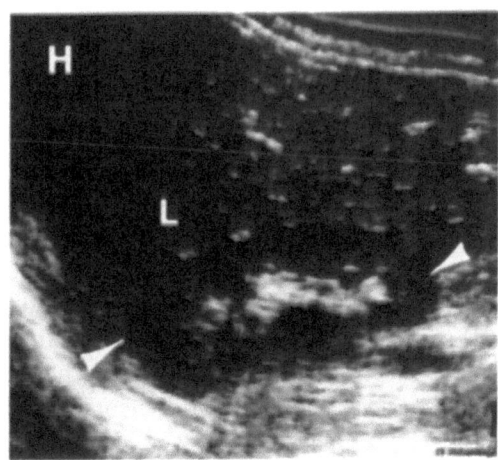

Fig. 1.4. Effect of respiration on organ size. Single sweep parasagittal scans through liver (*L*) and right kidney (*arrowheads*) demonstrating difference in kidney size depending upon whether patient breathes or suspends respiration during scan. **A** During expiration. Kidney appears short because transducer moves in a superior to inferior direction as kidney moves in an inferior to superior direction. **B** During suspended respiration. Transducer movement same as in **A**. True length of kidney is revealed.

pathologic collections such as abscesses or seromas.

4) Fetal motion. The presence of such motion is positive proof that the fetus is alive. The earliest type of fetal motion detectable is intracardiac motion which can be seen as early as the eighth week of life (1). Later in gestation, fetal limb and body motion can also be identified.

B. Abdominal Surveying

Large areas can be rapidly examined to demonstrate normality or to locate areas of pathology. The time required for an examination can be markedly reduced by using the real-time instrument to first generally scan the region of interest. If pathology is detected and it can be satisfactorily demonstrated with the smaller field of view of the real-time scanner, the examination is performed only with the real-time scanner. About 50% of our patients are so examined. Such studies mainly involve the gallbladder, kidneys, uterus, and ovaries. If, however, the abnormal region involves a larger field of view than can be fully encompassed with real-time scanners, then the real-time scanner is used to locate the plane of interest and a limited number of contact scans are obtained to better delineate the abnormality. In this way the real-time scanner helps the operator to obtain the best plane for the contact scan and the time required for contact scanning is reduced. The ability to rapidly survey the abdomen is especially important in the acutely ill patient who cannot tolerate lying on an examination cart for the time required to perform the usual contact scan (20 to 40 min). In such patients, a real-time examination can often be performed in under 10 min.

C. Optimizing Beam Orientation to Organs

The ability to visualize organ surfaces and mass interfaces depends upon the orientation of the ultrasound beam to the surface of the particular structure. Visualization is best when the beam is oriented perpendicular to the surface since in this orientation the intensity of signal reflected back to the transducer is greatest. A change in beam orientation of even several degrees from the perpendicular will produce a very significant decrease in intensity of returning signals. Since the orientation of the real-time beam can be freely changed, it is easier to orient such a beam to the surface of any organ or mass than the beam of the articulated arm contact scanner. In a like manner, real-time scanners facilitate the determination of the size and configuration of organs that can be encompassed entirely within their limited fields of view because the image plane can be readily oriented to both the true long and short axis of the particular organ.

D. Vascular Identification

A given vessel can be identified by establishing its relationships to other known vessels. In vessels that have a tortuous course, e.g., the bile ducts, portal venous system, celiac axis, and ectatic aorta, the real-time transducer is invaluable for tracking the course of the vessel so as to determine its origin and/or termination.

E. Differentiation of Solid from Cystic Masses

To accurately determine if a mass is solid or cystic, the complete width of the beam should fall within the diameter of the mass. A cyst can appear solid if the ultrasound beam goes partly through the cyst and partly through the adjacent solid tissue because echoes from the surrounding solid tissues can be projected within the cyst cavity to give it a solid appearance. Such slight changes in beam orientation that can make the difference between correctly and incorrectly characterizing a mass, especially a small one, are more easily and rapidly made with real-time than with articulated arm contact scanners.

F. Continuous Scanning of Organ Volume

Since many frames per second are obtained with real-time scanning, an almost infinite number of closely spaced scans through a given organ are obtained as the transducer is slowly swept through the organ. Because of the closeness of the adjacent scan planes, lesions that are within the resolving power of the instrument are not missed. By comparison, a contact scanner produces a series of discrete sections that are separated by a predetermined interval, usually a minimum of 0.5 to 1.0 cm. Therefore, it is possible that a small lesion can be missed between adjacent scans on a contact scanner while it will not be missed during the continuous slow sweep through the same organ with a real-time scanner. Small renal cysts and gallstones are two examples of lesions that are often better detected with real-time than with contact scanning (Fig. 1.5).

G. Imaging Difficult-to-reach Regions

Certain regions of the abdomen are difficult to examine with a contact scanner because of limitations of movement of the scanner arm assembly, inability of the patient to change position, or a combination of both. It is almost impossible, for example, with a contact scanner to obtain a long-axis view of the kidneys in the supine patient who has gas-filled bowel obscuring a view of the kidneys on a true parasagittal scan and who cannot change position. In such a situation, a long-axis view of the kidneys can only be obtained by scanning in a coronal plane through the flanks. However, most contact scanners lack the mechanical range of movement to permit the arm to rotate into the coronal plane (Fig. 1.6A). By comparison, with the real-time scanner most of the long-

axis examinations of the kidney are preferentially done with the patient supine and the transducer oriented in a coronal plane (the beam entering through the flanks or between rib interspaces) (Fig. 1.6B). In the recently post-operative patient suspected of having an abscess, it is often difficult to adequately image the surgical area with a contact scanner because the unremoved sutures, partially open wounds, and drainage tubes limit the field of view. However, with the compact and freely maneuverable sector scanner head, the ultrasound beam can easily examine deep structures via the regions of intact skin between sutures and drains (2).

Scanning patients in the erect position, in both transverse and sagittal planes, is difficult or sometimes impossible to perform with articulated arm contact scanners but simple to do with real-time equipment. Erect organ scanning is extremely useful, especially for imaging the pancreas when it is obscured by the gas-filled stomach or colon in supine position. In the erect position the bowel may be caudally displaced by the liver as it descends over the pancreas. Likewise, the liver and kidneys that are partially hidden by the overlying ribs in the supine position may descend below the rib cage in the erect position.

3. RECORDING REAL-TIME IMAGES: PHILOSOPHICAL CONSIDERATIONS

How to record real-time images is easily answered. Still frames can be photographed on Polaroid or x-ray film using a variety of cameras either while the images are in motion (using a fast shutter speed) or after they are first electronically frozen at the frame of interest. Motion recordings can be made with videotape recorders since many real-time scanners display images on conventional television monitors.

What to record is more difficult to answer

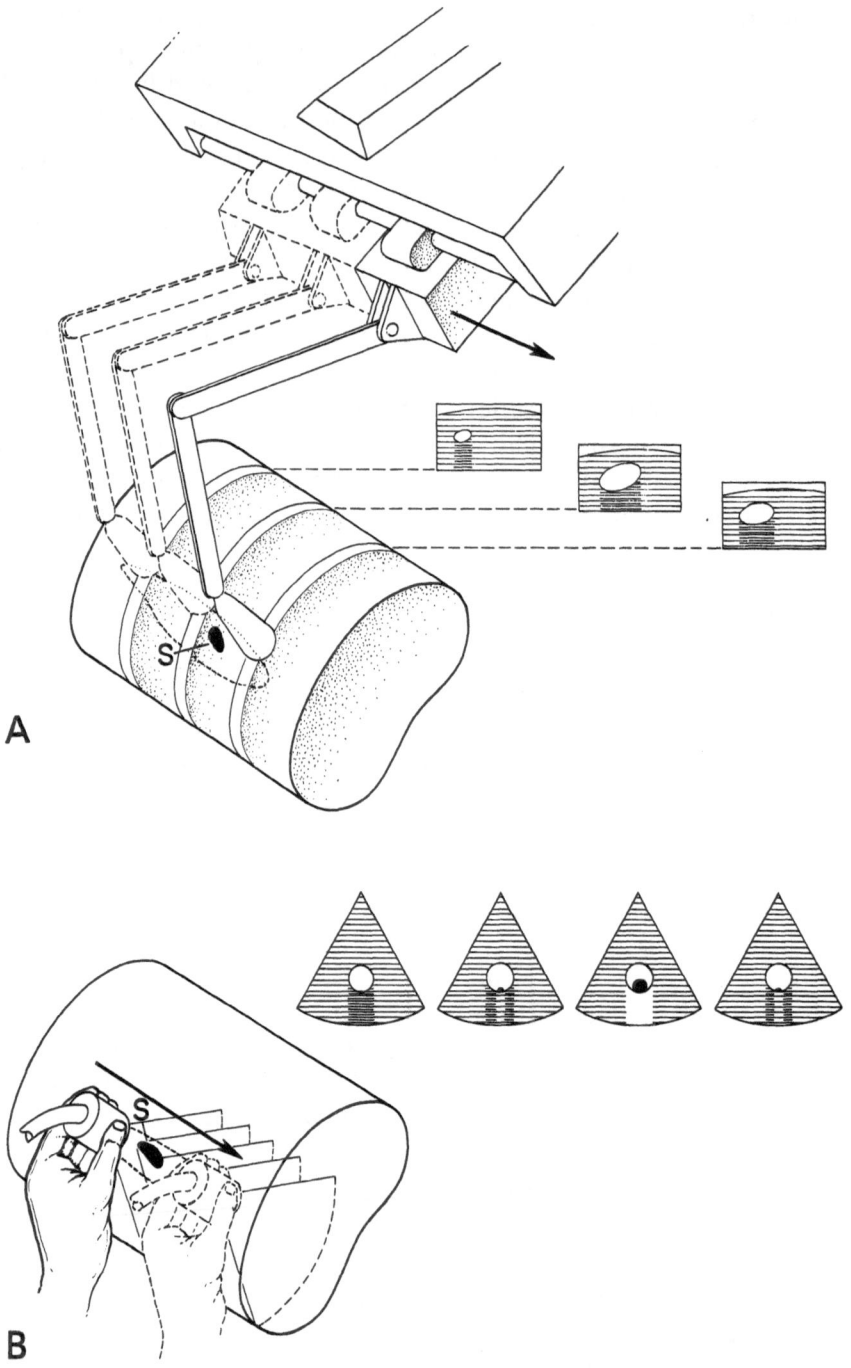

Fig. 1.5. Transverse scanning through gallbladder containing small stone (S). **A** Articulated arm contact scanner. Scanned planes are parallel to each other but separated by a minimum of 0.5 cm. Stone is missed between the planes. **B** Real-time scanner. Beam is continuously swept through gallbladder to produce overlapping or very closely spaced (less than 1 to 2 mm apart) images. Stone seen (in varying cross-sectional diameters) in several scans.

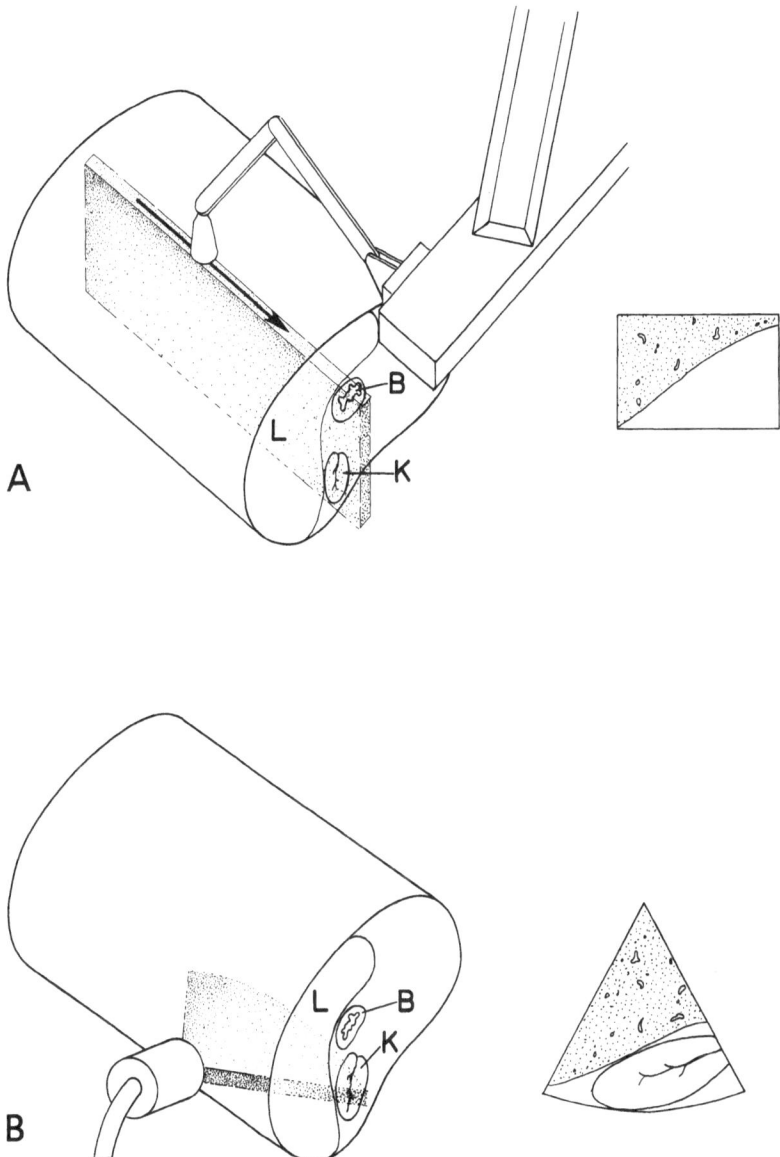

Fig. 1.6. Patient with gas-filled bowel (*B*) interposed between liver (*L*) and kidney (*K*). **A** Right parasagittal scan with articulated arm contact scanner. Kidney obscured by gas-filled bowel. **B** Coronal scan using real-time scanner. Kidney is imaged by beam traversing through liver lateral to bowel.

since the answer is related to who is performing the study. If the examiner is the physician who will interpret the study, the permanent recordings can be still frames showing representative images of normal organs and regions of pathology. The emphasis is placed on the word "representative." A detailed recording of structures is not neces-

sary because the examiner is experienced enough to know what is normal and pathologic. The diagnosis is basically made as the real-time study is performed. Still frames are recorded to document the immediate impression of the operator and to allow him to appreciate more subtle abnormalities upon review of the still recordings. The recording process is analogous to the way a radiologist performs a gastrointestinal fluoroscopic study and uses spot films to record crucial observations or to document regions of normal anatomy. Motion recordings of ultrasound examination on videotape are mainly reserved for cases too complicated for the physician to diagnose during the actual examination, or for teaching purposes.

If the examiner is not the person with the final responsibility for interpreting the study but either a trainee physician or technologist, then the approach to image recording may be different; how different depends upon the confidence that the physician in charge has in the individual performing the study. Many additional still images may be recorded of both normal areas and pathologic regions so that the physician interpreting the case is assured that the entire region of interest has been examined. The routine videotaping of the entire study by the operator for review by the interpreting physician, we believe, is a waste of time. The purpose of having someone other than the interpreting physician do the study is to save him time. That saving is lost if the physician has to review the videotape. He can probably do the study faster himself. However, videotaping can be used to advantage in a more limited application if, after the operator has examined the patient and recorded the still images, a 1- to 2-min rapid video recording of the region of interest is performed. This motion study will help assure the interpreting physician that the entire region has been adequately examined.

4. LIMITATIONS OF REAL-TIME IMAGING

Size of the field of view and image resolution are the two major limitations of real-time scanning. Once again, the analogy between fluoroscopy and real-time imaging is quite applicable. Both modalities produce small fields of view. Although the experienced radiologist can, for example, perform a diagnostic barium enema examination by using only a 4-in. image intensifier and record all images on spot films, it may be difficult for the less experienced radiologist to do so because of the small field of view. Put another way, real-time imaging is very much like viewing a room through a keyhole. In order to appreciate the sights seen through the keyhole, one must first be thoroughly familiar with the contents of the room. Any rearrangement of the furniture that may have occurred between peeks through the keyhole can then be easily appreciated because of the prior knowledge of the total room arrangement. Thus, real-time imaging demands of the operator a highly sophisticated understanding of intraabdominal anatomy. Furthermore, it demands that the operator be familiar with this anatomy when seen in a variety of standard and nonstandard imaging planes. Since it is so easy to apply the real-time transducer assembly to the abdomen in any anatomic orientation that the user desires, a variety of nonstandard image projections can be displayed and the user must be thoroughly familiar with the anatomy in these planes in order to get the greatest advantage from real-time instrumentation. It is often the nonstandard view that makes the real-time instrument so useful since it allows one to image the abdomen through windows often not accessible by the contact scanner.

The second major limitation of real-time scanning is usually the lower image resolution usually obtained as compared to contact scanning. Lower resolution is mainly the result of a lower line density (see Chapter 2). The limitations of image resolution are becoming less significant as improvements are being made in instrument design, and soon they will probably approach the resolution of static scanning systems.

References

1. Winsberg F (1979) First trimester use of ultra sound. In Hobbins JC (ed) Diagnostic ultrasound in obstetrics. Churchill Livingtone, New York

2. Skolnick ML (1980) Clinical applications of abdominal ultrasound—part 1. Surg Rounds 3:24–30

2
Instrumentation

Real-time scanners fall into two basic groups: the true real-time systems with a frame rate greater than the flicker fusion rate of the eye (over 16 frame/s) and what we are defining as quasi–real-time scanners with a frame rate below the flicker fusion rate of the eye. All of the true real-time ultrasound scanners are hand-held and freely moveable scanning assemblies. The quasi–real-time scanners usually have larger and heavier scanning assemblies that require support from an overhead arm.

All of the various generic types of real-time scanners described in this chapter are available from one or more manufacturers for abdominal use. However, most of the illustrations in this book were obtained on a prototype sector-scan system[1] designed and built by Terrance Matzuk, Ph.D. (Pittsburgh, Pennsylvania, U.S.A.).

The use of photographs of specific commercial instruments to illustrate the different generic types of scanners is in no way an endorsement of these products. Rather, these pieces of equipment were chosen either because they were used to produce the clinical illustrations for this book or because they represent well-known examples of that generic system, or both.

1. IMAGE QUALITY

Before describing the various types of instrument design, it is important to discuss certain factors common to all real-time instruments that affect image quality. These factors are line density, pulse repetition rate, depth of image, and frame rate. Since this

---

[1] All clinical ultrasound images not designated as being made on a specific manufacturer's system were produced on Dr. Matzuk's prototype system located in the Ultrasound Laboratory of the Department of Radiology at Presbyterian-University Hospital, Pittsburgh, Pennsylvania.

book is written for people who have a basic understanding of ultrasound imaging, we are assuming that the reader is familiar with the basic physics of ultrasound image formation.

A. Line Density

Line density refers to the number of vertical lines per field of view. These lines can be parallel to each other (linear arrays) or can radiate from a point (sector scanners) (Fig. 2.1). The greater the number of such lines per field of view, the higher the resolution of the image, provided that each line contains new information (Fig. 2.2). In the initial designs of certain linear array systems a relatively low number of lines of new information were used and the echoes displayed on each line were electronically duplicated next to the original line to produce twice the number of lines. The maneuver made the image aesthetically more pleasing but contributed no additional information. However, in more recent designs, this is no longer the case. Each line represents a new line of information and since the total number of lines has increased, electronic line duplication for aesthetics is not necessary.

B. Pulse Repetition Rate

Pulse repetition rate refers to the number of times per second that the transducer is electrically activated to produce a burst of ultrasound. After each burst is produced, the transducer acts as a receiver and detects echoes returning from the tissues that were insonated. The minimum interval between adjacent pulses is the length of time it takes for the ultrasound beam to travel from the transducer to the deepest tissue being imaged and back to the transducer. The distance between the transducer and the patient's skin can be an important factor affecting pulse repetition rate because for a given tissue depth the total length of travel of the beam is less when the transducer is adjacent to rather than offset from the skin (Fig. 2.3).

C. Maximum Image Depth

Maximum image depth refers to the distance that the ultrasound image penetrates into the body from the skin surface. The greater the depth of the image, the longer it takes for the sound wave to reach the deepest structure and return to the transducer. Thus, when the image depth is great, a lower pulse

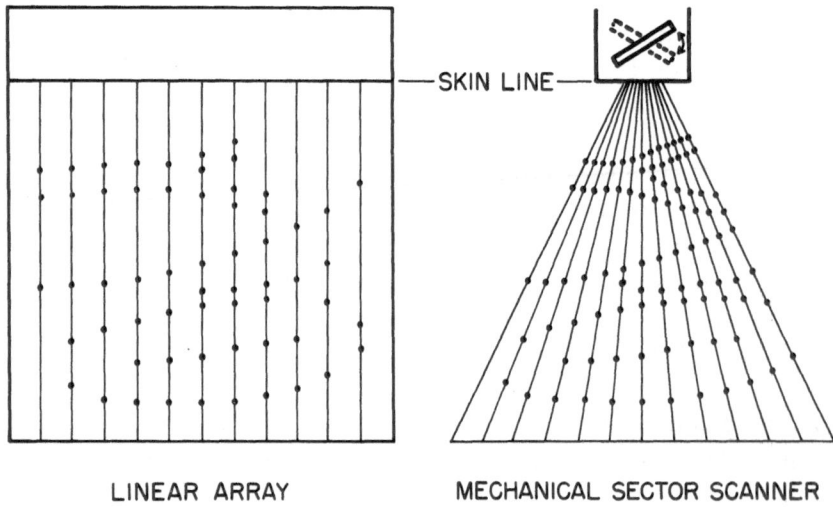

LINEAR ARRAY   MECHANICAL SECTOR SCANNER

Fig. 2.1. Line density versus shape of image.

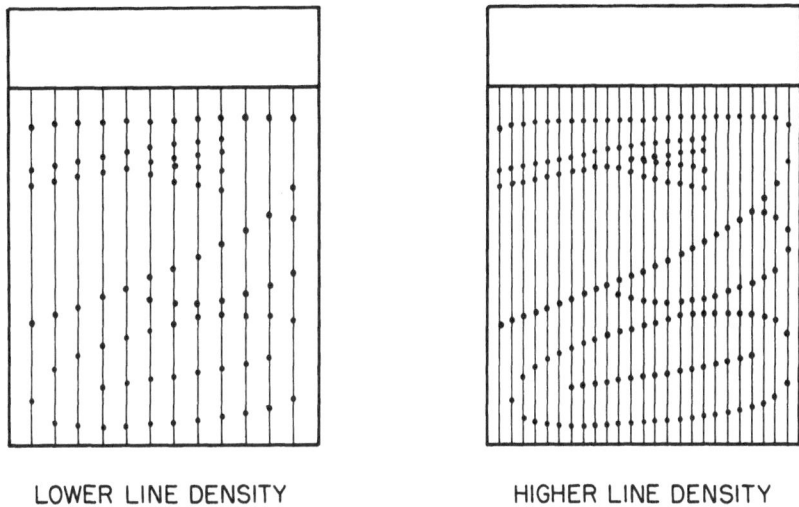

LOWER LINE DENSITY   HIGHER LINE DENSITY

Fig. 2.2. Effect of line density on image definition. Increasing line density improves image definition.

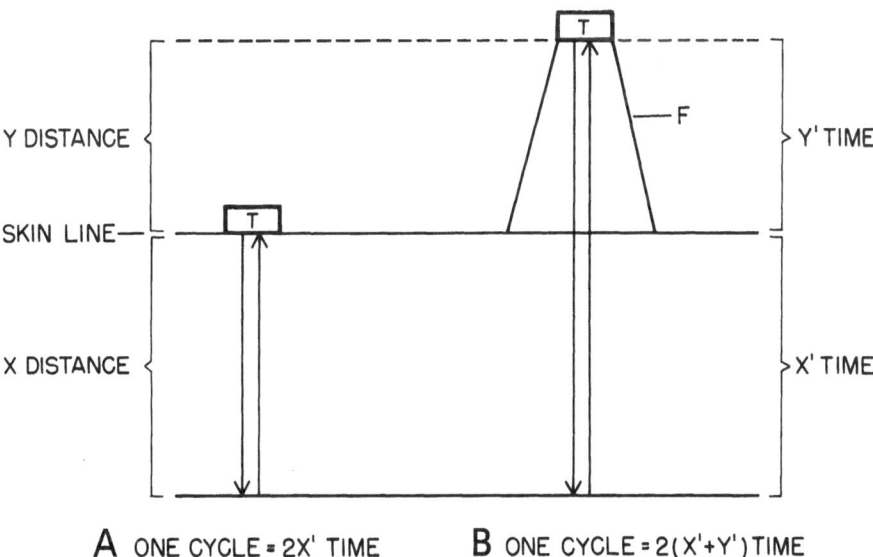

A ONE CYCLE = 2X' TIME   **B** ONE CYCLE = 2(X'+Y') TIME

Fig. 2.3. Effect of distance between transducer and maximum tissue depth on pulse repetition rate. **A** Transducer (T) on skin. **B** Transducer displaced from skin by fluid standoff (F). An increase in distance produces a longer interval between the emission of sound from and its return to the transducer and thus results in a slower pulse repetition rate.

repetition rate is required than when the depth is shallower. Or put another way, the less deep the image, the faster the pulse repetition rate can be.

D. Frame Rate

Frame rate refers to the number of images that the instrument produces per second. The higher the frame rate, the less likely is the image to flicker, and the more clearly defined will be the rapidly moving structures.

E. Combined Effects

Now let us examine how the line density, pulse repetition rate, image depth, and frame rate affect image quality. Assume the transducer beam pattern and therefore axial and azimuth resolutions are constants. If we fix the image depth, then it follows that we know the maximum usable pulse repetition rate because we know the maximum distance needed for the ultrasound beam to travel

from the transducer to the deepest part of the image and back to the transducer. Our two remaining variables, frame rate and line density, are inversely related to each other for any given depth. Each of these factors affects image quality in different ways. The faster frame rates are better for appreciating changing patterns of motion in rapidly moving structures. When image detail within the individual frame is the prime requisite, high line density is more important than high frame rate (Fig. 2.4).

If the image depth were reduced, then the distance and, therefore, the time for a round trip travel of the ultrasound beam is reduced, and the pulse repetition rate can be increased. The increase in pulse repetition rate produces an increased line density and thus an improvement in image quality.

Another variable affecting image quality that is found in sector scanners is the angle of the sector image. The smaller the sector angle, the smaller the field of view. However, sector angle and line density are intimately related. For a given pulse repetition rate and frame rate, reducing the sector angle increases the line density because, for the same

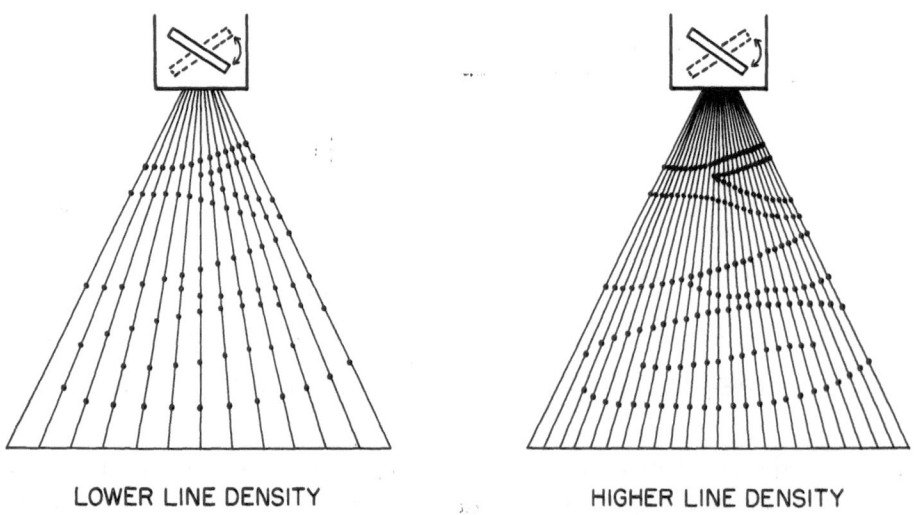

LOWER LINE DENSITY   HIGHER LINE DENSITY

Fig. 2.4. Factors affecting line density in mechanical sector scanner with constant scan angle. Lower line density produced by increasing frame rate or decreasing pulse repetition rate. Higher line density produced by decreasing frame rate or increasing pulse repetition rate.

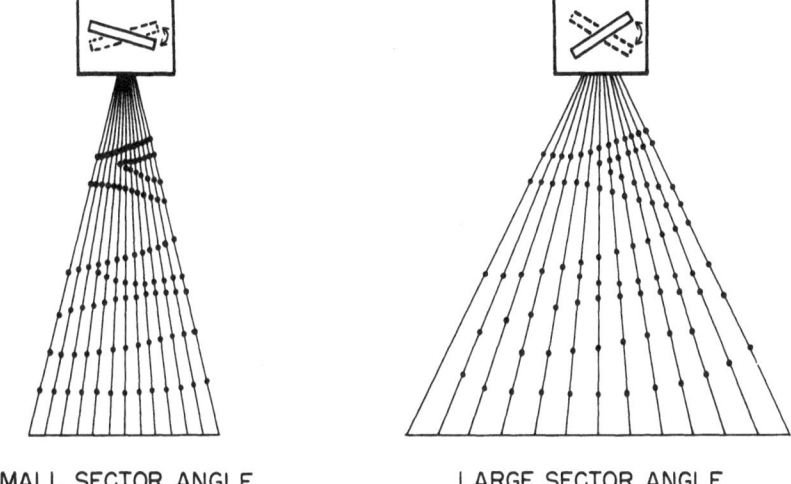

SMALL SECTOR ANGLE   LARGE SECTOR ANGLE

Fig. 2.5. Effect of sector angle on line density in mechanical scanner. Frame rate and pulse repetition rate are constant. Smaller sector angle gives greater line density. Larger sector angle gives lesser line density.

time, the beam travels through a smaller arc and the distance that the beam rotates between adjacent individual lines become closer together (Fig. 2.5).

Image quality is also affected by the axial and azimuth resolutions of the ultrasound beam which are in turn related to the shape and the frequency of the beam. In the hand-held sector scanners which utilize a single-element, mechanically moving transducer to produce the ultrasound beam, both frequency and focus are fixed for a given transducer. Focus is determined by the curvature ground into the transducer element, by the use of a plastic lens placed in front of the transducer, or by both. Frequency and focus can be changed by changing the transducer assembly or sometimes just the transducer element. In some systems, in order to improve the gray scale dynamic range, the frequency of the pulser and the receiver are changed when the transducer frequency is changed.

Among the hand-held real-time instruments, there are two basic varieties: mechanical scanners and electronic arrays.

2. MECHANICAL SCANNERS

Although there are several variations in design, the common features of all these instruments are (1) the image is displayed in a sector format encompassing an arc between 45° and 90°; and (2) the image is produced by a single-element transducer that physically is moved through this arc (either directly in contact with the skin or within a fluid-filled case).

A. Overview

The advantages of the mechanical scanners are (1) a relatively large-diameter transducer can be used for a good beam focus; (2) the amount of electronics is minimized since only one transducer is energized at any one time; (3) the design and construction of the transducer head is relatively simple, especially in those systems utilizing a single transducer; and (4) the ease in some instruments, especially the servo-controlled enclosed sector scanner, with which frame rate and the sector angle can be varied so as to optimize equipment parameters to specific clinical conditions. For higher resolution, a smaller sector angle is indicated, and to obtain the maximum field of view a larger angle is needed.

The major disadvantage of hand-held mechanical sector scanners is that the beam pattern is fixed for a given transducer. Since the transducers are single element crystals (rather than multielements as in the phased or annular arrays) the only way to change beam pattern is by connecting a different transducer to the scanner.

B. Oscillating Transducers—Unenclosed Crystal

A single transducer crystal is oscillated through a predetermined angle. The rate of oscillation (frame rate) and angle of oscilla-

tion may be varied by the operator. The transducer is oscillated by an external motor that is connected to the transducer by gears and/or levers (Fig. 2-6A) (1). In these designs, the oscillating transducer is in direct contact with the patient's skin. During operation, both the patient and operator feel vibrations from the instrument—the patient from the transducer oscillating on his skin and the operator from the vibrations of the motor and drive mechanism that cause the transducer to reverse its direction many times a second. These vibrations may produce discomfort in some patients and hand fatigue in some operators. The vibrations can be somewhat reduced by placing a fluid-filled thin plastic bag resembling a blister in front of the oscillating transducer to dampen its movements. Because the transducer element is exposed, it is easy for the operator to change frequencies or focal lengths just by changing transducer ele-

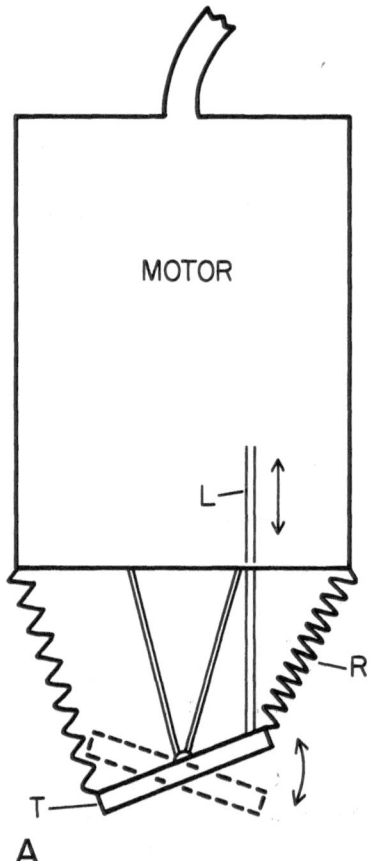

MOTOR

L —

R

T —

A

Fig. 2.6. Oscillating transducer; unenclosed crystal. **A** Rotatory movement of motor is converted to oscillatory transducer motion by mechanical linkage (*L*) connecting motor to transducer (*T*). Rubber boot (*R*) protects drive mechanism from ultrasonic coupling agents. **B** Example of commercial system: Picker sector view (Picker Corporation, Northford, Connecticut). **C** Sagittal section, upper abdomen (sector view scanner). *L*, liver; *K*, right kidney; *D*, diaphragm; *H*, direction of patient's head. **B** and **C** Courtesy of Picker Corporation. (**B** and **C** on page 19.)

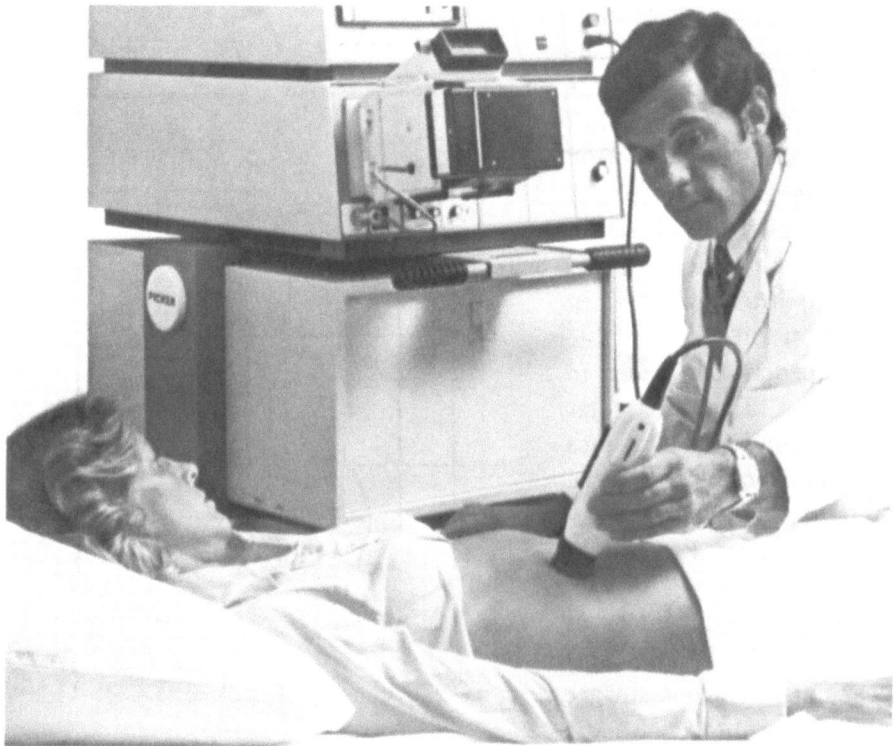

B

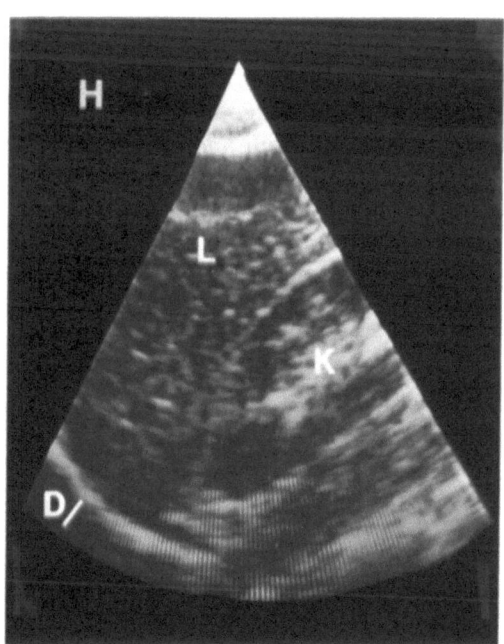

C

C. Oscillating Transducers—Enclosed Crystal

Another variation of a sector scanner is one in which the transducer is enclosed in a fluid-filled container. It may be driven by an external motor or the transducer, and its backing may form the armature of the motor that actually oscillates the transducer. In this latter situation there is no external motor to move the transducer. The transducer is attached to a disk of rubber permanent magnet material that is mounted across the poles of an electromagnet. By changing the direction of the current flowing through the coils of the electromagnet, the magnet disk and transducer are made to oscillate. A position-sending device (servo control) is attached to the back of the transducer, which indicates to the electronic drive circuits controlling the motor the exact position of the transducer at every instant in time. The servo-

ments. An example of such equipment and the images it produces are shown in Fig. 2.6B and C.

control system ensures that the transducer moves at a uniform velocity throughout its entire arcuate path and also allows the operator to stop the transducer at any point in the arc in order to obtain a time-motion display from that ray (Fig. 2.7A). Castor oil, rather than water, is used as the fluid within the container so as to reduce the intensity of the reflections at the interface between the fluid and skin. Castor oil is preferable because its acoustic impedence is closer to tissue than that of water. This particular system was designed and built by Terrance Matzuk, Ph.D., of Pittsburgh, Pennsylvania, and the first prototype was installed at Presbyterian-University Hospital, Pittsburgh, Pennsylvania.[2]

The geometry of the ultrasound image in this system depends upon the distance between the transducer and the front surface of the case (the surface in contact with the patient). When the transducer is placed just behind the front surface, a sector image is produced. When the transducer is placed several centimeters behind the front surface, a trapezoid image is produced which gives a larger area of view in the near field since the apex of the sector is now significantly displaced above the surface of the skin (Fig. 2.7B–D). The diameter of the front surface of the case is greater in this configuration in order not to reduce the sector angle of the image.

This system is vibration free, both to the patient and to the operator. The patient feels no vibration because the transducer element does not touch the skin. The operator feels no vibration because the only moving part is the transducer and its mass is too little compared to the mass of the case to produce vibrations. The entire system is illustrated in Fig. 2.7E.

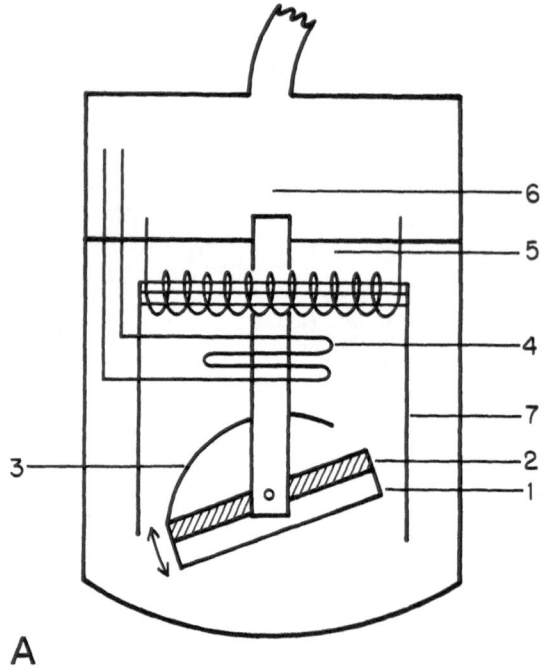

A

Fig. 2.7. Oscillating transducer; enclosed crystal. **A** Schematic diagram. Transducer element (*1*) is mounted on permanent magnet disc. (*2*) that rotates on bearings attached to column (*6*). Wire coil (*5*) and magnetic pole pieces (*7*) form field magnet of motor. Varying the strength and direction of current through coil (*5*) changes the speed and direction of movement of the transducer. The position of the transducer at every locus in its arc is monitored by a tapered and curved aluminum vane (*3*) that induces a voltage in a position-sensing coil (*4*) which varies with the position of the vane (servo-control system). **B** Field of view; sector versus trapezoid transducer. **C** Sector transducer assembly (*S*); trapezoid transducer assembly (*T*). **D** Sagittal images of right kidney (*K*) and liver (*L*) produced by sector and trapezoid assemblies. *H*, direction of patient's head. **E** Prototype servo-controlled sector scanner in use at Presbyterian-University Hospital, Radiology Department, Pittsburgh, Pennsylvania. System designed and built by Terrance Matzuk, Ph.D.

---

[2] One version of this transducer is commercially available from Philips Medical Systems, Shelton, Connecticut, for abdominal applications.

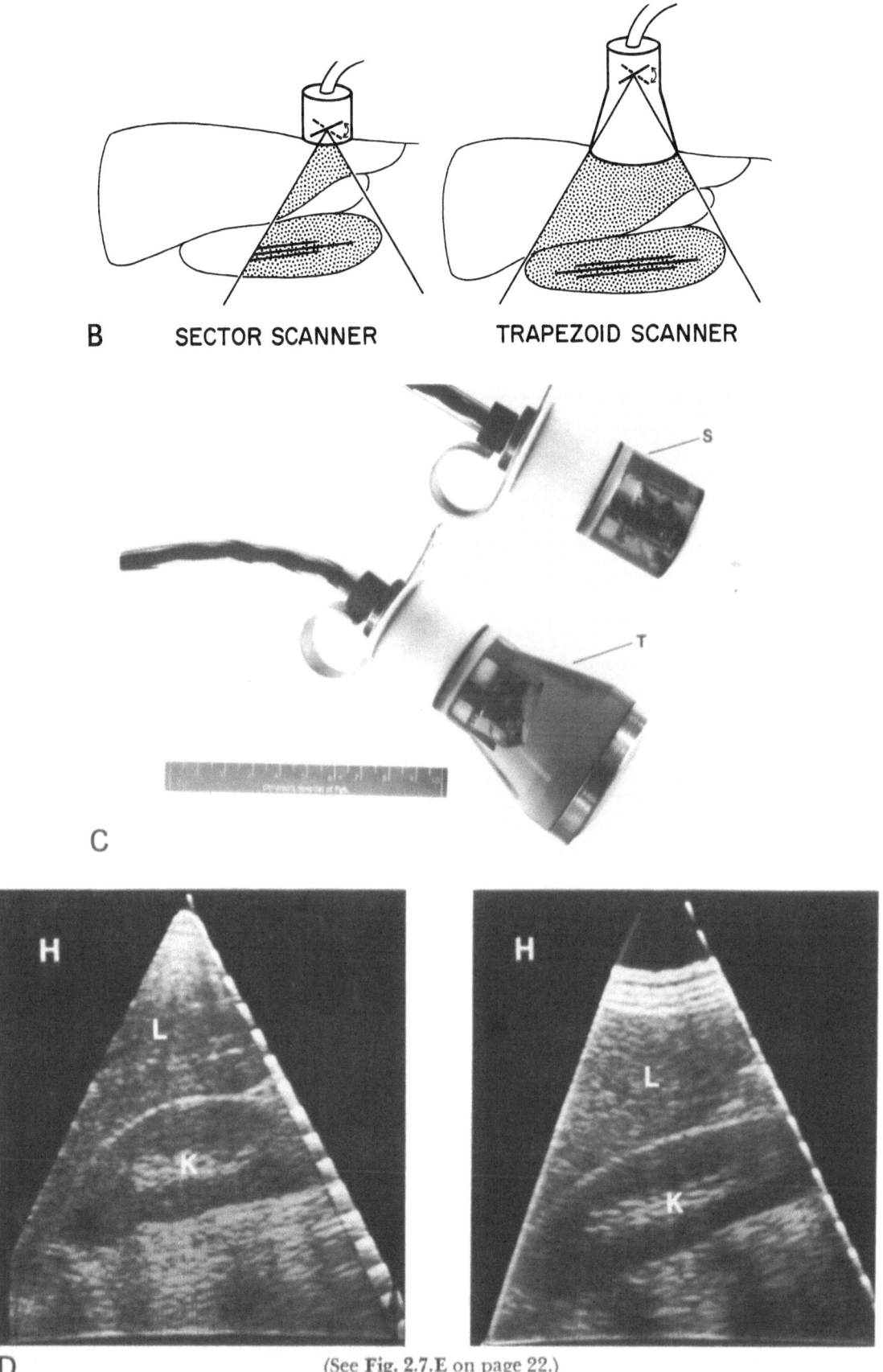

B   SECTOR SCANNER   TRAPEZOID SCANNER

C

D   (See **Fig. 2.7.E** on page 22.)

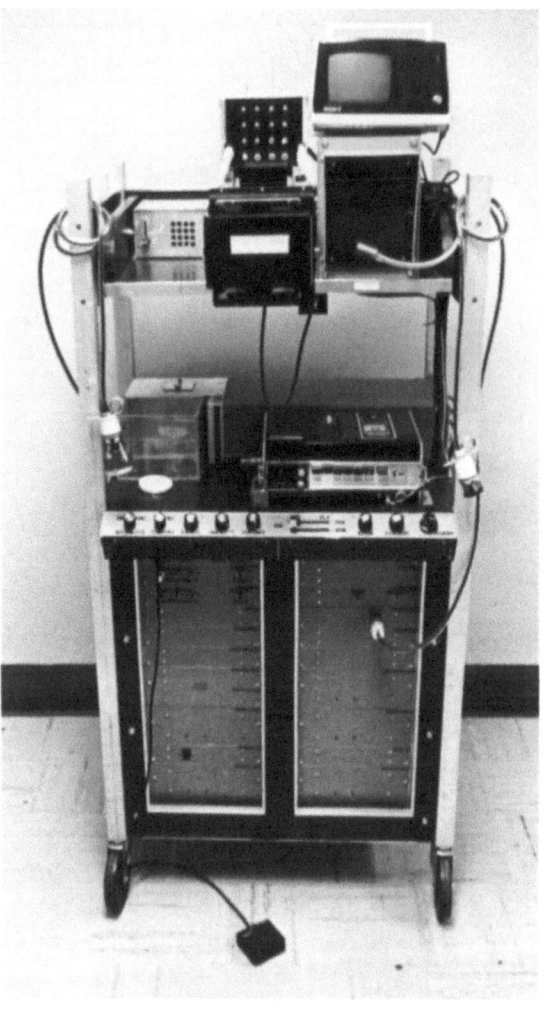

Fig. 2.7.E.

D. Rotating Wheel Transducer

In this design three to four transducer elements are mounted on a wheel and spaced either 120° or 90° apart. The wheel is between approximately 2 and 5 cm in diameter and rotates within an enclosed case in one direction, being driven by an external motor. The ultrasound beam emerges through an acoustically transparent window along the lower surface of the case enclosing the wheel. As the wheel rotates, an electric switching mechanism allows only the transducer behind the acoustic window to transmit and receive ultrasound waves. Thus, each transducer is active for one-third or one-fourth of the time that is necessary for one rotation

of the wheel. Since the wheel rotates in one direction, the transducer housing has no perceptible vibration and is comfortable both to the patient and the operator.

There are several variations in design of this transducer assembly. The rotating wheel upon which the transducers are mounted can be mounted in line with the drive motor, oriented 90° to the axis of the motor, or offset but still parallel to the motor (Fig. 2.8A). An example of a commercial unit and the image it produces are presented in Fig. 2.8B and C.

3. ELECTRONIC ARRAYS

In these systems many small rectangular transducer elements (approximately 2×10 mm per element) are arranged adjacent to each other within the transducer head. The individual elements do not function as discrete transducers. Rather, groups of elements are electronically fired at or almost at the same time so as to approximate the characteristics of a single larger-size element. However, by rapidly changing the sequence for pulsing elements within a group, or by changing the pulsing of adjacent groups, the beam can be rapidly shifted through a plane without the need to actually mechanically move the transducer crystal.

There are two basic types of arrays: linear and phased.

A. Linear Arrays

A series of discrete transducer elements are arranged adjacent to each other along their narrow dimension to form a transducer assembly about 4 to 10 cm in length. Depending upon the design, the individual number of elements can vary between approximately 64 and 200. The width of the field of view produced by the linear array is equal to the

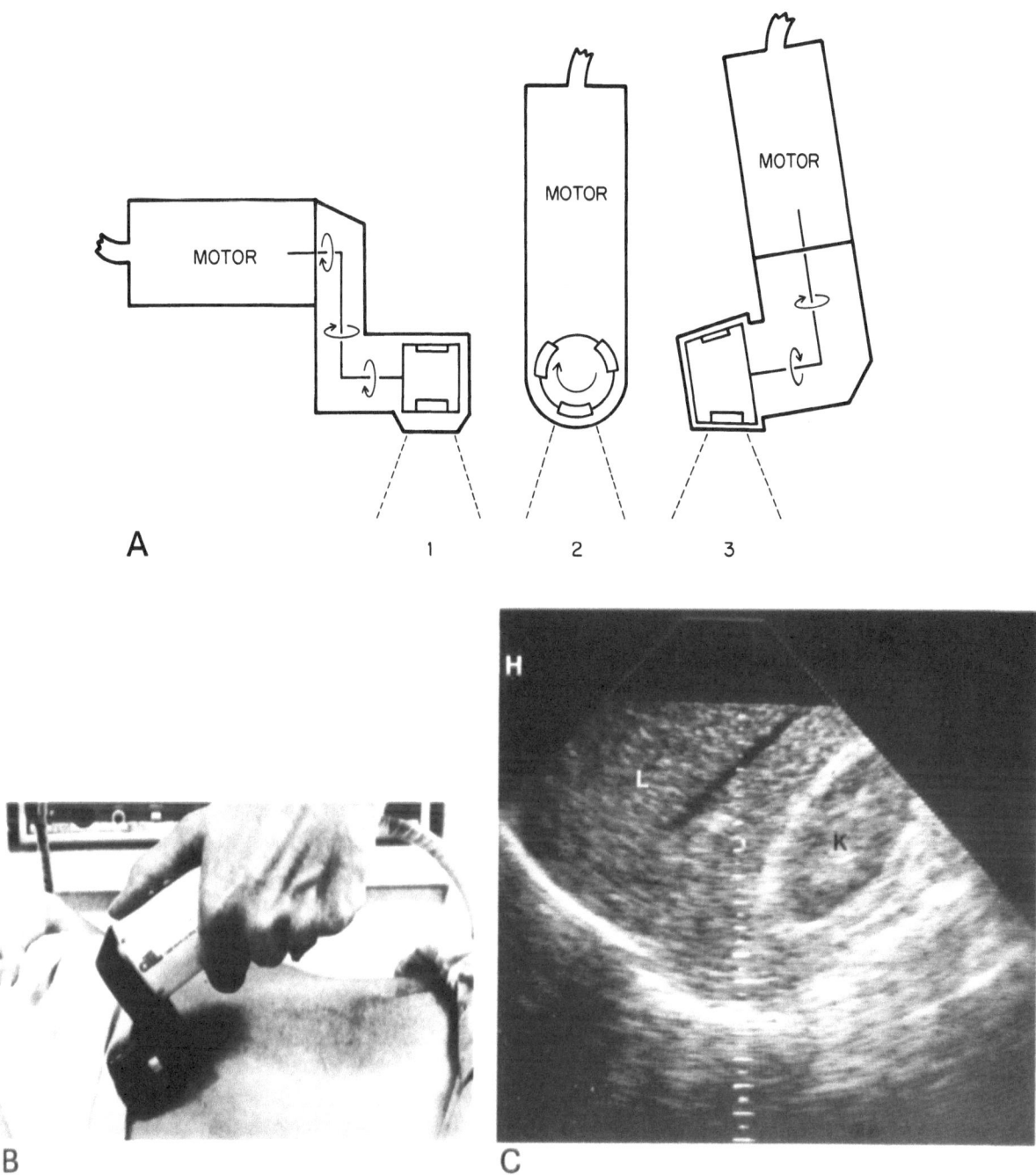

Fig. 2.8. Rotating wheel transducer. Multiple transducers are mounted on a rotating drum driven by an external motor. A sector or trapezoid display is formed as the transducers sweep a beam through an acoustic window. **A** Variations in transducer design: *1,* drum offset but parallel to motor; *2,* drum mounted in line with motor; *3,* drum oriented 90° to motor. **B** Commercial example of scanner assembly manufactured by ATL (Advanced Technology Laboratories, Inc., Seattle, Washington). **C** Sagittal scan through right lobe of liver (*L*) and right kidney (*K*). Apex of image electronically blanked off the monitor (ATL scanner). **B** and **C** Courtesy of ATL, Inc.

physical length of the array. Each array operates at a single frequency, but arrays can be constructed at different frequencies for different applications.

If each element of the array were fired individually, a very poor beam pattern would result because the narrower the width of the element, the more the beam disperses. Therefore, several elements are pulsed at one time in order to produce a beam pattern similar to that obtained from the pulsing of a larger single-element transducer (Fig. 2.9A) (3). For example, the first three transducers are electrically pulsed together, then the second through fourth are pulsed, then the third through fifth, and so on. In other words, groups of individual transducers are fired together to form larger functional elements (Fig. 2.9B). The entire array is pulsed in approximately 1/20 to 1/50 s so as to produce between 20 and 50 frames/s, depending upon the circuitry. The line density of the linear arrays depends upon the number of discrete elements within the array, the number of elements pulsed at one time, and the sequence of pulsing.

The beam produced by the linear array is usually focused with a cylindrical lens placed in front of the transducer elements. This fixed-focus lens determines the azimuth resolution in the plane perpendicular to the

image plane and determines the thickness of the image slice (Fig. 2.9D). The azimuth resolution in the image plane is determined by the number of elements pulsed together and the transducer frequency.

To improve the azimuth resolution in the image plane, the method of pulsing the individual transducer elements within each group is changed. When all elements in a group are pulsed at the same time, the resultant wave front behaves like a nonfocused single-element transducer equal in diameter to the width of all the elements in the group (Fig. 2.9A). However, when the central elements in a group are pulsed several nanoseconds (10^{-9} s) after the elements on either side, then a focused beam is produced (Fig. 2.9C and D) (4). This time delay is much shorter than the time it takes for the ultrasound beam to make a round trip from the crystal into the patient and back to the crystal, which is approximately 260 μs (10^{-6} s) for a 20-cm tissue depth. By comparison, the interval between the pulsing of adjacent groups of elements is between 300 and 1000 μs. The depth at which the beam focuses and the sharpness of focus are related to the delay between the pulsing of the central and outer elements of the group. Thus, the time interval between the pulsing of individual transducer elements within a group to focus the

Fig. 2.9. Linear arrays. **A** Pulsing a single element (*E*) gives a wider beam pattern than the simultaneous pulsing of multiple adjacent elements (*E-E-E-E*) since when the group of elements is pulsed it behaves similar to a single larger element whose width equals the four elements. **B** Pulsing of a nonfocused array. A group of elements (*E*) is simultaneously pulsed (*1*). After the echoes return to this first group then the next group (*2*) is pulsed, and so on until all the elements of the array are pulsed. **C** Pulsing of an electronically focused linear array. The individual elements (*E*) in each group (*1, 2, 3,* etc.) are *not* simultaneously pulsed. The central elements of each group are pulsed several nanoseconds after the lateral elements so as to focus the beam. By comparison the interval between the pulsing of adjacent groups is several hundred microseconds.

(Figure continued on pages 25-27.)

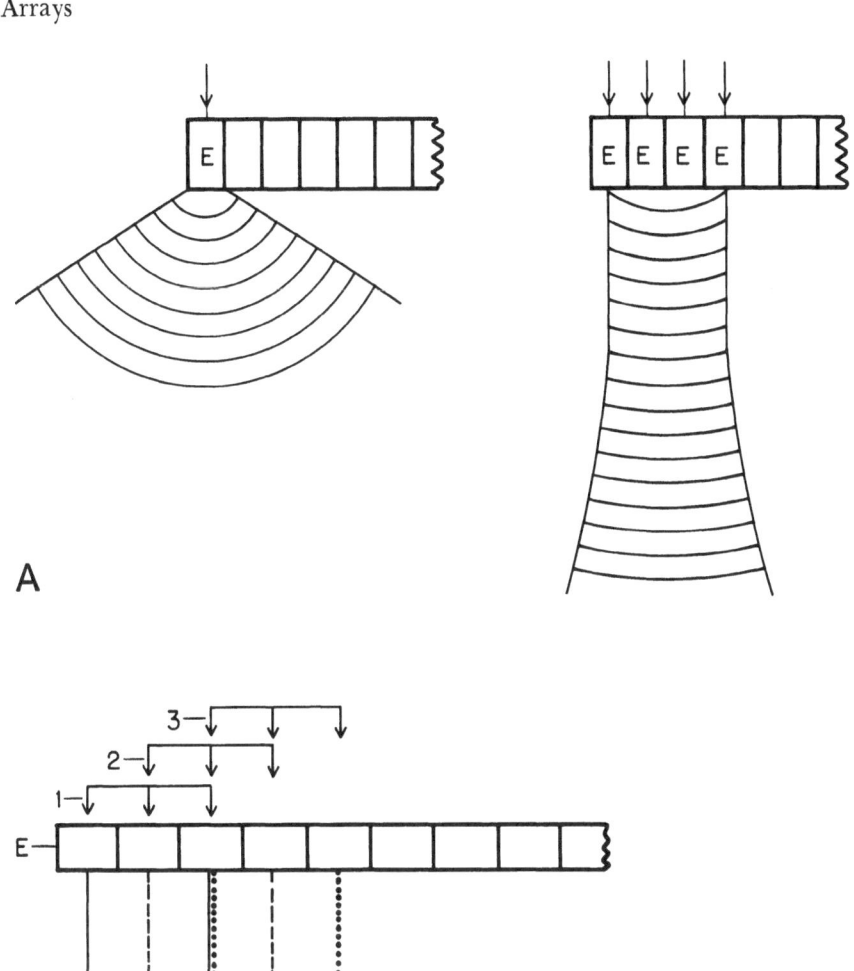

A

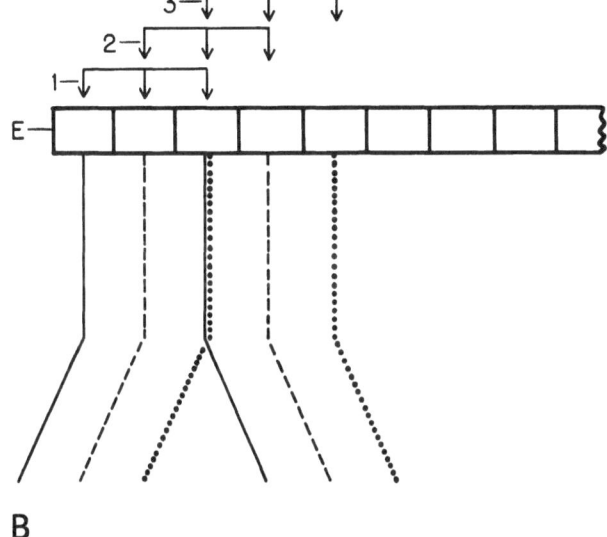

B

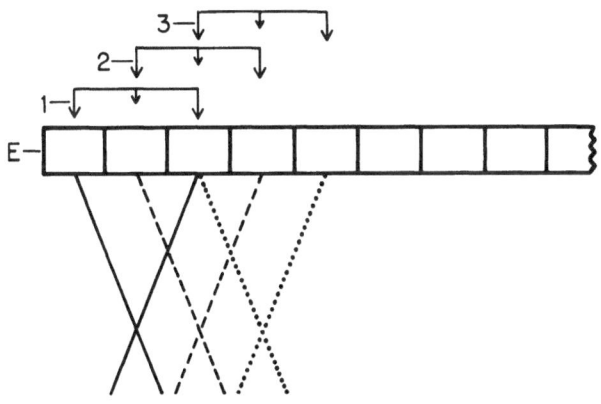

C

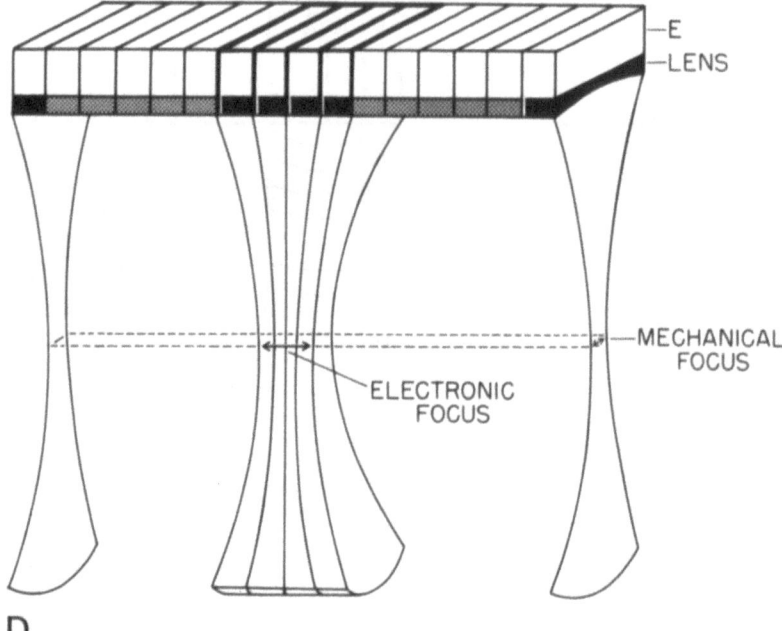

Fig. 2.9. (cont.) **D** Dual focusing. Focus in the plane perpendicular to the image plane is achieved mechanically using a lens placed in front of the elements (*E*) of the array while within the image plane focus is electronically produced. **E** Example of commercial system. ADR (Advanced Diagnostic Research Corporation, Tempe, Arizona) linear array with an electronically focused 3.5-MHz transducer. **F** Image produced by ADR system. Right lobe of liver, transverse scan. *HV*, hepatic veins; *PV*, portal veins; *R*, right side of patient. **E** and **F** Courtesy of ADR Corporation.

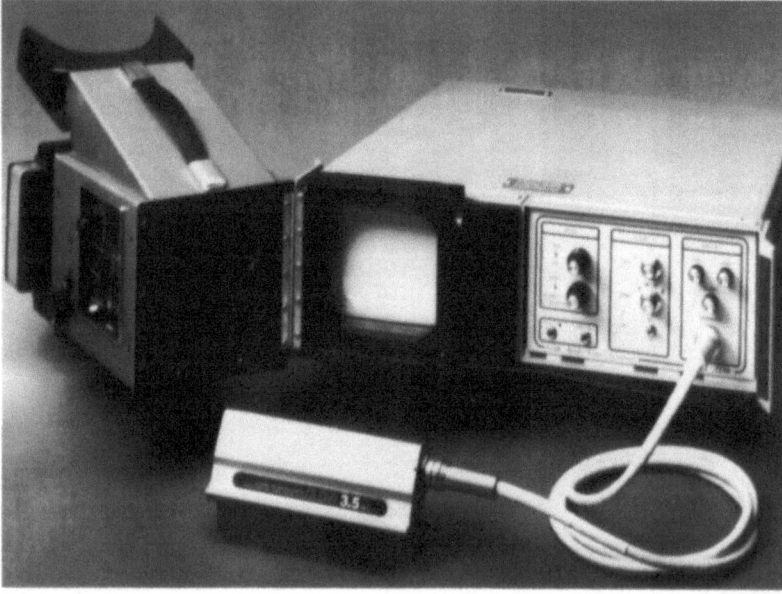

beam is a small fraction of the time interval between the pulsing of adjacent groups of elements. In some systems the operator can select the depth at which the focus is best so as to optimize focus for the region within the scan of greatest interest. An example of a currently manufactured linear array and the images it produces are shown in Fig. 2.9E and F.

B. Phased Arrays

The phased array also contains a series of small transducer elements arranged in a row, but the length of the transducer array is much smaller than the maximum width of the ultrasound beam pattern. The image produced is sector in shape.

In the phased array *all* the transducer ele-

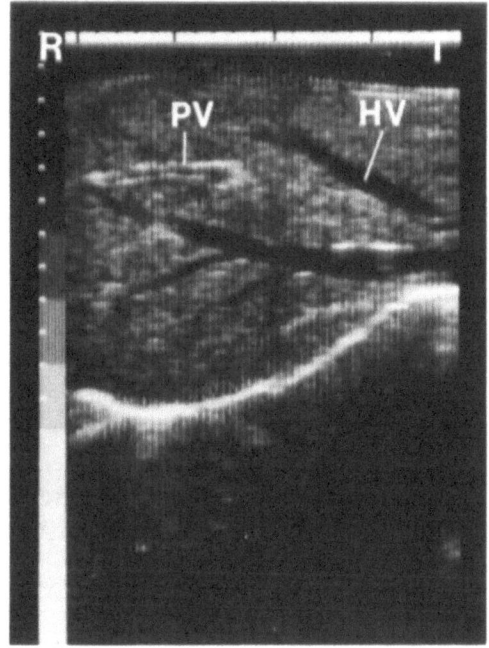

Fig. 2.9.F

ments must be pulsed for the formation of *each line or ray* of the image, whereas in the linear array only a *small group of elements* is required to produce a *given line* of the image. However, all the elements of the phased array are not pulsed at the same time. They are pulsed with a slight (several nanoseconds) lag between elements to shape the beam in a manner similar to the beam shaping used for electronically focusing groups of elements in the linear array. In the linear array the delay pattern for pulsing individual elements within a group is constant since each group produces only one line of the image. However, in the phased array, since all elements participate in the formation of each ray of the image, the sequence for pulsing the individual elements and the extent of the delay between elements constantly change in order to electronically move the beam through an arcuate pattern (Fig. 2.10A). Thus, with the phased array one can electronically sweep the beam to produce a sector display similar to that of the mechanical transducer without the need

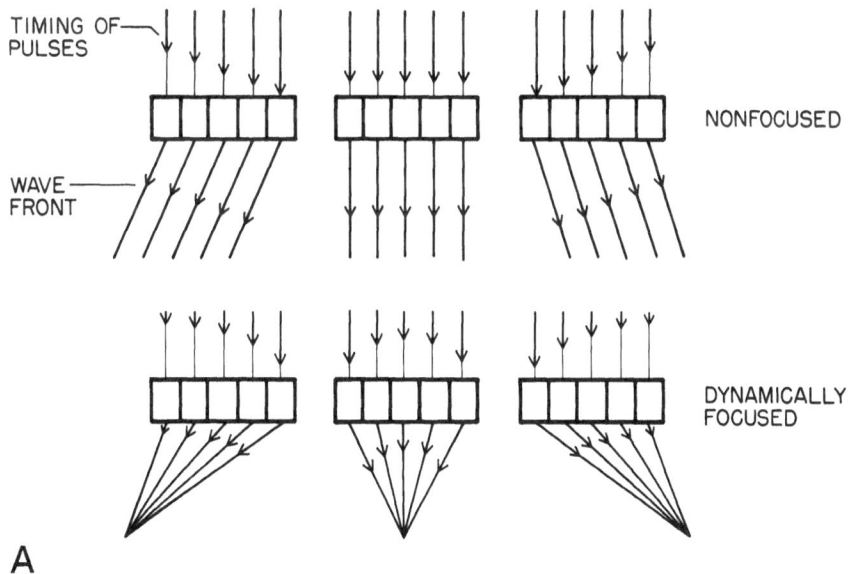

A

Fig. 2.10. Phased array. **A** Beam steering; nonfocused and focused transducers. Shape and direction of beam determined by the timing of pulses to each of the elements. For simplicity of illustration dynamic focusing is shown only at one depth. (Figure continued on page 28.)

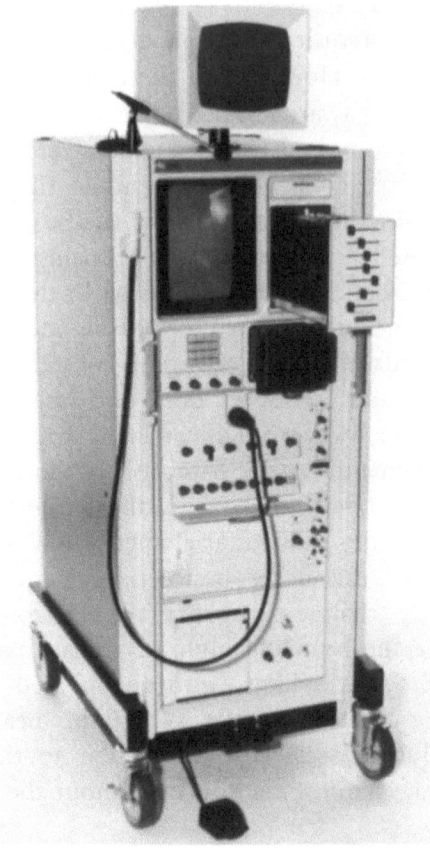

B

Fig. 2.10. (cont.) **B** Example of a commercial system: Varian Phased Array Ultrasonograph (Varian Associates, Palo Alto, California). **C** Close-up of Varian phased array transducer. White spaces between black lines are the individual transducer elements. **D** Sagittal scan, right lobe of liver (Varian system). **B–D** Courtesy of Varian Associates.

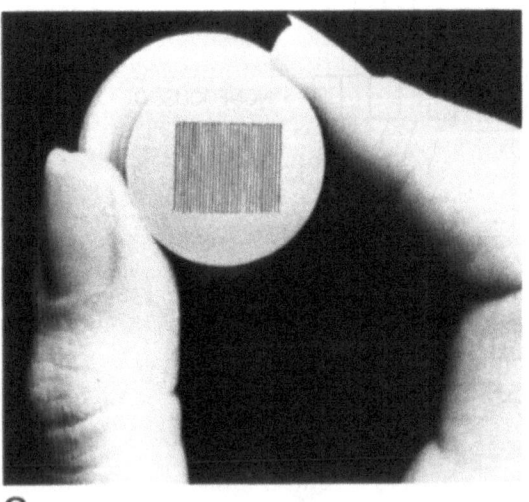

C

D

Fig 2.10. (cont.)

for a mechanically moving transducer. A similar pattern of delay is introduced into the received signals to enable the array to be sensitive to returning echoes only along the same beam direction (5). An example of a commercial phased array scanner and a typical image are shown in Fig. 2.10B–D. In some of the more elaborate phased array systems, the beam can rapidly change its zone of focus along the axial direction during the time that the echoes from a single pulse are received by the transducer so as to produce a beam with a very narrow but very long zone of axial resolution (dynamic focusing) (6).

The phased array has the advantage over the mechanical sector scanner of theoretically producing much higher resolution because the beam can be dynamically focused at multiple depths to produce a long, narrow beam. The frame rate and angle width can also be varied electronically. Some phased array systems have in addition the advantage of being able to produce a time-motion tracing from any single ray of the sector image while simultaneously displaying the sector image. Although this feature is more useful in cardiac than abdominal scanning, it is helpful in the abdomen for critically evaluating arterial pulsations. The major disadvantage of the phased array is the high cost of systems because of the extensive computer-controlled electronics necessary to control the beam steering and focusing for each receiver channel within the array. In addition, the beam pattern may not be uniform across the entire sector angle and the resolution may be better in the center than at the edges (7). This problem does not occur with mechanical sector scanners because the movement of the beam corresponds to a physical displacement of the transducer element, and the beam configuration does not change as the transducer moves. Although it is also possible to change transducer frequencies with the phased array, the cost per transducer usually is greater than with linear arrays or mechanical sector scanners.

4. QUASI-REAL-TIME SCANNERS

A. Multitransducer Mechanical Scanner

In this system three transducers mounted in a row are enclosed within a rectangular case, one end of which is rounded (Fig. 2.11A). The transducer case can either be used as a freely moveable hand-held scanner or can be attached to a telescopic overhead arm. Since the case is larger and heavier than most hand-held real-time scanners, use of the telescopic arm partially counterbalances the weight of the case and facilitates its movement. In addition, the arm contains position-sensing devices so that as the transducer attached to the arm is moved, the position of the transducer on the patient is graphically displayed in one corner of the image as a bar within an outline of the human body. When all three transducers are oscillated and pulsed, a large trapezoid display is produced. The width of the trapezoid at the skin surface equals the length of the case (Fig. 2.11B). The beams from the three transducers do not overlap or compound, but the images are electronically gated so that the image produced by one transducer stops at the boundary of the next one. When only the middle of the three transducers is used, a sector display is obtained (Fig. 2.11C). When only the transducer at the rounded end of the case is used, a much wider arc sector display is produced (Fig. 2.11D) because the transducer swings around the side of the case.

This system has two modes of operation: quasi-real-time at 7.5 frames/s; and high resolution at 1 frame/s with improved resolution produced by the slower frame rate (Fig. 2.11E).

B. Annular Array Scanner

This design (Fig. 2.12A) utilizes a water delay, mechanically operated scanning system incorporating a 10-cm diameter stationary annular array transducer. The beam is swept through a trapezoid field of view by a mirror oscillating within the water container. Since the water path from the trans-

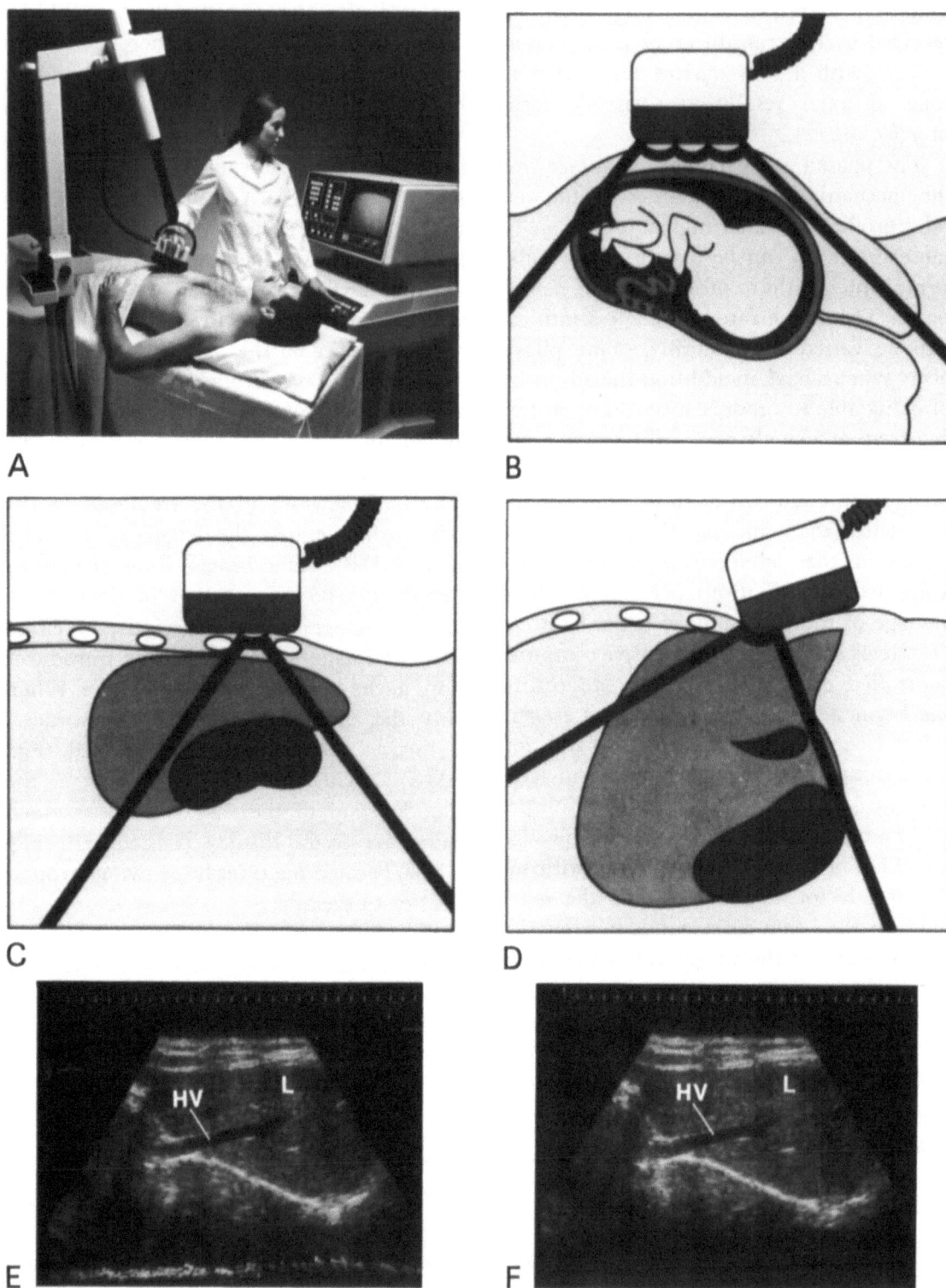

Fig. 2.11. Multitransducer mechanical scanner. **A** Commercial system, model RA-1, manufactured by Diasonics, Inc., Sunnyvale, California. **B** Broad trapezoid display; all three transducers utilized. **C** Narrow trapezoid display; only central transducer utilized. **D** Wide sector arc using single transducer at one end of case. **E** and **F** Quasi–real-time (**E**) at 7.5 frames/s versus high resolution image (**F**) at 1 frame/s. Both images are scans of right lobe of liver (*L*). *HV*, hepatic vein, **A–E** Courtesy of Diasonics, Inc.

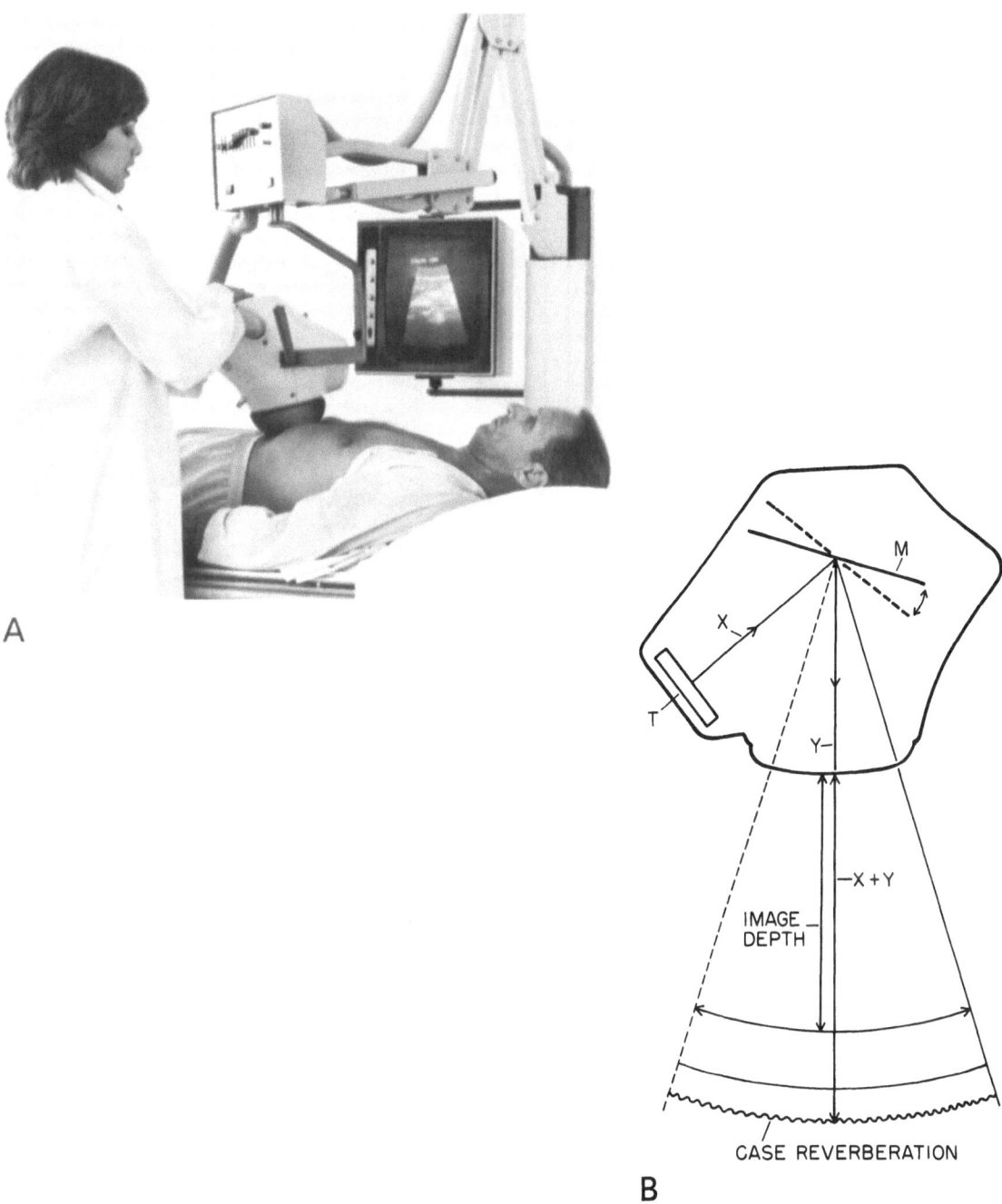

A

B

Fig. 2.12. Annular array scanner. **A** Example of commercial system: Xerox model 150. Courtesy of Xerox Corporation, Pasadena, California. [This system is no longer marketed by Xerox but a similar system is now marketed by Smith Kline Industries, California.] **B** Length of water path (*X* and *Y*) in transducer assembly is slightly greater than maximum depth of displayed image so as to eliminate the projection of the case reverberation into the field of view. *T*, transducer; *M*, mirror. (Figure continued on page 32.)

ducer to the skin is greater than the maximum depth of view within the patient, no reverberations produced by the reflection of sound between the patient's skin and the face of the transducer appear within the field of view (Fig. 2.12B). As a result of the long ultrasound beam path, the pulse repetition rate is slower than that with hand-held real-

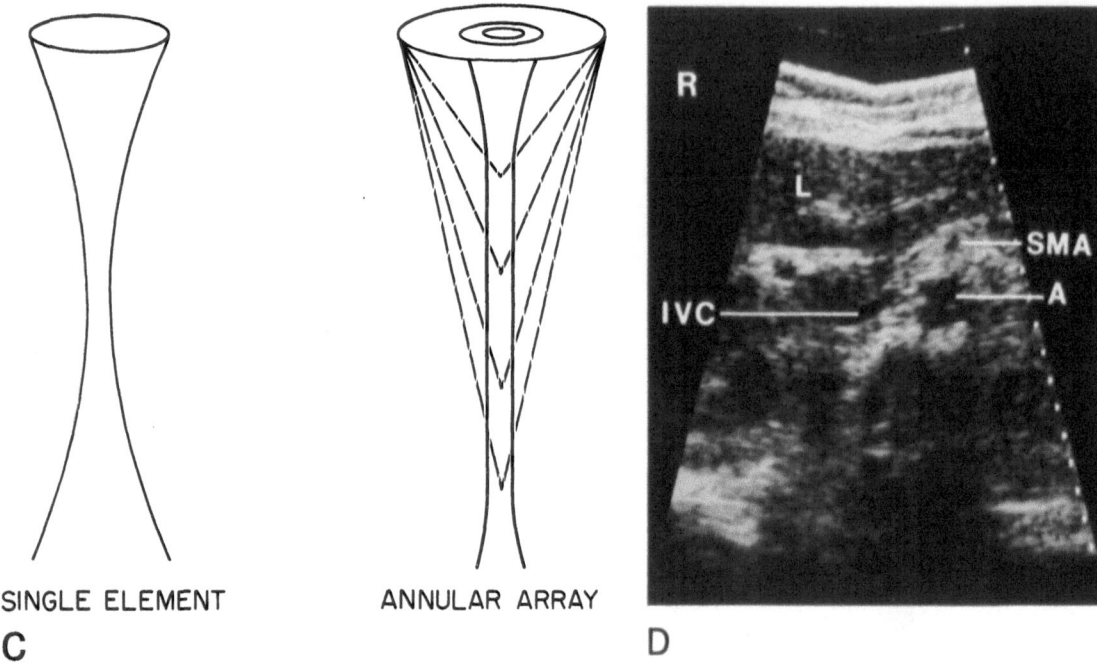

SINGLE ELEMENT   ANNULAR ARRAY

C   D

Fig. 2.12. C Single element versus annular array beam pattern. Beam pattern fixed in single element transducer. Beam pattern variable in annular array by electronically changing zone of maximum focus. Thus, a longer zone of fine focus can be obtained in an annular array as compared with a single crystal transducer. **D** Quasi–real-time image from Xerox system. Transverse section of upper abdomen, 12 frames s. *L*, liver; *IVC*, inferior vena cava; *A*, aorta; *SMA*, superior mesenteric artery; *R*, right side of patient. **E** Same region as in **D**, high resolution scan, 1 frame/s. **F** Quasi–real-time operation. Annular array focused at one depth (which is operator selectable) to produce fixed beam pattern. Beam sweeps through tissue (ray 1 to ray 2, and so on) as mirror (*M*) oscillates. Transducer (*T*) is fixed. **G** High resolution operation. For each ray of the ultra-sound beam, the transducer electronically refocuses itself at each of six different depth zones. At each zone of focus, the transducer is pulsed and reflected echoes are received before the transducer refocuses itself at the next depth. Thus, the transducer is pulsed six times at each ray before the mirror advances the beam to the next ray. (For simplicity, only three zones are shown.)

time scanners (containing transducers adjacent to the skin). Thus, to obtain an adequate number of lines per image in real time (128 lines), the frame rate must be less than that in hand-held scanners.

An annular array transducer consists of several ring-shaped elements mounted concentric to each other. By sequentially pulsing the rings so that the pulses to the more central rings are delayed electronically (by several nanoseconds) as compared to the pulses to the more peripheral rings, the beam can be focused at a given depth. The depth of the focus can be changed by varying the delay between the pulsing of the rings, and the focal depth can change from pulse to pulse (Fig. 2.12C). This method of focus is basically the same as that used in the phased array scanner except that in the annular array system only the depth of focus is electronically varied while beam position is mechanically varied by moving the mirror. In

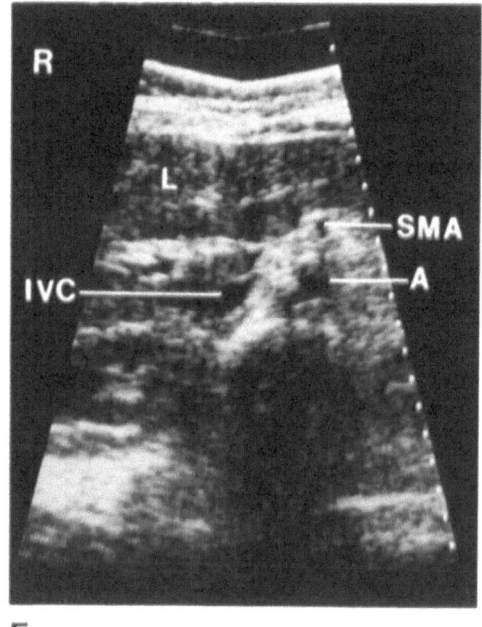

E

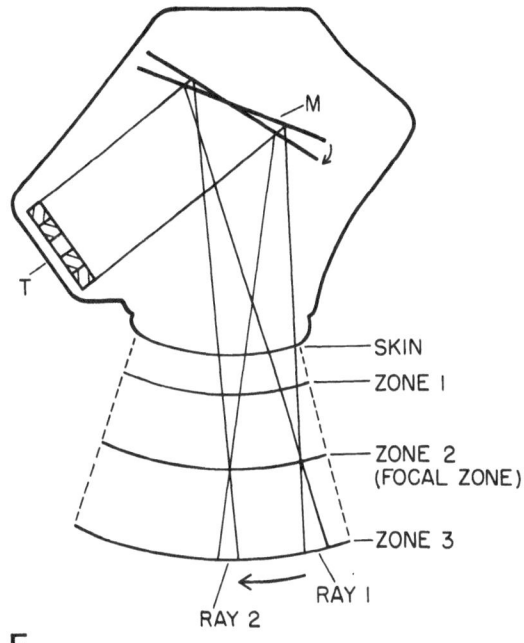

F

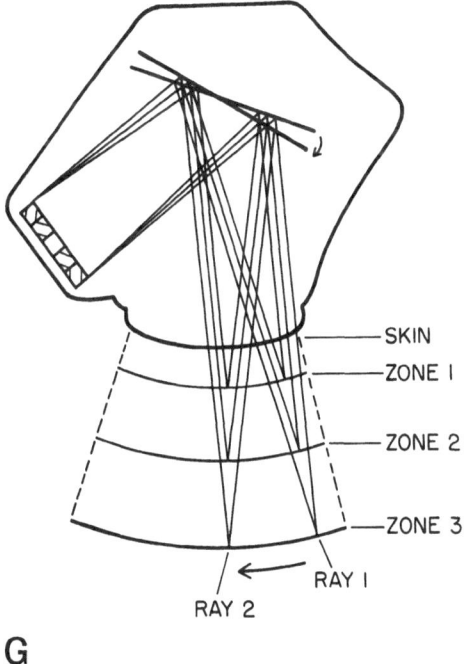

G

the phased array both the beam focus and beam position can be electronically varied.

This water delay system has two frame rates: 12 frames/s which produces a quasi–real-time image containing 128 lines (Fig. 2.12D); and 1 frame/s which gives a higher resolution image (Fig. 2.12E) containing 256 lines. At 12 frames/s the transducer array is focused at one of six possible depth zones of focus. The operator chooses the desired zone of focus. Each ray of the sector image is pulsed only one time and then the transducer advances to the next ray position (Fig. 2.12F). At the 1 frame/s mode, a uniformly fine zone of focus is produced that encompasses all six focus levels. The transducer is pulsed six times for each ray so that the focus can be electronically changed to sequentially focus at each depth zone in each ray. Only the image in the zone of focus is displayed so that the image in each ray is the composite of images from six different zones of focus. After the six pulses, the beam advances to the next ray, and the sequence is repeated (Fig. 2.12G). For this high resolution scanning mode a much slower frame rate is required because six times the number of pulses are needed.

5. INSTRUMENT DESIGNS VERSUS FIELDS OF VIEW

Each of the ultrasound beams produced by the various scanners—sector, trapezoid, or rectangular—has certain advantages and disadvantages.

The advantage of the sector scanner is that a small skin area is required for contact with the transducer. As the beam enters the patient, it diverges to produce a larger field of view. Thus, one can image structures under the ribs by placing the transducer over an interspace between ribs (Fig. 2.13), or one can maneuver the transducer in a narrow subcostal region to image deeper upper abdominal structures. The concavity or convexity of the patient's skin surface is of little consequence to the sector transducer. The

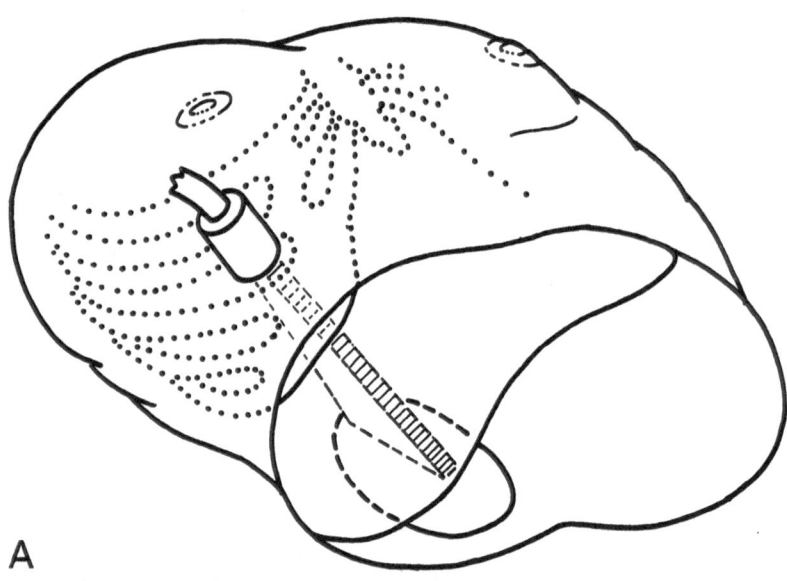

A

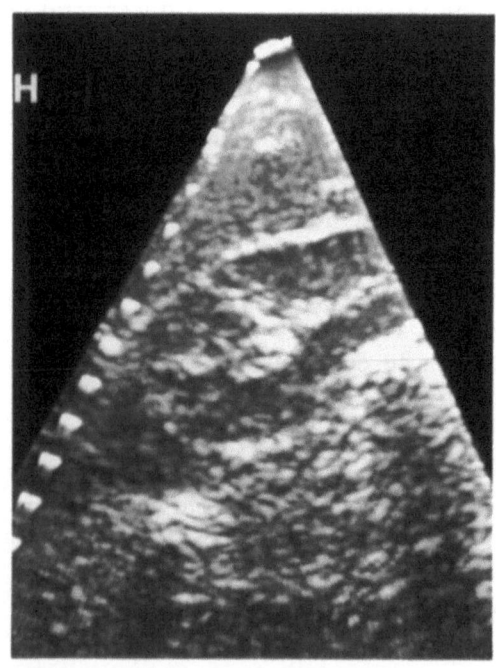

B

Fig. 2.13. Scanning between ribs with sector transducer. **A** Small size of transducer head allows it to fit easily between ribs while diverging pattern of sector image increases the image area with increasing depth. **B** Sagittal image of right kidney through rib interspaces (Matzuk prototype system).

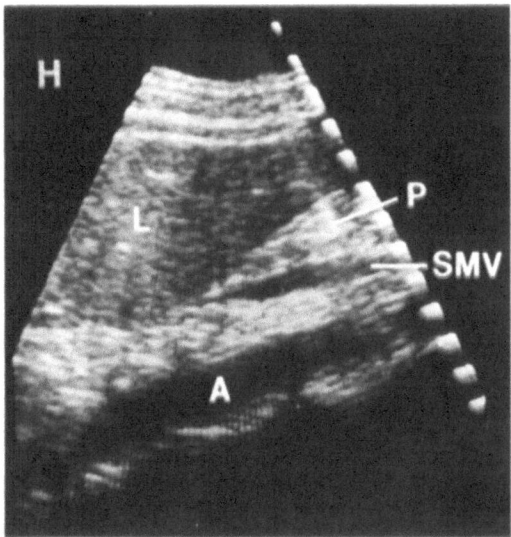

Fig. 2.14. Trapezoid format image. Midsagittal view of liver (*L*), pancreas (*P*), superior mesenteric vein (*SMV*), and aorta (*A*). Trapezoid format provides a greater area of the near field while maintaining the same far field width as the sector scanner (Matzuk prototype system).

is displayed several centimeters above the skin. The individual rays at the skin surface are not overly clustered together to distort the image, and the useable image can be obtained from the skin surface downward.[3]

The linear arrays and large-field transducer systems produced by incorporating several mechanical sector scanners in one case have the advantage of producing a larger image area close to the skin surface. This larger field of view is especially useful in examining the abdominal aorta and the fetus. However, the disadvantage of these array or bar-shaped transducers is that their length sometimes limits their accessibility to certain areas of the abdomen. For example, while the array is very useful for imaging a patient with a flat contour to the anterior abdomen (Fig. 2.15A), it is difficult to examine structures deep to ribs because of the shadows cast by the ribs (Fig. 2.15B). In certain anatomic configurations the transducer does not make complete skin contact because the region being examined has either a concave (Fig. 2.16A) or convex configuration (Fig. 2.16B). The former situation can occur with the transducer oriented transversely in the epigastric region of a thin patient with a protruding rib cage, and the latter can be seen during the scanning of the kidneys through the flanks. In either case, an incomplete or inadequate field of view is obtained. These deficiencies of the linear array or bar-type transducer can be partially overcome by orienting the transducer along planes that provide more complete skin contact or that eliminate overlying ribs (Fig. 2.17), such as orienting the long axis of the transducer between ribs or placing the transducer just below and parallel to the rib cage in the subcostal region and angling the beam toward the patient's head.

main drawbacks of the sector transducer, whether it is a mechanically operated one or a phased array, are (1) the first few centimers of the image are really of little diagnostic value since this is the area where the individual lines or rays of the image are so close together as not to produce a useful image; and (2) the area of image seen in the near field is much less than that seen in the far field. However, structures in the far field are well seen. In one rotating wheel sector format system (Fig. 2.8C) the first few centimeters of image are blanked off the display screen so that the apex of the sector image is not displayed.

A compromise beam pattern has been achieved in one mechanical sector scanner (Matzuk design) by recessing the oscillating transducer several centimeters from the front of the fluid-filled case to obtain a trapezoid field of view (Figs. 2.7 and 2.14). There is a larger entrance beam than that in the sector scanner since the apex of the sector beam

---

[3] Similar trapezoid-shaped images can now be obtained with recently designed rotating wheel and oscillating sector transducers commercially available from several manufacturers.

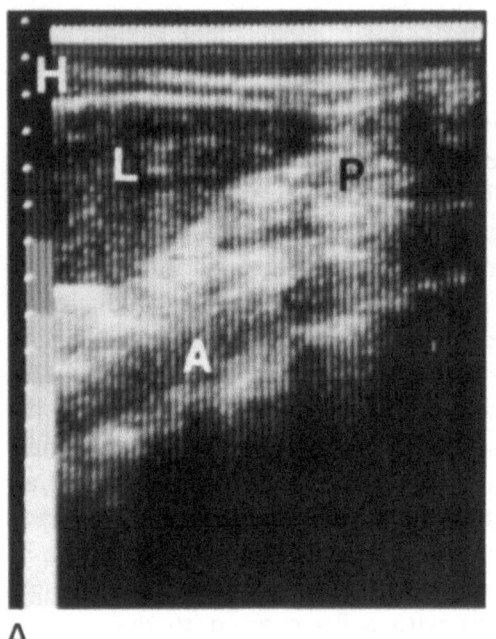 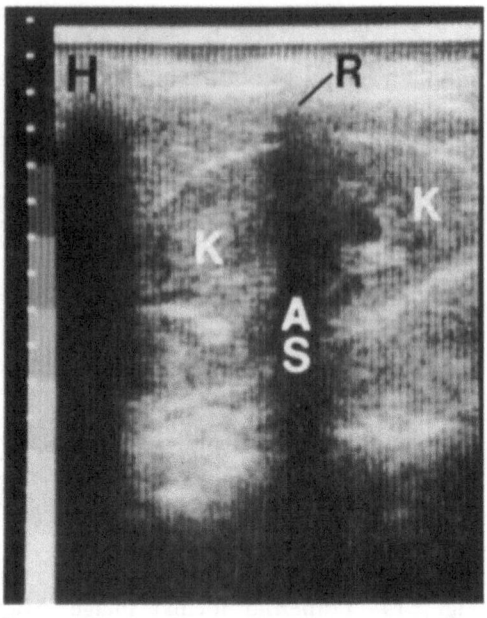

Fig. 2.15. A Application of linear arrays: imaging a large area of tissue close to the skin. The length of the image equals the length of the array. Midsagittal view of liver (*L*), pancreas (*P*), and aorta (*A*). **B** A limitation of linear arrays: organ below ribs (*R*) is partially obscured by rib acoustic shadows (*AS*). Coronal plane, right kidney (*K*). (Beam enters through right posterior axillary line.) (Images produced by ADR system.)

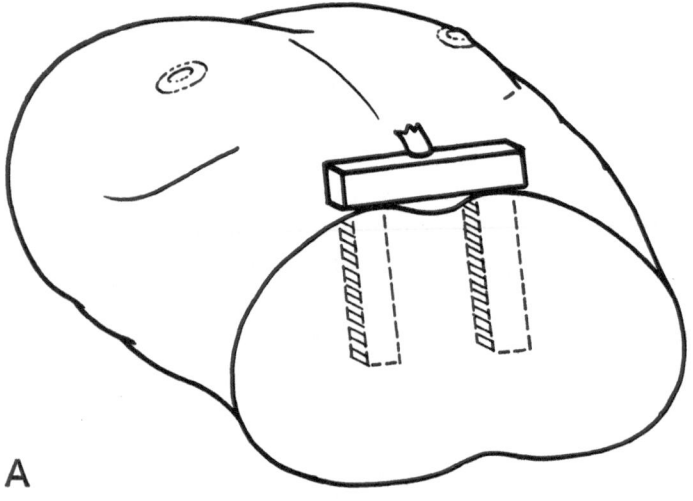

Fig. 2.16. Limitations of linear arrays. Reduced image area (hatched) resulting from incomplete skin contact with transducer. **A** Concave configuration of anterior abdomen. In transverse plane lateral aspects of array make skin contact but central area does not.

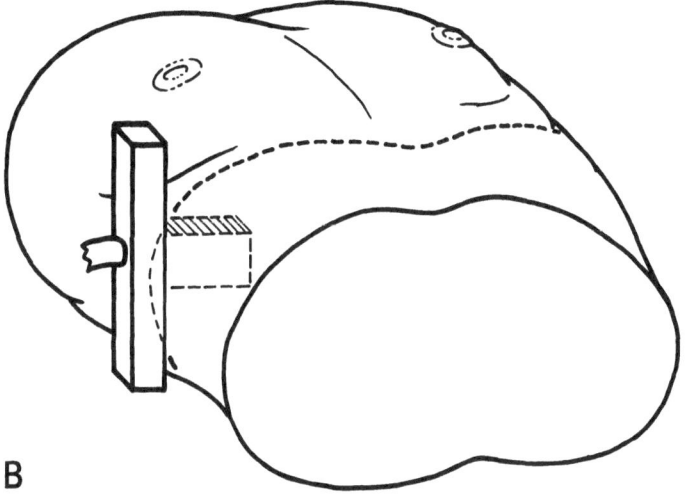

B

Fig. 2.16. B When transducer is placed over convex skin surface (as in transverse scanning through flank) only central portion of transducer makes skin contact.

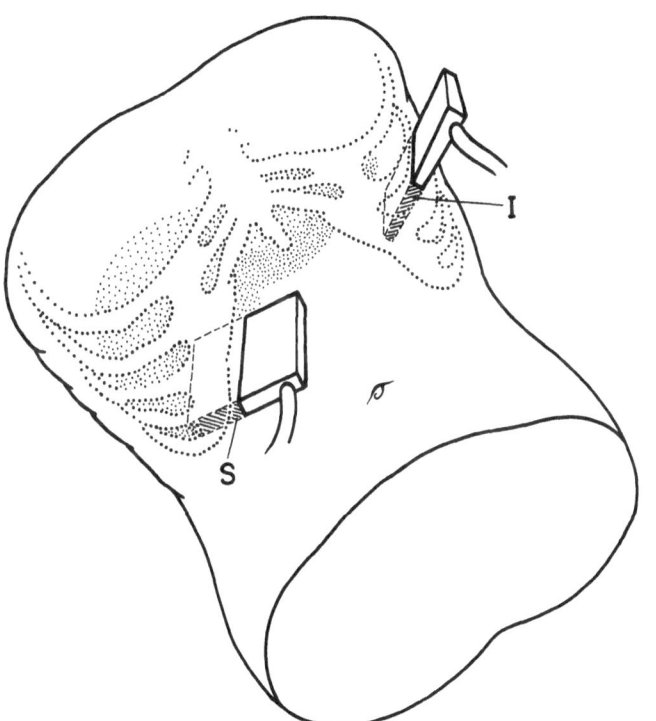

Fig. 2.17. To alleviate difficulties of rib shadowing and incomplete skin contact when using a linear array, subcoastal (*S*) and intercostal (*I*) transducer placement can be used for examining upper abdominal organs, especially the liver and kidneys. However, in using these approaches, one must realize that the anatomic planes are diagonal rather than the more familiar sagittal and transverse ones.

6. EQUIPMENT COSTS

The field of ultrasound instrumentation is undergoing extremely rapid change. Although the generic types of real-time systems described above will probably be available for several years to come, the individual designs and the manufacturers producing them may show considerable change. At present, the phased array systems are the most expensive. They range from approximately $65,000 to over $100,000. The mechanical sector scanners and the linear arrays overlap in price. Linear arrays range from approximately $15,000 to $40,000, and the mechanical sector scanners range from approximately $20,000 to $50,000.

References

1. Griffith JM, Henry WL (1974) A sector scanner for real-time two-dimensional echocardiography. Circulation 49:1147

2. Matzuk T, Skolnick ML (1978) Novel ultrasonic real-time scanner featuring servo-controlled transducer displaying a sector image. Ultrasonics 16:171–178

3. King DL (1973) Real-time cross-sectional ultrasonic imaging of the heart using a linear array multi-element transducer. J Clin Ultrasound 1:196–200

4. Ligtvoet, CM, Ridder J, Lancée CT, Hagemeijer F, Vletter WB, Gussenhoven WJ (1977) A dynamically focused multiscan system. In: Bom N (ed) Echocardiology with doppler applications and real-time imaging. Martinus Nijhoff Medical Division, The Hague, The Netherlands, pp 313–323

5. Somer JC (1968) Electronic sector scanning for ultrasonic diagnosis. Ultrasonics 6:153

6. Thurstone FL, Von Ramm OT (1974) A new ultrasound imaging technique employing two-dimensional beam steering. In: Booth N (ed) Acoustical holography. Plenum Press, New York, Vol 5, p 249

7. Personal communication, Terrance Matzuk, Ph.D., P.E.

3
Scanning Techniques
and Anatomic Considerations

Abdominal ultrasound imaging with real-time instrumentation makes greater use of the operator's cross-sectional anatomic knowledge than does large-field static ultrasound imaging. This greater exercise of anatomic knowledge results from two characteristics of ultrasound real-time imaging: the smaller field of view of the instruments and the complete flexibility and mobility in placing the transducer at any site on the abdomen.

1. SCANNING METHODS

To obtain the greatest benefits of real-time instrumentation, the operator should de-velop logical methods of examining the abdomen, and in addition should be familiar with specific scanning techniques and maneuvers that will enhance the diagnostic information obtained with the real-time scanner. Real-time abdominal scanning is more than just placing the transducer on the abdomen and watching the image. Although the chances of producing artifacts are less with real-time scanning than with contact scanning (because the image is automatically produced), there are certain manipulations that the user should perform which could either enhance or degrade the diagnostic information obtained.

A. Regional Imaging

When examining a region with the small field of view of a real-time scanner, one must be able to identify the structure or structures being imaged, even if total organs are not seen. To illustrate this concept, a series of views of the upper abdomen comparing real-time fields of view with the large areas seen with the contact scanner is shown in Fig. 3.1. The secret to working with a small-field-of-view scanner is to sweep the scanner through an area of interest and mentally integrate multiple rapidly changing small fields of view so as to appreciate a larger anatomic region. Although structures on individual views with the real-time scanner may not be completely discerned, when multiple adjacent fields are sequentially examined, the

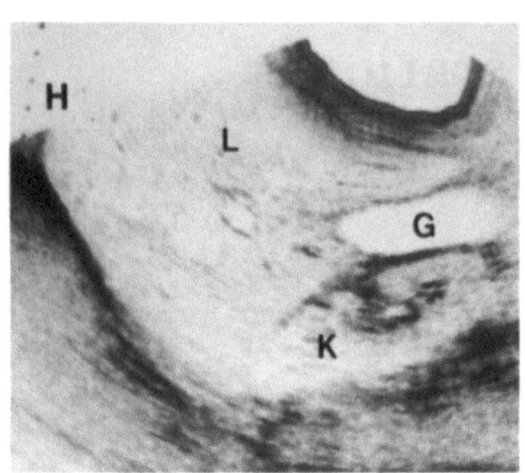

A

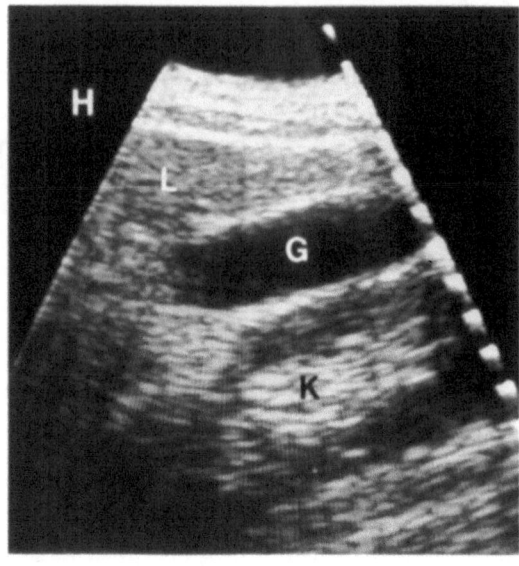

B

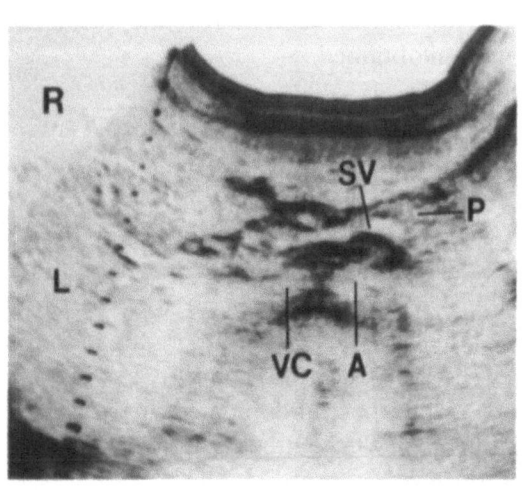

C

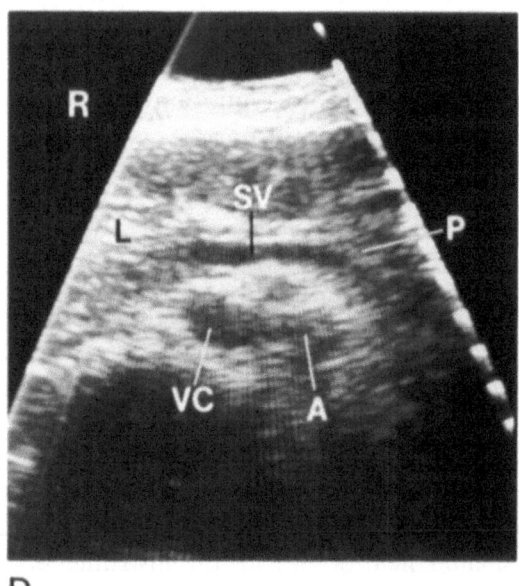

D

Fig. 3.1. Comparison fields of view of a contact and a real-time trapezoid scanner (Matzuk system). **A** and **B** Sagittal view through right upper quadrant. *L*, liver; *G*, gallbladder; *K*, right kidney. **C** and **D** Transverse view through upper abdomen. *L*, liver; *P*, pancreas; *SV*, splenic vein; *A*, aorta; *VC*, vena cava.

anatomic structures become more readily appreciated.

Because of the limited field of view of the real-time scanners, the approach should be that of regional imaging as distinguished from total cross-sectional imaging which is frequently employed in contact scanning. When the specific region has been defined clinically, first one examines the key organ within that region and then the surrounding structures as they relate to the specific organ. The prime task is to locate the key organ. The operator should be able to mentally visualize the key organ through the intact abdomen, or at least to mentally visualize the usual location of that organ, and then be able to place the transducer on the skin overlying the approximate region of that organ.

For example, in imaging the gallbladder, the transducer is usually placed in the right subcostal region. With the patient's respiration suspended in deep inspiration, the instrument is moved in arcuate sweeps until the gallbladder is located. Then long and short axis images through the gallbladder are obtained. Next the liver should be briefly scanned, specifically to see if any dilated intrahepatic bile ducts are identified, and the common duct should be identified as it crosses the portal vein, and its diameter measured. If no abnormalities are seen in these related structures, then the examination can be terminated. If any abnormality is seen in the adjacent structures, then the area of interest should be enlarged to further clarify that abnormality. If the common duct is dilated, then the pancreas should be examined to see if a mass is present within the head and if the pancreatic duct is dilated. In addition, a more careful examination of the liver and periportal regions should be performed to see if any metastatic lesions are identified.

Before beginning the real-time examination, the operator must be familiar with the patient's clinical problem and specifically what information the referring physician seeks to obtain from an ultrasound examination. Most often the referring physician is requesting that a particular clinical problem be clarified and, therefore, he is concerned with a specific organ or region within the abdomen. Sometimes, unfortunately, the referring physician is not clear as to what information he wishes to obtain from an ultrasound study. Instead he requests a search of the entire abdomen hoping to find the cause of some perplexing clinical situation that other diagnostic studies have not discovered. Except for a situation where an intraabdominal abscess is suspected but not clinically localized, a complete search of the abdomen for occult disease is, in our opinion, not an indicated procedure.

Now we shall discuss specific scanning techniques for imaging abdominal structures with real-time instrumentation.

B. Organ Axis Identification

Certain organs (kidney, pancreas, gallbladder, uterus) may not be oriented along a true transverse or sagittal plane in the abdomen. When abdominal scans are obtained in sagittal or transverse planes, these organs may be visualized in diagonal sections thus making it difficult to assess their true size and configuration. For accurate evaluation, it is essential that the organ be seen both in its true long and short axes. In order to do so, the operator should slowly rotate the transducer over the organ until its long axis is actually imaged. After the organ is examined in its long axis, then the transducer should be rotated 90° to that axis and the organ scanned in its true short axis (Fig. 3.2). It is helpful to actually look at the patient's abdomen and see the orientation of the transducer when in true long axis before rotating it to the true short axis to know at what position the 90° rotation should be. If the operator determines the degree of rotation only by the image on the screen, he may mistake a diagonal view of the organ for a true short axis view.

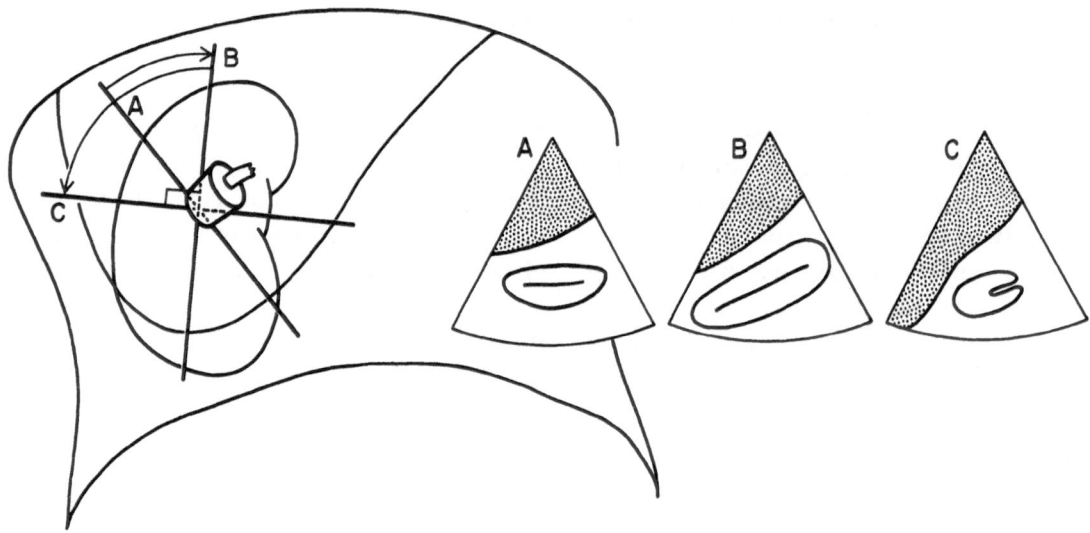

Fig. 3.2. Rotating transducer over organ to determine true long and short axes. **A** and **A′** Image plane when transducer is initially placed over kidney, a plane in no specific axis. True long and short axes can only be determined by rotating transducer until first longest image is seen (**B** and **B′**) and then in a plane 90° to **B** to visualize the shortest axis (**C** and **C′**). *L*, liver; *K*, kidney; *VC*, vena cava.

C. Scanning Entire Organ Volume

Once the true long or true short axis of the organ is determined, then it is important to continuously image the entire volume of that organ so as not to miss small focal lesions. Since the real-time scanner continuously produces images as the operator moves the instrument from one margin of the organ to the other, a series of closely spaced images of the organ will be displayed. Scanning in both axes is required for a complete examination. The more slowly one sweeps through the organ, the more closely spaced are the individual scans, and the better chance one has of detecting small lesions. A continuous sweep scan through the kidney or gallbladder should take several seconds. In organs that are long and narrow, such as the kidney, gallbladder, or uterus, different methods of continuously sweeping the transducer through the organ are recommended for long and short axis imaging. For long axis scanning, the central plane is first found. Then the transducer is pivoted so as to sweep the beam from the central plane to one edge of the organ and then in the other direction to the opposite edge (Fig. 3.3A). Arcuate movements should not be used for short axis scanning because of the greater length of the organ in this axis. Rather, it is best to actually move the transducer over the skin from one end of the organ to the other in an orientation perpendicular to the long axis so as to fully visualize the short axis (Fig. 3.3B).

D. Capsular and Surface Identification

Organ capsules, major intraorgan reflecting surfaces (such as renal pelvis and calyces and infundibula), and walls of blood vessels are best visualized when the beam is perpendicular or almost perpendicular to these surfaces. The operator can readily make changes in transducer position to improve the beam orientation to the organ under examination so as to enhance the chances of seeing the organ capsule or major interface (Fig. 3.4).

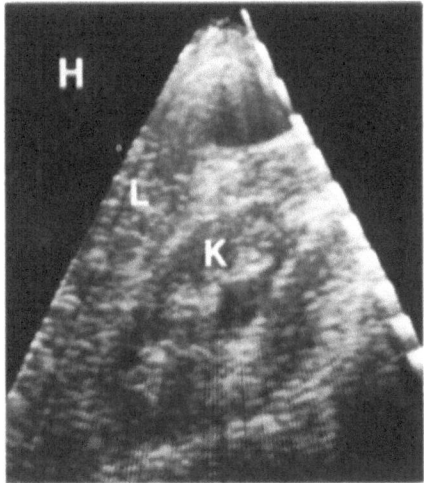

A'

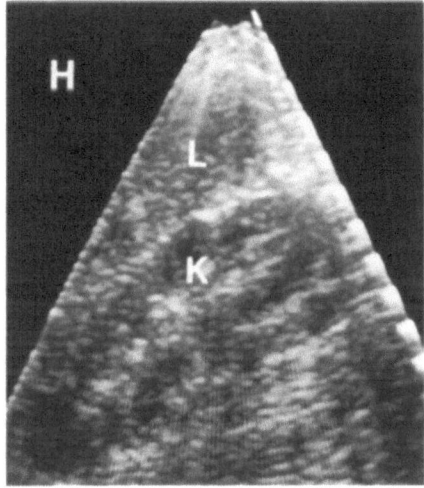

B'

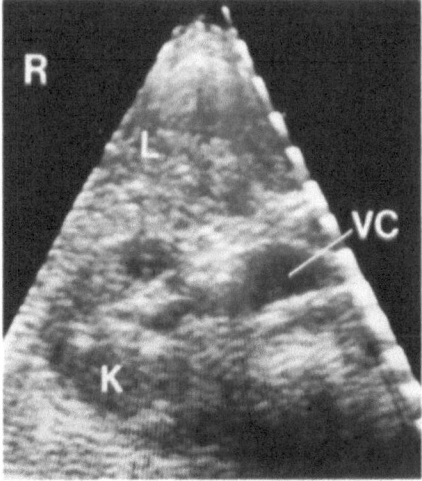

C'

Fig. 3.2. (cont.)

At times even minimal changes in position can make the difference between good and poor imaging of a specific organ. Thus, after the examiner has identified the organ of interest, he should slightly rock the transducer back and forth on the skin to attempt to improve its visualization (Fig. 3.5).

E. Mass Differentiation: Cyst Versus Solid

In order to characterize a mass, especially one under 2 cm in diameter, it is important that (1) the ultrasound beam should be perpendicular to the surfaces of the mass so as to optimally image these interfaces; and (2) the entire width of the beam should fall within the mass.

When the mass in question is a cyst and the beam goes partly through the cyst and partly through the adjacent solid tissue, reflections from the adjacent solid tissue are displayed as if they came from within the cyst. The cyst may appear as if it is a solid mass containing internal echoes. This effect occurs because at any given beam depth the strongest reflection occurring within the beam width is the reflection displayed on the oscilloscope. In addition, when the beam passes only partially through the cyst, the intensity of reflections produced by the tissues deep to the cyst will be less than if the beam is centered within the cyst (because of attenuation of that part of the beam going through the solid tissue) and the typical zone of increased reflectivity behind the cyst will not be seen (Fig. 3.6A) (1). For the cyst to appear echo free and cast a zone of acoustic enhancement, the beam width must be completely within the cyst (Fig. 3.6B). Since the narrowest region of the beam is at the focal zone, the greatest chances for detecting small cysts occurs when the focal zone of the beam is at the depth of the cyst.

Since the real-time transducer is freely maneuverable, the beam can be readily swept continuously through the entire volume of the mass from several different angles in

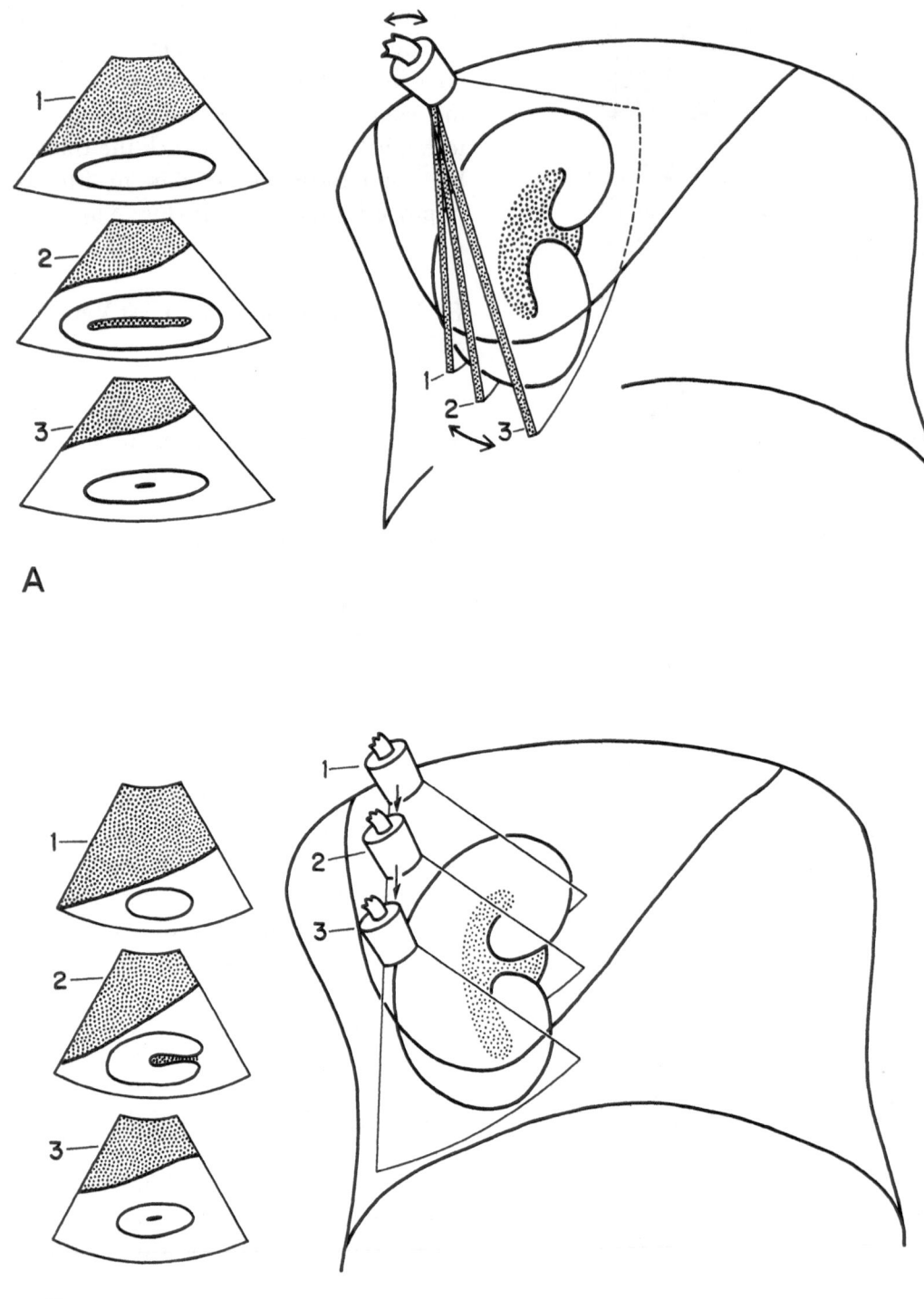

Fig. 3.3. Sweeping through entire organ volume. **A** Long axis. Transducer pivoted to sweep beam from lateral edge (*1*), through central plane (*2*), to medial edge (*3*) of kidney. **B** Short axis. Transducer is slid over kidney from superior pole (*1*), through center (*2*), to inferior pole (*3*).

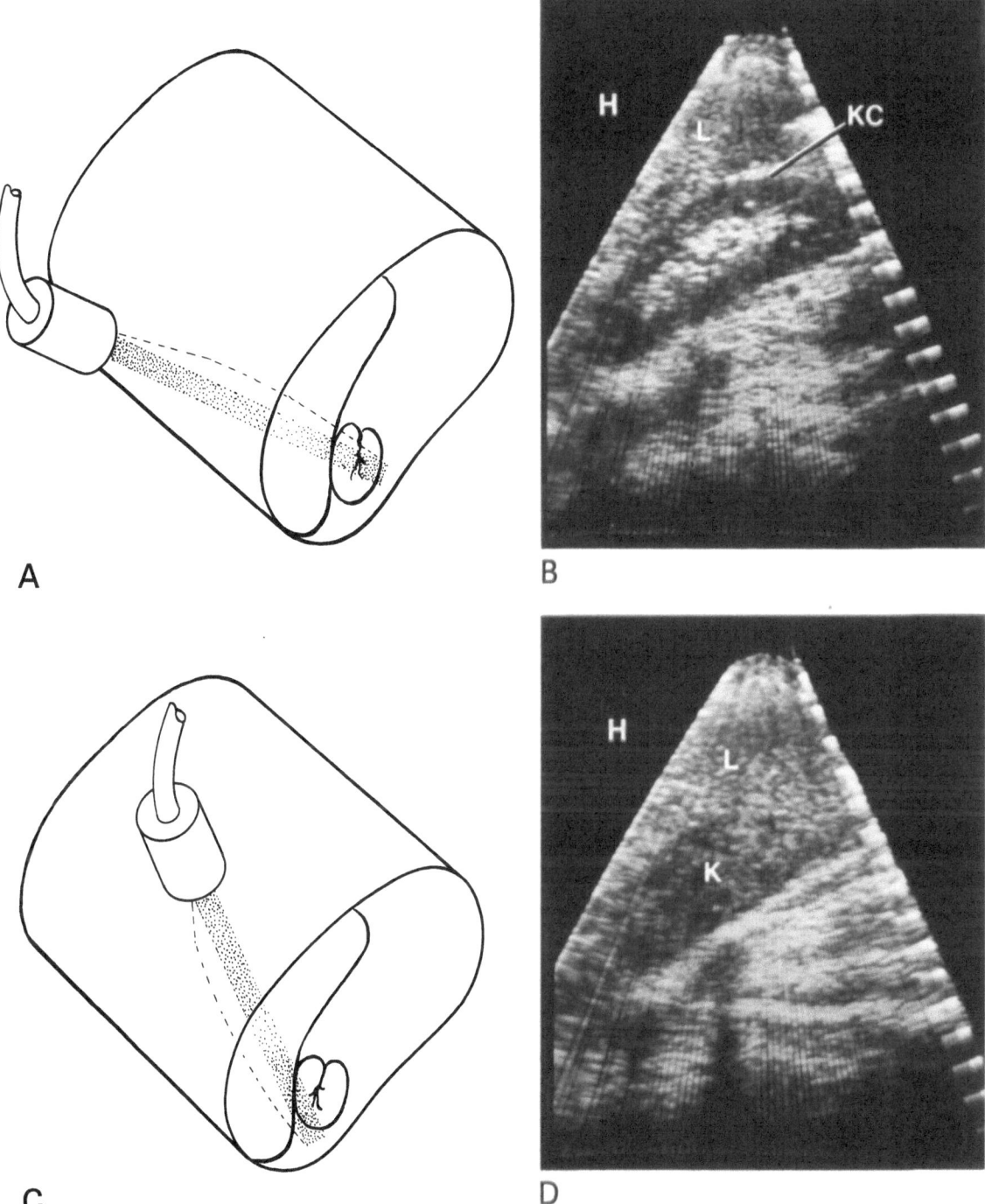

Fig. 3.4. Effect of beam orientation upon capsular visualization. **A** and **B** Beam perpendicular to kidney capsule (*KC*). Capsule visualized. **C** and **D** Beam not perpendicular to renal capsule. Capsule not seen. Liver (*L*) parenchyma blends into kidney parenchyma (*K*).

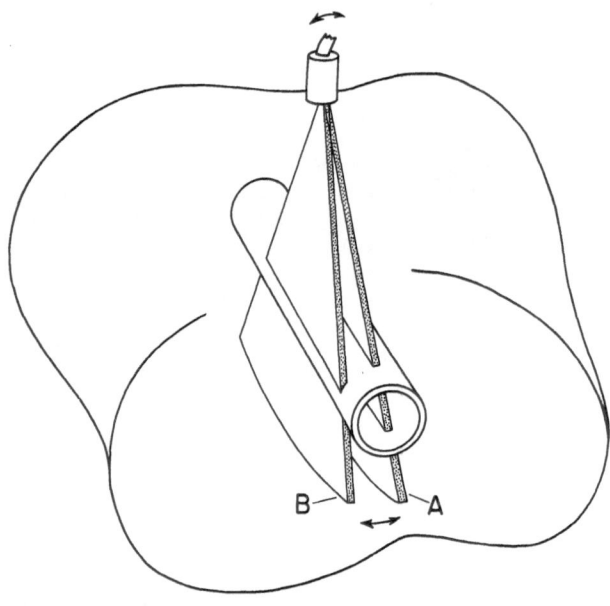

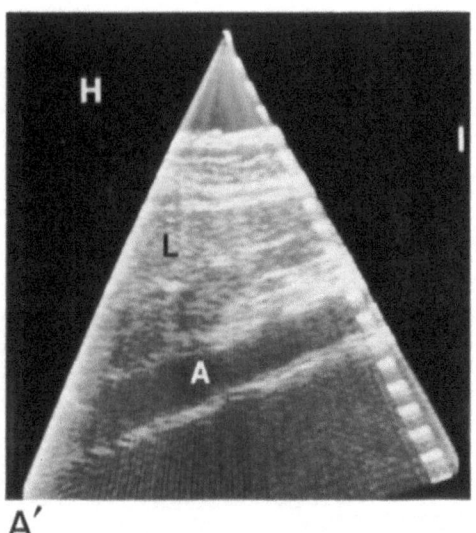

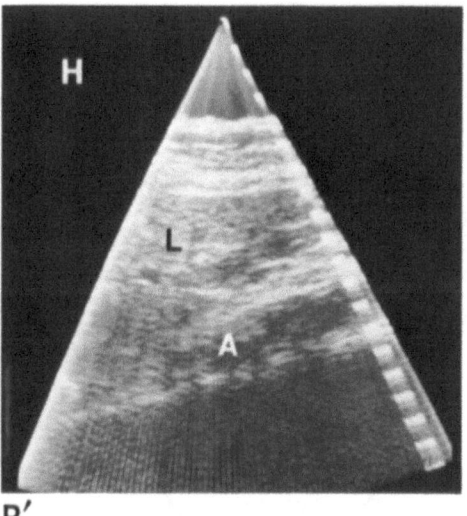

Fig. 3.5. Minimal change in beam orientation significantly affects visualization or organ surface. **A** and **A′** Beam is perpendicular to aorta (*A*). Aortic walls and lumen clearly seen. *L*, liver. **B** and **B′** Beam is several degrees off the perpendicular. Aorta is not distinctly imaged.

order to ensure that the beam is perpendicularly oriented and centered within the mass on one of the sweeps. Using such maneuvers, cysts can be readily differentiated from solid masses more rapidly and more accurately than can be achieved with articulated arm contact scanners.

F. Identifying Vascular Structures

Vascular structures may be identified by demonstrating the vessel from which it origi-

nates or into which it terminates. At times when a vessel is initially imaged its identity may not be clear because only a short segment is seen in the field of view. To identify such a vessel, the operator should track its course to its juncture with a more readily identified larger vessel so as to determine which smaller branch this vessel is. Since the vessel being tracked may take a tortuous course, the probe may have to be rotated or angled as it is moved in order to continuously image the vessel. The patient should suspend respiration during this maneuver (Fig. 3.7).

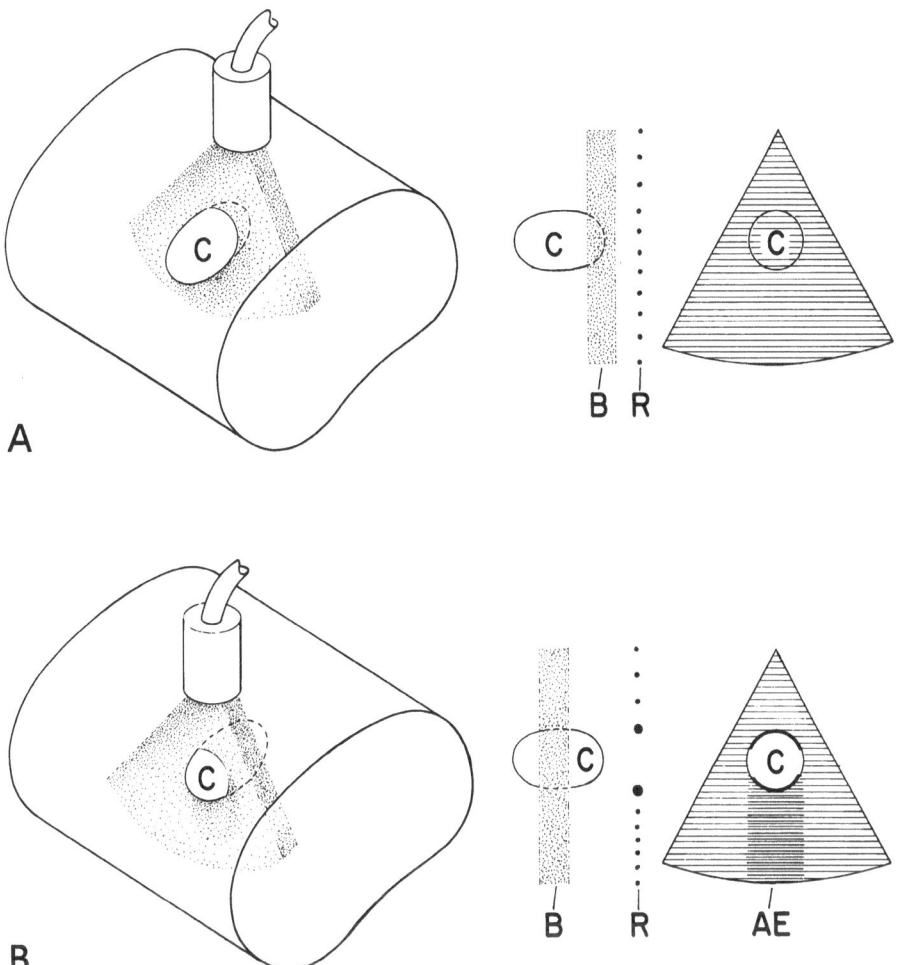

Fig. 3.6. Effect of beam position upon identification of cyst. **A** Beam width (*B*) partially through cyst (*C*) and partially through the adjacent solid tissue. Echoes appear within cyst. No acoustic enhancement produced deep to cyst. Dots represent the intensity of reflected echoes (*R*) from tissues at each depth within the ultrasound beam that are displayed on the screen. **B** Beam width (*B*) that is located entirely within cyst (*C*). Cyst appears echo free. Strong reflections are produced by front and back walls. A zone of acoustic enhancement (*AE*) appears deep to the cyst.

The three major vascular structures used as references in the upper abdomen are the aorta, the vena cava, and the portal vein. By determining whether the vessel in question either originates from or terminates into one of these three vessels, one could determine if it is an artery, a branch of the portal system, or a vein draining into the vena cava.

Vascular structures may also be identified by their constant relationship to a known structure. Sometimes it is not possible to determine the origin or termination of a vessel because the course cannot easily be traced. However, one can often identify the vessel because it maintains a constant relationship with another more easily identified structure. For example, the tubular structure seen crossing anterior to the portal vein (Fig. 3.8) in the right parasagittal plane in which the vena cava lies deep to the portal vein is the common bile duct.

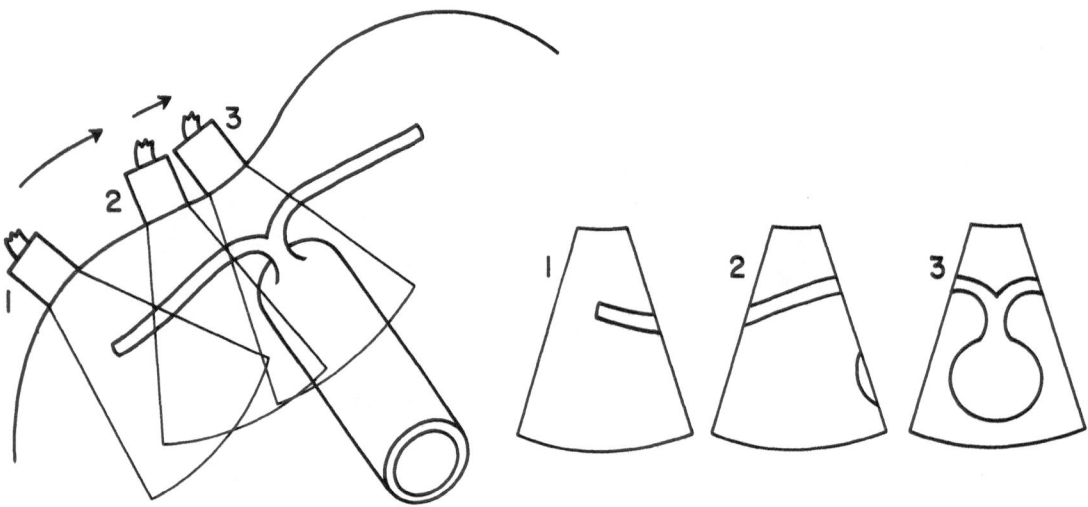

Fig. 3.7. Tracking of tortuous vessel by rotating and angling the transducer as the transducer is slid on the skin overlying the vessel.

Another method of identifying vascular structures is by observing characteristic motions. The easiest artery to identify is the aorta because it normally demonstrates pulsatile movements of its walls, especially the anterior one, that are synchronous with the pulse. These pulsations may be diminished when clot lines the wall of an aneurysm. Veins can be identified by a change in caliber during phases of respiration (Fig. 3.9). Smaller arteries and veins may be difficult to identify by their intrinsic movements because it may be hard to determine whether these movements originate within that vessel or are referred pulsations from the aorta. This distinction can sometimes be made if the real-time scanner also has a time-motion display. By orienting the beam perpendicular to the walls of the vessel in question, one may be able to identify arterial pulsations producing expansion and contraction of walls of the vessel as distinct from transmitted pulsations which show both walls of the vessel moving in the same direction, or from respiration-induced changes.

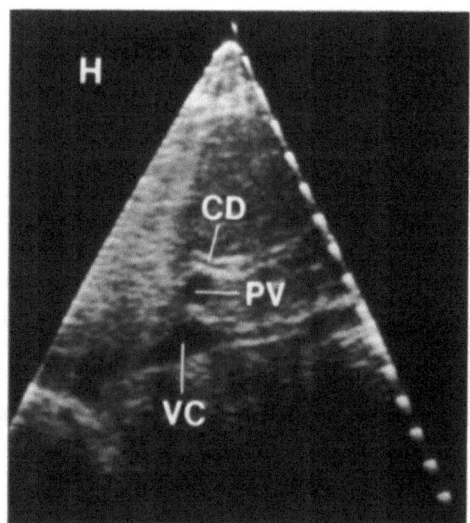

Fig. 3.8. Common duct (*CD*) is identified because of its constant relationship anterior to the portal vein (*PV*) in the sagittal plane in which the portal vein is situated above the vena cava (*VC*).

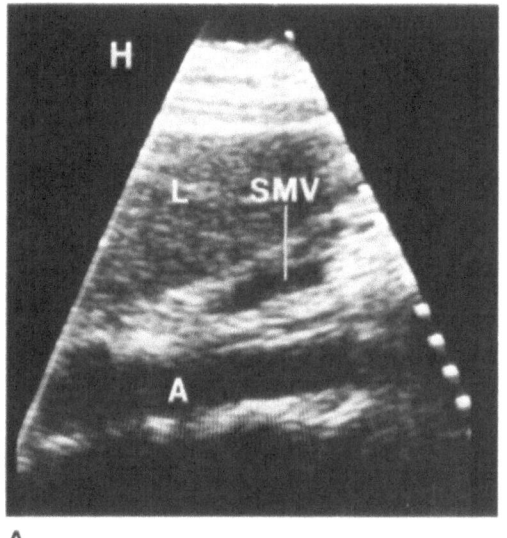
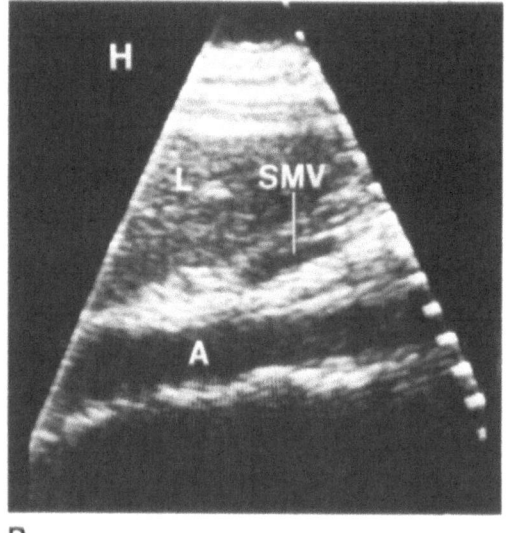

A   B

Fig. 3.9. Vessel anterior to aorta (*A*) identified as vein (superior mesenteric vein; *SMV*) because it changes caliber during respiration, expanding during inspiration (**A**) and decreasing in caliber with expiration (**B**). *L,* liver.

G. Bowel Versus Extraluminal Masses

Loops of bowel are best identified when one can see a change in their caliber and contours or movement of their contents. All of these changes are indicative of peristaltic activity. Although it is best to have food or fluid within bowel to identify it, even a changing pattern of acoustic shadows produced by moving intraluminal gas is indicative of bowel (Fig. 3.10). Occasionally when bowel is dilated, the identifying valvulae conniventes (Fig. 3.11) or haustral markings of small or large bowel can be seen. If these markings are present, then one does not have to demonstrate peristaltic activity to prove that the structure is actually bowel rather than an extraluminal fluid collection. Another method of identifying bowel is by introducing fluid or air intraluminally, and observing the unknown fluid-filled structure to see if a change in the pattern of its fluid content occurs as a result of the introduced material. In general, when the patient's condition permits we prefer the introduction

of fluid rather than gas. To clarify an unknown left upper abdominal fluid-filled structure, the patient may be given water to drink, and the change within the mass is observed as the water is swallowed. To distinguish a retrovesical pathologic mass from stool in the colon, a tap water enema may be given. The colon can be differentiated from an abnormal mass because the former changes both in caliber and in pattern of internal echoes as the water is introduced (see Chapter 9). By comparison, pathologic fluid-filled masses show no change in contour or internal echo pattern either during observation over a period of time or following the introduction of fluid orally or rectally.

Occasionally, in patients who have been fasting for some time, loops of small bowel containing partially digested food may be seen that show no peristaltic movement. It may be difficult to differentiate such bowel loops from enlarged paraaortic nodes or retroperitoneal masses by their appearances alone. However, one additional maneuver may be used—that of varying the amount of

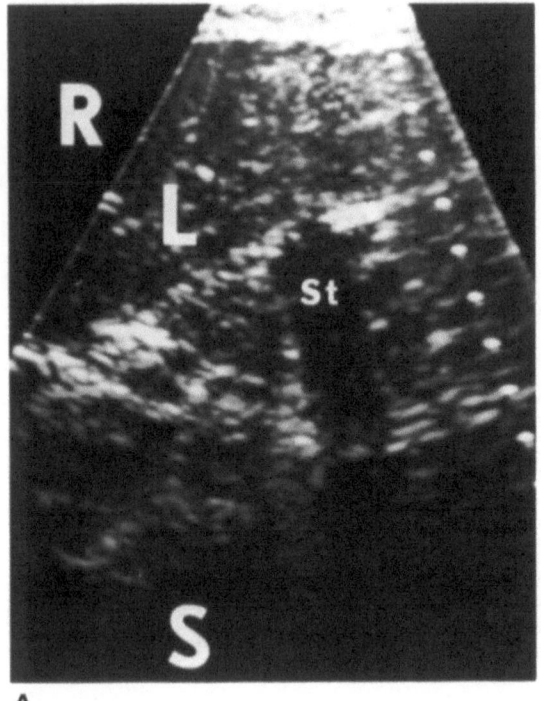

A

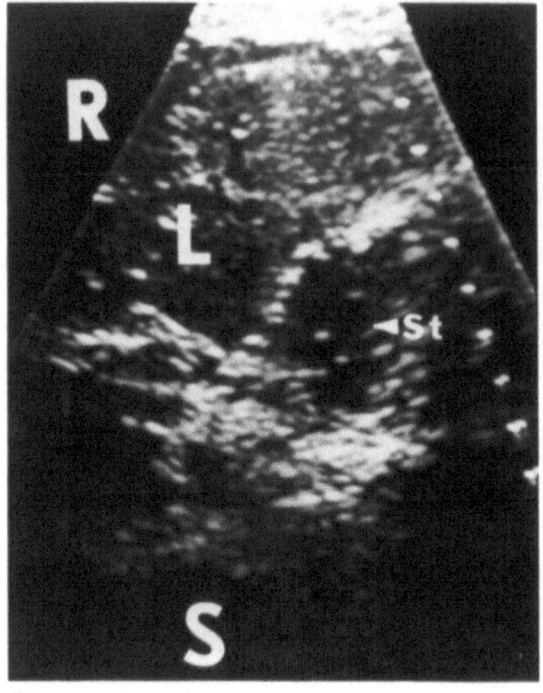

B

C

Fig. 3.10. Identification of mass as loop of bowel because peristalsis produces a changing pattern of gas and fluid within the mass. **A** Stomach (*ST*) filled with gas. **B** Fluid mixed with food particles replaces the gas. **C** Food particles change pattern. *L,* liver; *S,* lumbar spine; *R,* right side of patient.

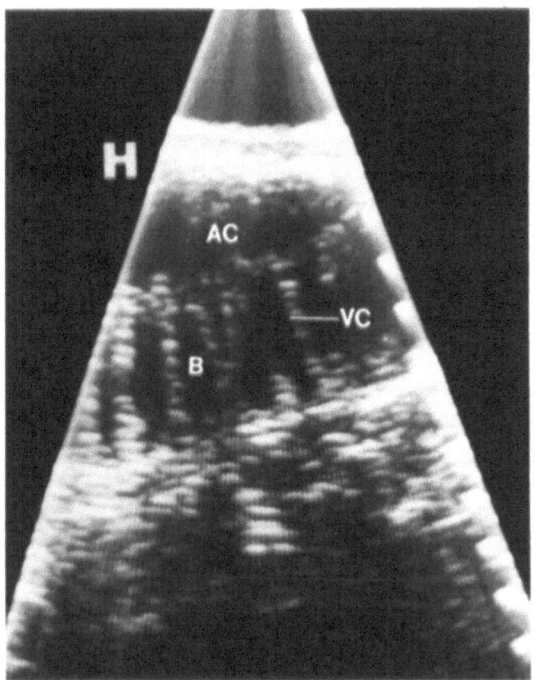

Fig. 3.11. Sagittal view of dilated small bowel (*B*) identified by presence of valvulae conniventes (*VC*). Ascites (*AC*) is adjacent. *H,* direction of patient's head.

pressure with which the transducer is applied to the anterior abdomen—to see if the caliber of the mass in question changes as a result of the varied pressure. A loop of bowel can be compressed with increased pressure whereas a solid mass will not change diameter under similar circumstances (Fig. 3.12).

H. Effect of Transducer Pressure

The quality of a real-time image can be improved, especially in obese patients, by applying greater pressure to the transducer. The increased pressure compresses the overlying tissues, particularly the fat that is interposed between the skin and organ of interest, thereby shortening the travel path of the beam and reducing its scatter and absorption in tissue (Fig. 3.13).

I. Change in Patient Position

Changing patient position can be used to better define organs or organ abnormalities by (1) demonstrating movement of a pathologic structure within an organ and (2) eliminating overlying ribs or gas-filled bowel.

The gallbladder is the most common organ in which a change in position is used to definitively identify pathology—mobile intraluminal stones. Either the decubitus or the erect position can be used, but we prefer the erect position if the patient can tolerate it because a greater shift in the position of the stone can occur when the patient goes from supine to erect than from supine to decubitus (see Chapter 6).

To eliminate the effect of overlying ribs or bowel, the erect position is again preferable to the decubitus position and is especially useful in examining the pancreas. In the erect position the liver often descends anterior to the pancreas thereby producing a gas-free window by which to visualize it. At the same time, portions of the liver that may have been obscured because of overlying ribs now become visible. In cases where it is difficult to see the upper poles of the kidneys, the erect position can facilitate scanning these regions as well. In patients unable to assume the erect position, the decubitus position with the left side down is helpful in imaging the right lobe of the liver since the liver rotates inferiorly and anteriorly and thus more of the organ lies below the rib cage.

Pancreatic imaging is less predictable in the decubitus position. If the pancreas cannot be seen with the patient supine, then both decubitus views should be attempted to better visualize it.

J. Fluid-filled Stomach: an Ultrasound Window

As a further aid to the examination of the pancreas, the stomach can be filled with

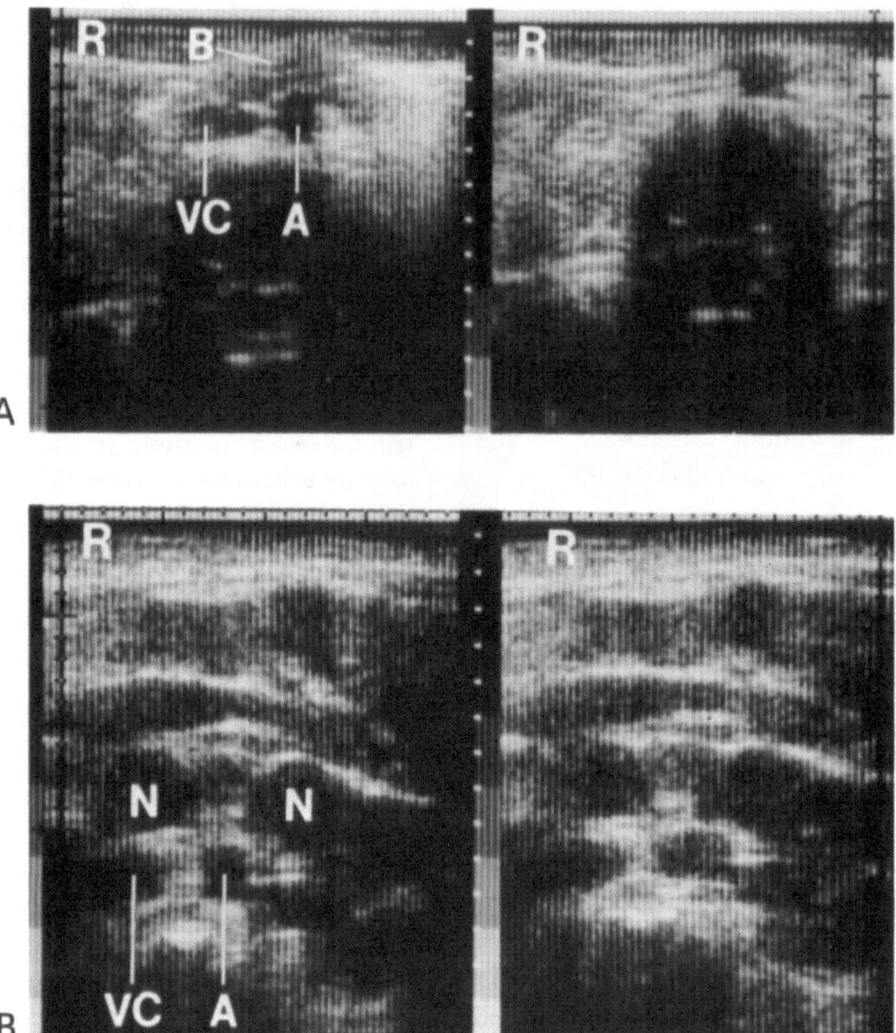

Fig. 3.12. Differentiation of food-filled bowel from enlarged lymph nodes by compressing the abdomen with linear array transducer (manufactured by Advanced Diagnostic Research Corporation). Transverse scans, midabdomen. **A** Loops of bowel (*B*) decrease in caliber with compression. *A,* aorta; *VC,* vena cava. **B** Enlarged paraaortic nodes (*N*) show no change in size with compression.

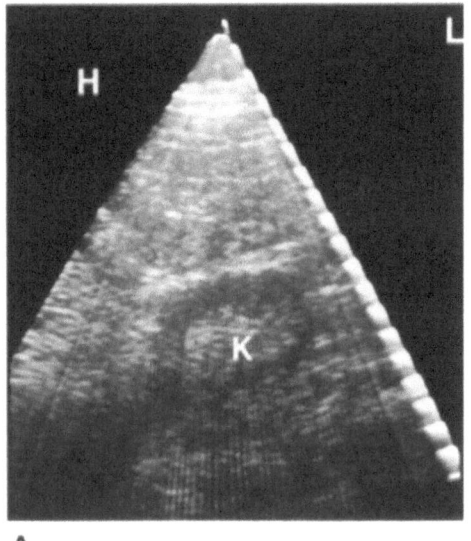
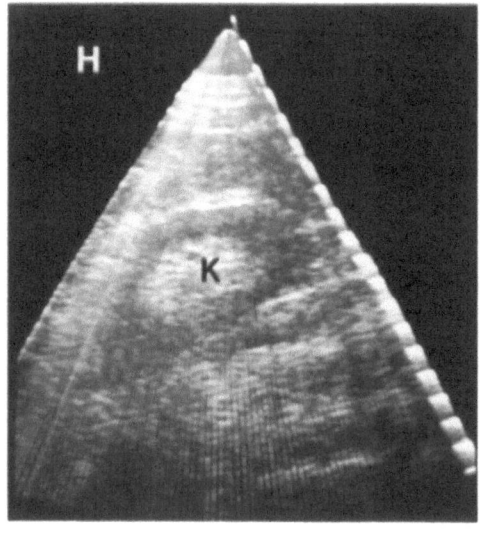

A   B

Fig. 3.13. Improved visualization of deeper tissue by increasing transducer pressure on abdomen to compress intervening tissues. Sagittal view of left kidney (*K*). **A** Without compression. **B** With compression.

fluid to create an ultrasonic window (also see Chapter 9). A fluid with more acoustic absorption than water—milk, eggnog, or tomato or orange juice—is recommended so that the intensity of the sound beam behind the fluid-filled stomach will be similar to the intensity of beam behind the liver. However, when the gallbladder is also to be examined, milk or eggnog should not be used since these fluids contain fat and will contract the gallbladder. Although sometimes filling the stomach with fluid is useful for visualization of the pancreas with the patient supine, this maneuver is most useful in conjunction with the erect position, especially for visualization of the pancreatic tail which is usually obscured by the gas-filled stomach. In the erect position the horizontal beam traverses through the fluid-filled dependent part of the stomach that lies anterior to the tail of the pancreas. In the supine position even if the stomach is fluid filled, a gas bubble almost always remains above the fluid and stops the vertical ultrasound beam from reaching the tail (Fig. 3.14).

K. Effects of Respiration

Identification of respiration-induced change in organ position is an important criterion for demonstrating normality of certain structures within the abdomen. The major applications are in identifying change in diaphragm position and in the appreciation of movement in organs that are normally free to move with respiration, i.e., the liver, spleen, gallbladder, and kidneys. Failure to demonstrate movement with respiration in these organs may be indicative of an inflammatory or neoplastic process binding the organ to adjacent structures (provided there has been no previous surgery in the area). The recording of respiratory motion on still films can be obtained by double exposing during maximum inspiration and maximum expiration (Fig. 3.15).

Organ imaging during normal respiration can be useful in ways other than demonstrating range of organ motion. If the operator holds the transducer on one location on the skin as the organ below moves during res-

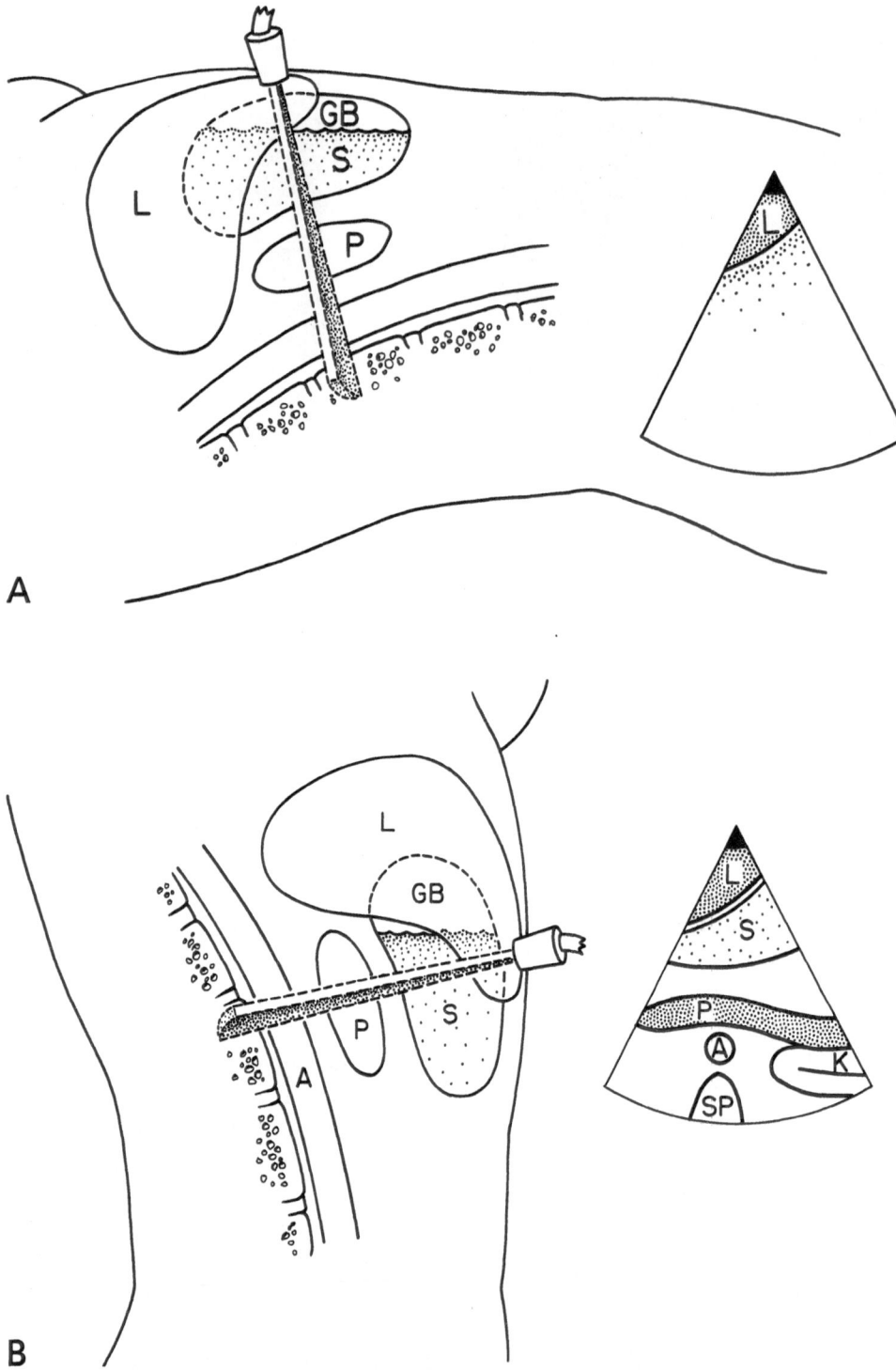

Fig. 3.14. Effect of patient position on usefulness of fluid-filled stomach as acoustic window for pancreatic imaging. **A** Supine position. Gas bubble (*GB*) over fluid blocks ultrasound beam. **B** Erect position. Gas bubble rises to superior portion of stomach leaving fluid window in lower part through which ultrasound beam can pass. *L,* liver; *P,* pancreas; *A,* aorta; *S,* stomach; *K,* kidney; *SP,* spine.

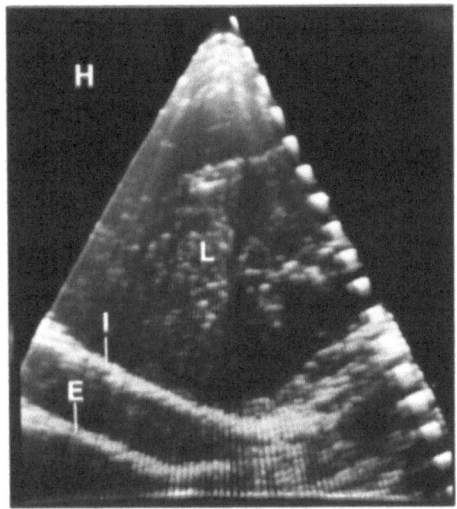

Fig. 3.15. Recording range of diaphragm motion by double exposing image during inspiration (*I*) and expiration (*E*). Right parasagittal view, upper abdomen. *L,* liver.

piration, the examiner can survey the organ without having to move the ultrasound instrument. This maneuver is quite useful in situations where portions of an organ are obscured by overlying bowel or ribs. The examiner can, for example, place the transducer in a rib interspace and survey the liver and kidney as they move back and forth beneath the ultrasound beam (Fig. 3.16). If

instead the operator had the patient suspend respiration and moved the transducer over the skin, portions of the liver and kidney would be obscured by the overlying ribs that cast acoustic shadows. Organ scanning during respiration is also a useful technique when examining a patient who is too ill or uncooperative to suspend respiration.

2. RECORDING OF STILL IMAGES

A. Freeze Versus Nonfreeze Frame

Still photographs are usually made with the patient in suspended respiration. Some instruments possess freeze frame circuitry that facilitates image recording because a given image can be electronically frozen and then photographically recorded later. Freeze frame may produce a degraded image as compared to the one our eyes view during real-time display or to that obtained by photographing the display tube without freeze frame. When freeze frame is used, only a single frame is displayed. In nonfreeze frame photography the shutter speed of the camera is usually set at 1/10 to 1/15 s so that two or three frames are photographically integrated. Our eyes

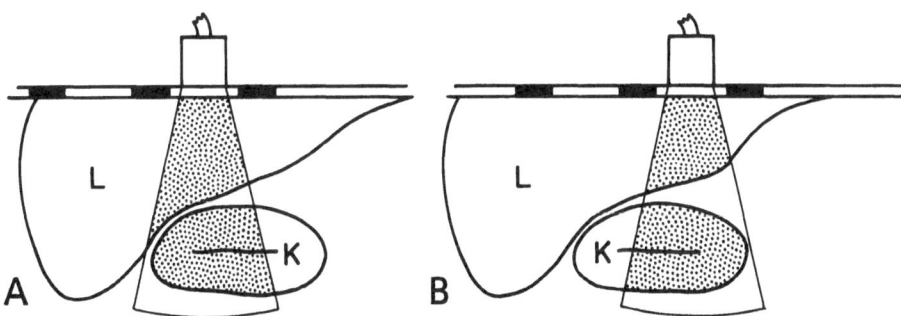

Fig. 3.16. When ribs limit acoustic accessibility to underlying organs, transducer may be held fixed in one interspace and respiratory motion used to sweep organ through ultrasound beam. Sagittal view. *L,* liver; *K,* right kidney. **A** Inspiration; upper pole of kidney visualized. **B** Expiration; lower pole of kidney visualized.

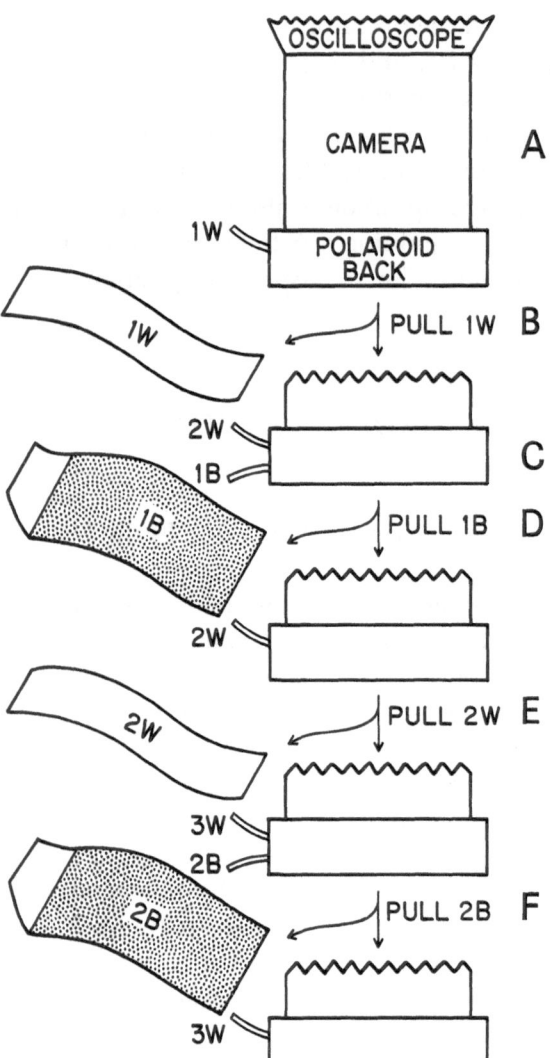

Fig. 3.17. Technique for rapidly exposing two Polaroid frames. **A** Take exposure #1. **B** Pull small white tab. **C** Take exposure #2. **D** Pull large black tab. Exposure #1 is removed from camera. Then pull second small white tab (**E**) and second large black tab (**F**). Exposure #2 is removed from camera.

also integrate images. Visual or photographic integration usually improves image quality because the signal-to-noise ratio of the image improves. System noise is random and so is not likely to fall in the same location on each frame whereas meaningful information repeats itself in the same locations and is thus enhanced. If, however, the image being recorded is that of a structure that significantly changes position between adjacent frames, photographic integration of two or three frames will give a less sharp image than the photographic recording of a single frozen frame.

B. Exposing on the Fly

In instruments not possessing freeze frame capacity, or in those instruments in which image quality during freeze frame display is degraded compared to image quality in real-time mode, the operator should develop rapid coordination between his eyes and his hand or foot that operates the shutter control button so as to record the image at the instant he sees the optimal one displayed. If the patient cannot suspend respiration for the length of the exposure (usually between 1/10 and 1/30 s), then the operator can usually get excellent images with no organ motion by timing his exposure to coincide with the end of the inspiratory or expiratory cycle of the patient.

C. Rapid Sequence (Polaroid) Film

When Polaroid film is used, it is helpful to have an assistant pull the film so as to facilitate the rapid recording of multiple images. If an assistant is not available, the operator, when using Polaroid film, can take two images in rapid sequence by pulling only the smaller paper tab after the first image is taken and then immediately taking the second exposure. The larger black tab is then pulled to develop the initial exposure and next the second small white paper tab and the larger black tab are pulled in sequence to advance and process the second frame (Fig. 3.17). This method *cannot* be used for taking *more* than two images in rapid sequence. If more than two images must be recorded in close proximity to each other, this method should not be used because of the time pause after the initial two exposures that is required to pull all the tabs. If the image is displayed on a television format, multiimage cameras can be used, of if funds are available, images can be initially recorded on video disc and subsequently transferred to film for permanent storage (2).

References

1. Jaffe CC, Rosenfield AT, Sommer G, Taylor KJW (1980) Technical factors influencing the imaging of small anechoic cysts by B-scan ultrasound. Radiology 135:429–433
2. Skolnick ML (1979) A new approach to ultrasound image recording using a video disc recorder. Radiology 133:530

4
Kidney

The kidney, because of its anatomic location in the flanks, can be imaged through more ultrasonic windows than any other abdominal organ. As a result, one has a greater chance of obtaining good images of this organ than of more central intra- or retroperitoneal organs which possess fewer ultrasonic windows and can more readily be obscured by overlying gas-filled bowel.

1. ANATOMY

The left kidney is normally several centimeters more superior than the right one. Their long axes are oriented diagonally with the upper poles lying closer to the vertebral column and more posterior than the lower poles. In cross section the kidneys are usually oval with the medial-lateral dimension being greater than the anterior-posterior measurement (Fig. 4.1). In some patients the lower poles of the kidneys, especially the right one, can be close enough to the anterior abdominal wall to be palpated and confused with a pathologic mass. Although they are retroperitoneal, both kidneys exhibit considerable mobility. They move several centimeters in a superior-inferior direction with respiration and when the patient changes position. In the shift from a supine to a decubitus position, the kidneys rotate medially to lie with their long axes more in a transverse plane. In the prone position, the diagonal orientation may increase compared to the supine position because the lower poles now

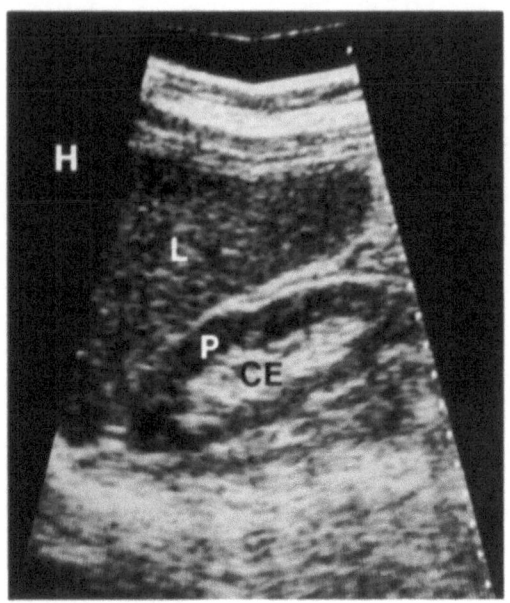

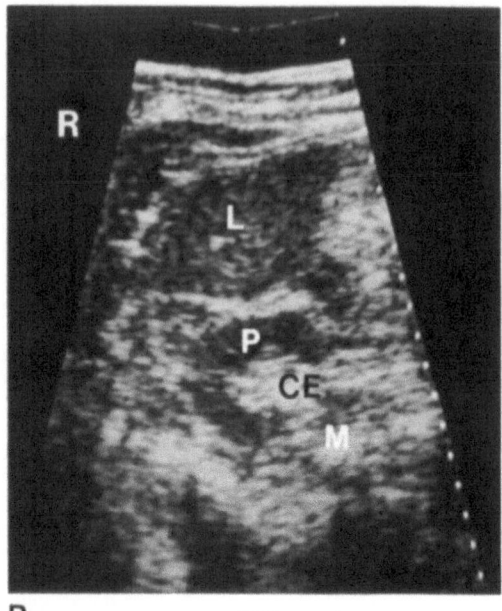

A   B

Fig. 4.1. Normal right kidney. Sagittal (**A**) and transverse (**B**) planes. *L*, liver; *P*, renal parenchyma; *CE*, central echo complex containing peripelvic fat, major vessels, and collection system; *M*, psoas muscle. (Xerox 150 scanner.)

become even more laterally positioned.

Although the renal capsule is usually smooth, fetal lobulation can produce a localized indentation of the capsule (Fig. 4.2).

Normal intrarenal structures that can be ultrasonically identified include (1) the central echo complex consisting of nondistended collecting system, major vessels, and peripelvic fat; (2) the pyramids; and (3) arcuate arteries which demarcate the corticomedullary junction (Fig. 4.3) (1). Although the normal calyces and infundibula usually lack enough urine to identify them as tubular structures, occasionally a normal calyx and infundibulum can be seen (Fig. 4.4) (2).

An envelope of highly echo-reflective retroperitoneal fat which varies in thickness depending upon the patient's habitus surrounds each kidney (Fig. 4.5).

The right kidney is covered anteriorly and laterally by the large mass of the liver (Fig. 4.1), while the left kidney is covered anteriorly by the stomach and bowel and only laterally by the spleen (Fig. 4.7).

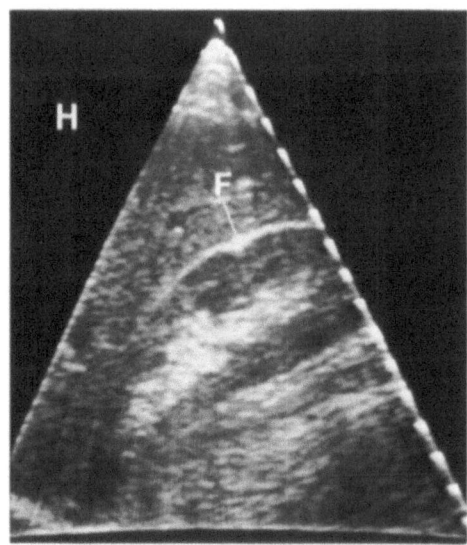

Fig. 4.2. Fetal lobulation (*F*) producing localized indentation of renal capsule.

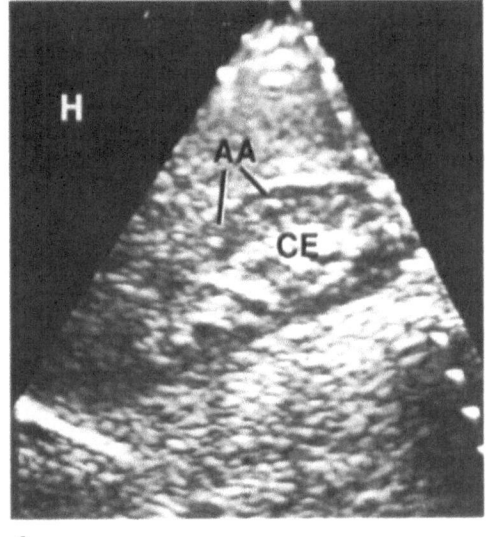

A

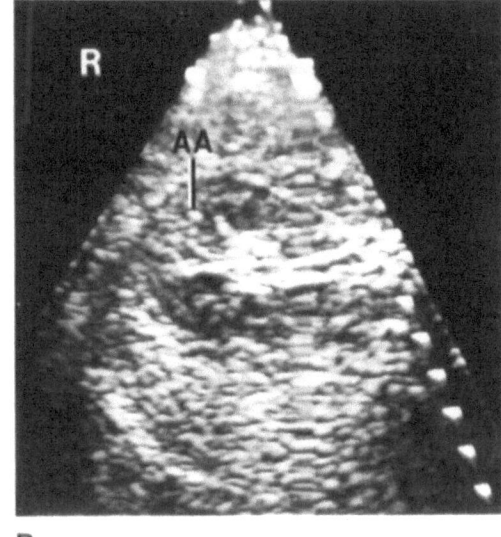

B

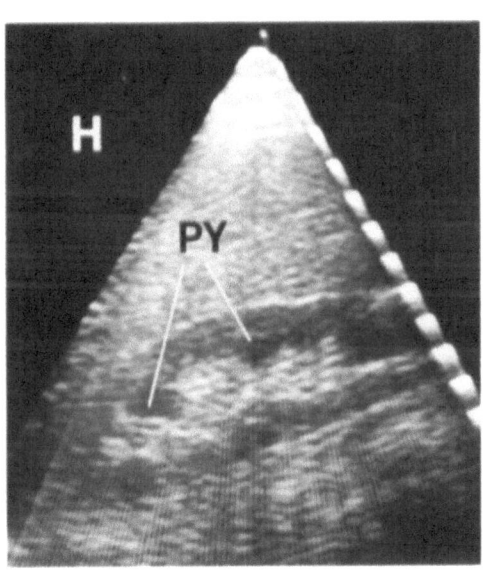

C

Fig. 4.3. Normal intrarenal architecture. Sagittal (**A**) and transverse (**B**) planes of same patient and sagittal plane of another patient (**C**). AA, arcuate arteries; *PY*, pyramids; *CE*, central echo complex.

2. SCANNING TECHNIQUES

A. Effect of Overlying Tissues

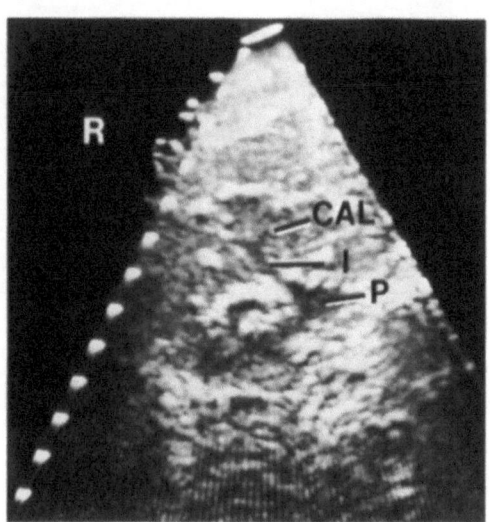

Fig. 4.4. Normal renal pelvis (*P*), infundibulum (*I*), and calyx (*CAL*). Transverse plane.

Before discussing specific transducer positions for imaging the kidney, there are two important principles relating to transducer placement to keep in mind. First, the path of the beam should be chosen so that the thickness of the tissue intervening between the skin and region of interest is minimal. Thus, the degradation that the ultrasound beam undergoes by scattering and attenuation as it traverses through the overlying tissue will be minimized so as not to reduce the image quality of deeper structures. In addition, when the overlying tissues are thin, higher frequency transducers which produce fine image resolution can be employed. Second, ultrasound does not pass equally well

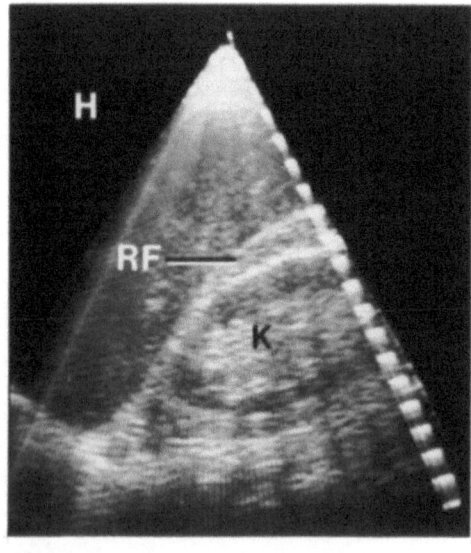

A

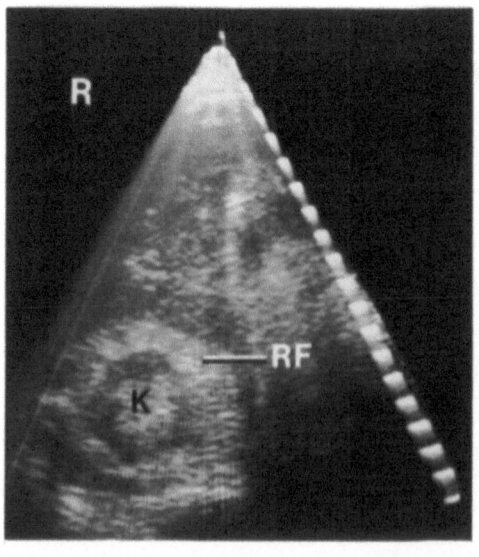

B

Fig. 4.5. Retroperitoneal fat (*RF*) surrounding kidney (*K*). Sagittal (**A**) and transverse (**B**) planes.

through all soft tissues (tissues free of bone, barium, or air). Therefore, the distortions that various types of intervening tissue impart to the ultrasound beam must also be considered. For example, certain thick muscles, especially those in the paravertebral region, distort the ultrasound beam to a much greater extent because of the scattering and reflecting effects of sound upon the layers of muscle and connective tissue than does a greater depth of more uniformly textured tissue such as liver. As a result, images of the kidney appear much more poorly defined when the overlying tissue is paravertebral muscle than when it is liver (Fig. 4.6).

B. Supine Imaging

Although the kidneys can be imaged from a multiplicity of directions—through the anterior abdomen, the flanks, and the back—certain ultrasonic approaches are preferable.

We usually begin the examination with the patient supine and the beam directed into the right kidney either from the anterior abdominal surface (sagittal plane) or through the flanks (coronal plane) (Fig. 4.7). Transverse scans can be obtained through either approach by rotating the transducer 90°. If the liver and kidney lie or can be projected on deep inspiration to lie below the costal margin, then the anterior approach is preferred especially when a linear array is used since there will be overlying ribs to produce artifacts. When the anterior approach is unsuccessful because gas-filled bowel is interposed between liver and kidney or because the liver and kidney are underneath the rib cage and the closely spaced anterior ribs limit the size of the ultrasonic window, then the flank approach is employed. The ribs continue to overlie the kidney in this approach but the interspaces are wider than over the anterior chest. A sector scanner is the preferred instrument in this approach since the transducer assembly can fit be-

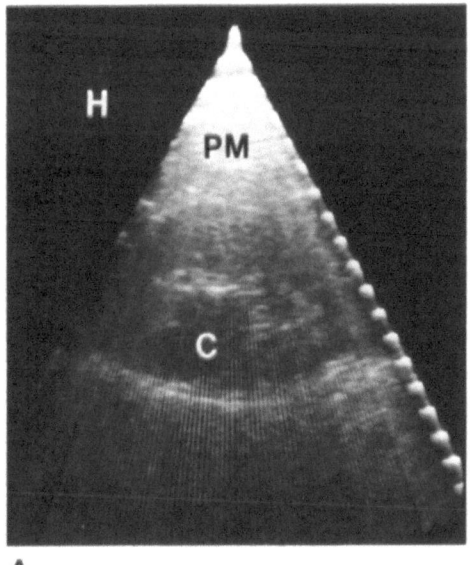
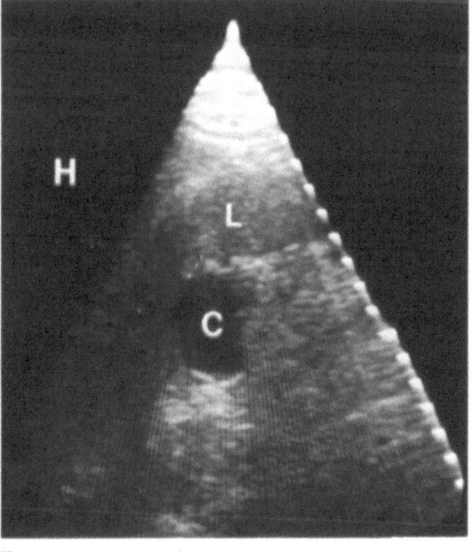

A   B

Fig. 4.6. Attenuating effects of different overlying tissues on visualization of deeper structures. Right kidney containing cyst (*C*). **A** Imaged through back with patient prone. Beam traverses paravertebral muscles (*PM*). Cyst is not clearly defined. **B** Imaged through flank with patient supine. Beam traversed lateral abdominal wall and liver (*L*). Cyst clearly seen.

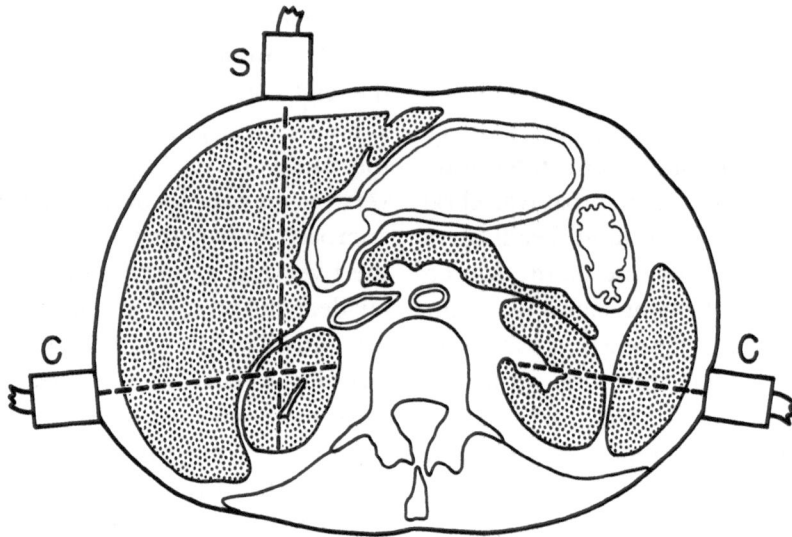

Fig. 4.7. Usual planes for imaging kidneys with patient supine. Right kidney: sagittal (*S*) and coronal (*C*) planes. Left kidney: only coronal plane.

tween ribs (Fig. 2.13). However, when the kidney is close to the flank, as in thin patients, the entire kidney may not be covered in one sector image because the kidney is too close to the apex of the sector. The entire kidney can still be adequately imaged with a sector scanner on two separate frames by first scanning the upper and then the lower pole. Alternately, by using a linear array (Fig. 4.8), the entire kidney can be imaged on one field.

The supine examination of the left kidney usually can best be performed through the flank (using the spleen as an acoustic window) because in the normal subject the stomach and bowel which lie anterior to the kidney are often gas filled (Fig. 4.7). When the spleen is enlarged, it projects anteriorly over the kidney and displaces the bowel to provide an acoustic window similar to that of the liver on the right to permit imaging from the anterior approach. The left kidney is usually closer to the left flank than the right kidney is to its flank because the thickness of the spleen is less than the liver. Therefore, a sector scanner may image an even smaller part of the left than the right kidney and multiple images may be required

to record the entire kidney in long axis. In spite of the artifacts that may be produced by overlying ribs, the linear array may be more satisfactory for imaging overall renal length.

Since the muscle layers in the intercostal

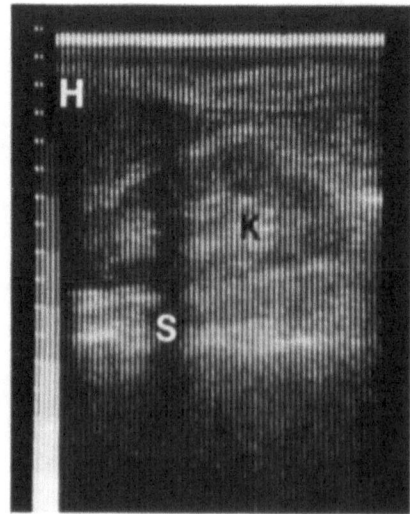

Fig. 4.8. Linear array. Superficially located kidney (*K*) seen in entirety. *S*, rib acoustic shadow. (Advanced Diagnostic Research Corporation scanner.)

and flank regions are much thinner and not as interlayered with connective tissue planes as the paravertebral muscle, they do not significantly impede the passage of sound. Imaging during breathing (Fig. 3.16) with the array held in one location may facilitate imaging through overlying ribs because portions of the kidney obscured by rib acoustic shadows in one phase of respiration will appear in the interspaces in another phase.

C. Decubitus Imaging

If the supine position does not allow for satisfactory renal imaging, especially on the left side, the decubitus view is the next choice. In this position the kidney moves medially and inferiorly so that more of the organ is located below the ribs and further from the flanks.

A pillow or roll of towels is placed under the flank of the side of the patient adjacent to the table in order to cause the body to arc over the pillow. The maneuver increases the distance between the ribs and the iliac wing on the side of the body away from the table to provide a longer bone-free region through which to examine the uppermost kidney (Fig. 4.9) and presses the kidney closer to the flank so as to reduce the thickness of intervening muscle and fat through which the beam must travel. It may be a little more difficult to find the true long and short axes of the kidney in this position as the location of the kidney can vary considerably depending upon the build of the patient and how loosely the kidney is attached within the retroperitoneal space. Since the kidney usually rotates medially, one should begin the scanning more anteriorly than one would if the patient were supine. Otherwise, the same maneuvers are applied as when the patient is supine.

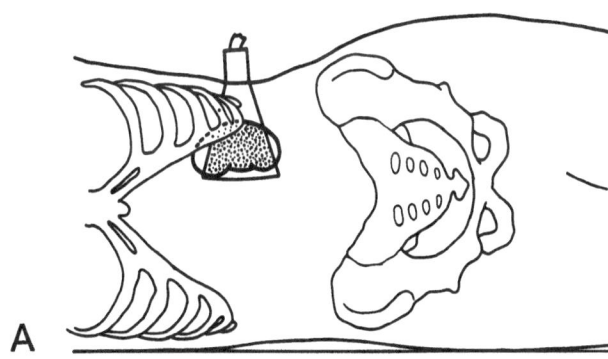

A

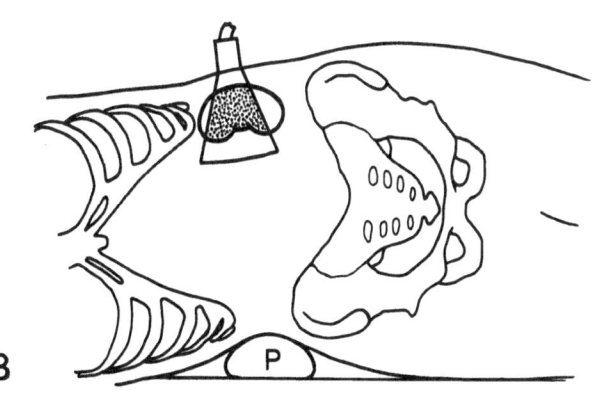

B

Fig. 4.9. Pillow facilitates renal imaging with patient in decubitus position. **A** Without pillow. Ribs closely approach iliac crest. Limited rib-free region for transducer placement. **B** With pillow (*P*) under flank. Space between ribs and iliac crest is widened and kidney is pushed closer to the flank, thereby decreasing thickness of intervening tissue that can attenuate sound.

D. Prone Imaging

The prone position is usually the least advantageous for examining the kidney because of the attenuating effects of the paravertebral muscles on the ultrasound beam which decreases image resolution. However, this position is used when the kidney is to be biopsied or when a cyst within it is to be punctured. The distance between the kidney and skin is shorter than with the patient supine, and there are no vital structures overlying the kidney that can be injured by the cutting biopsy needle. In addition, the kidney can be stabilized to facilitate the biopsy or cyst puncture by placing a firm pillow or pad underneath the patient's anterior abdominal wall at the level of the kidneys. This pad should be thick enough to produce mild discomfort to the patient and also to produce a slightly convex superior contour to the back. When the patient lies in this position, there should be no pillow under the head so as to exaggerate the effect of the pillow under the abdomen (Fig. 4.10). Usually the prone position is used after the diagnosis of an intrarenal mass lesion has been made in another position.

E. Erect Imaging

The kidneys can also be examined with the patient erect, although this approach is infrequently used. In the erect position, the kidneys may descend a greater distance below the rib cage than they could in a nonerect position, even with the patient suspending his breath in inspiration. Thus, the erect position can be useful when it is difficult to adequately examine the upper portions of the kidneys in other views because of the overlying ribs. The erect position has one other advantage: in patients in whom dilated collecting systems are identified, the failure to drain the collecting system in the erect position further substantiates the observation that the dilatation is probably secondary to obstruction rather than indicating dilatation secondary to urinary stasis which can occur in the supine position.

F. Effect of Respiration

The kidneys should be examined in both expiration and deep inspiration. Although inspiration projects more of the kidneys below the rib cage and may facilitate an anterior approach on the right, the lower poles may be obscured by overlying bowel. On the other hand, in expiration, although the kidneys are more covered by ribs, they are also more enveloped by liver or spleen and thus less likely to be obscured by bowel.

G. Finding the Axis

Regardless of the position used, we prefer to begin the study by attempting to image

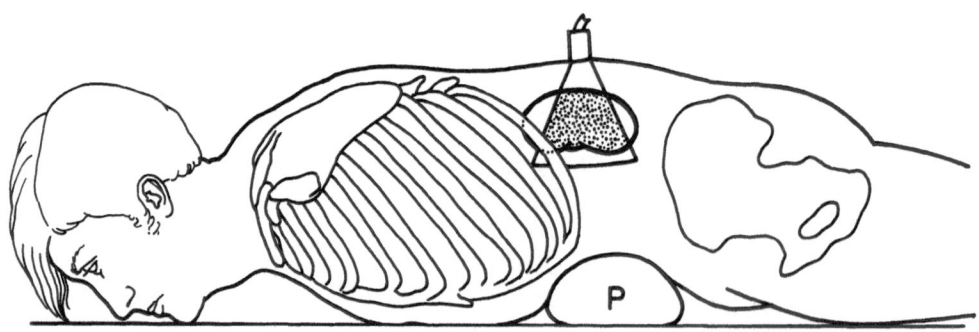

Fig. 4.10. Patient prone. Effect of pillow (P) similar to that in decubitus position.

the kidney in long axis. The transducer is initially placed in the sagittal or coronal plane. Once a portion of the kidney is identified within the ultrasound field, then the transducer is slowly rotated in order to obtain a true long axis view of the organ (Fig. 3.2). After this view is obtained and the midplane of the kidney identified by the appearance of the strong central echo complex, then the transducer is angled or swept first in one direction and then in the other to fully image the renal tissue on either side of the midplane (Fig. 3.3A). To image the kidney in the short axis, the transducer is rotated 90° to its long axis position and then swept up and down the kidney (Fig. 3.3B).

H. Visualizing the Surfaces

It is important for the operator to realize that long axis views of the kidneys in the sagittal plane (either obtained with the patient prone or supine) show different surfaces of the kidney than do long axis views obtained in the coronal plane (through the flanks). In the sagittal plane, because the anterior and posterior surfaces of the kidneys are perpendicular to the ultrasound beam, masses that project from these surfaces are well defined. By contrast, in the coronal plane, the medial and lateral surfaces of the kidneys become perpendicular to the beam and are clearly seen (Fig. 4.11) while the anterior and posterior surfaces are not. In the transverse plane, all four surfaces of the kidney are seen; therefore, it does not matter whether the transducer is positioned transversely on the sagittal or coronal plane (Fig. 4.12).

I. Correlating with Intravenous Pyelography

Before beginning a renal ultrasound examination, it is most important that the operator first examine the intravenous pyelogram to determine the size and location of any suspected masses within the kidney. This information will help the operator choose the optimal approach for imaging the mass. When a mass projects beyond the margin of the kidney, then the long axis view that shows the mass in profile should be used. If the mass is intrarenal, then either the coronal or sagittal plane can be used provided the plane transects the mass. It is also important to know the size of the mass on the intravenous pyelogram in order to correlate that size with the size of the mass seen by ultrasound. If there are discrepancies in size between the two studies, one may not be seeing the same structure on both examinations.

J. Perpendicular Views

In order to be sure that a mass actually exists in the kidney and to fully appreciate its size and configuration, ultrasound views in two perpendicular planes should always be obtained. If these two views are not always obtained, then for example, one could confuse a dilated renal collecting system with a renal cyst (Fig. 4.13). In the former situation, the configuration of the cystic mass is considerably different on the two views, appearing oval in one and showing the branching of dilated infundibula and calyces projecting from the pelvis in the other. In the latter case, the cystic mass is oval or spherical with a uniformly continuous margin on both views.

K. Beam Positioning Through Mass

In small masses the differentiation between cystic and solid is sometimes difficult if the beam is not properly positioned (Fig. 3.6). When the width of the beam is narrower than the diameter of the cyst, the entire ultrasound beam goes through the cyst and it appears as an echo-free structure (Fig.

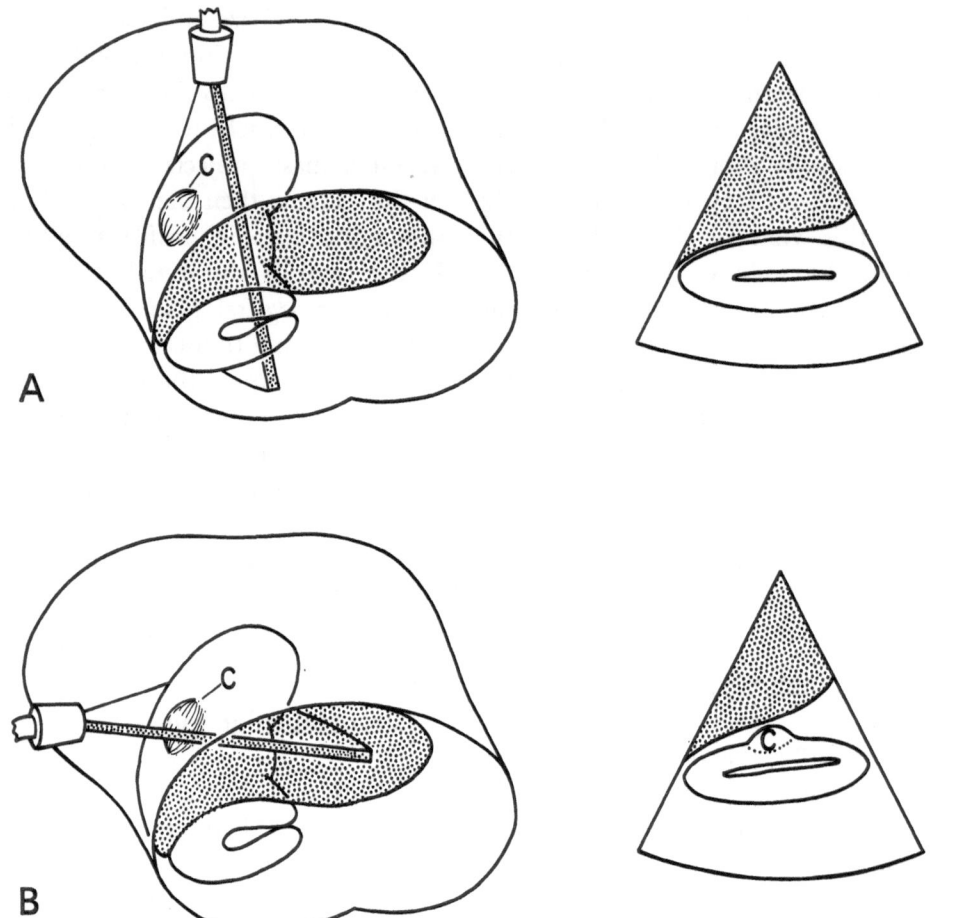

A

B

Fig. 4.11.

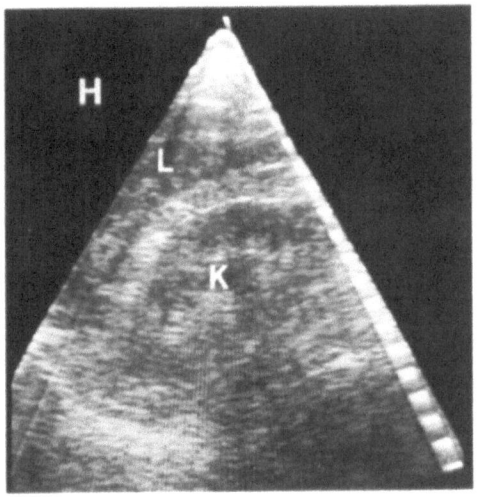

A'

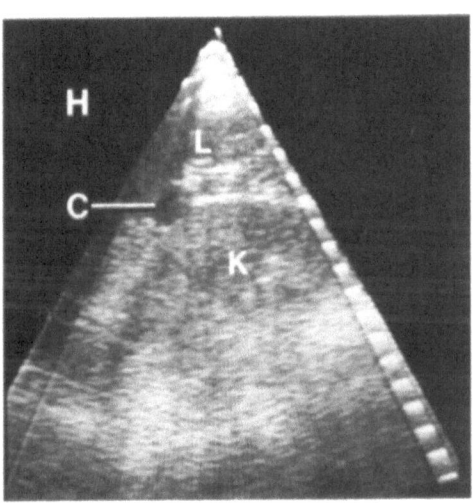

B'

Fig. 4.11. Cyst projects from lateral surface of kidney. **A** and **A'** Sagittal plane. Beam not in plane of cyst. Cyst not imaged. *L*, liver; *K*, kidney. **B** and **B'** Coronal plane. Beam traverses through and images cyst (*C*).

4.14A). If, however, a portion of the beam goes through the cyst and a portion goes through the adjacent solid tissue, then the echoes produced from the solid tissue may be projected within the lumen of the cyst to produce a confusing picture (Fig. 4.14B). This difficulty can be overcome by continu-

ously sweeping the beam through the mass with the patient in suspended respiration. Usually when the beam is traversing through the widest diameter of the mass, it will be entirely within the mass and a typical appearance of a cyst will be revealed. Thus, minimal changes in the orientation of the beam to the mass can have a significant effect on the appearance of the mass and the resultant diagnosis.

L. Gain Settings

The level of gain setting also affects the differentiation between solid and cystic masses. With too high a setting, low level echoes will appear within cystic masses (Fig. 4.15). At too low a setting, a solid mass will appear echo free (Fig. 4.16). Even though real-time scanners and contact scanners produce a gray scale that supposedly can show a wide dynamic range at a given gain setting, in clinical practice there is no one gain setting for all patients. Rather, the gain should be set with reference to a known cystic structure within the patient which is of approximately the same size and depth as the unknown mass (3). The urinary bladder, the gallbladder, or a dilated renal pelvis can be used as standards for fluid-filled cavities to compare against an unknown intrarenal mass. The appropriate gain level is the highest level at which the control fluid is echo free. Therefore, the control fluid should be imaged with increasing gain until echoes just appear within and then the gain is lowered slightly.

Sometimes, when the gain setting is relatively high and the parenchymal echoes are intense, a small cyst (1 to 3 cm) may appear echo free but the appreciation of acoustic enhancement behind the cyst may be difficult. Since the cyst is small, the degree of reduced attenuation through the cyst cavity relative to the adjacent solid tissue may not be enough to appreciate the zone of enhancement at a relatively high gain level.

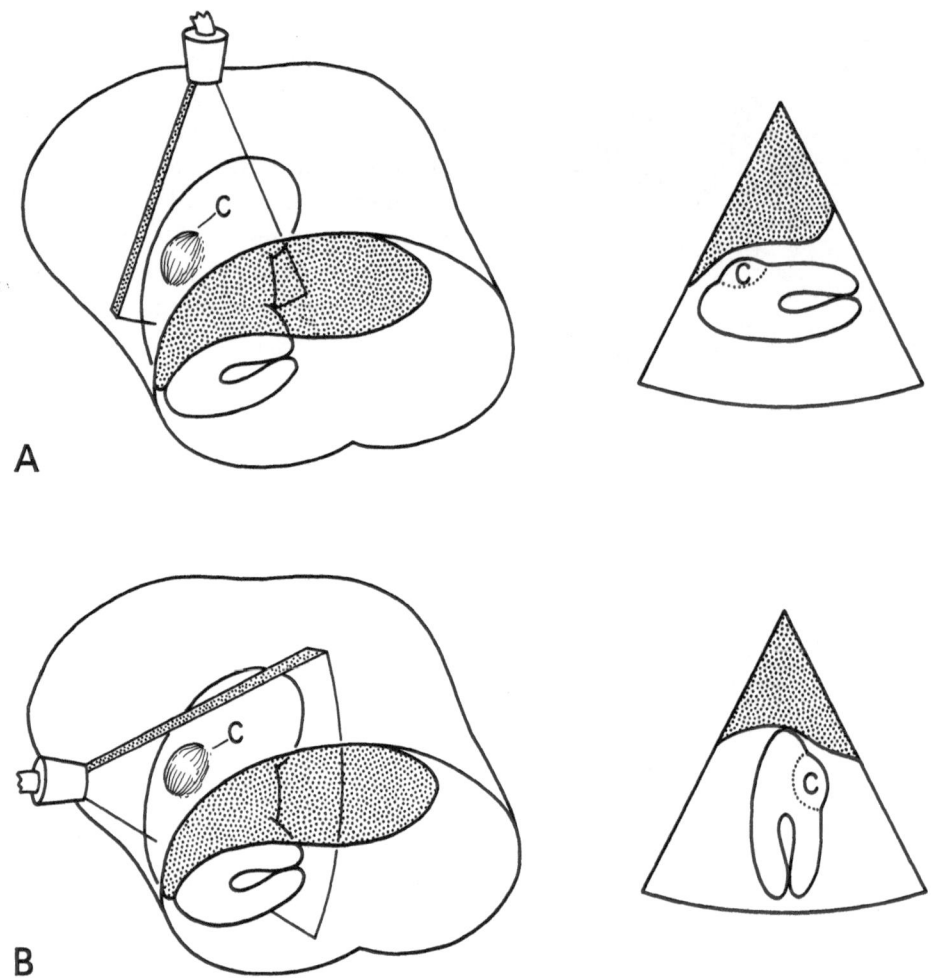

A

B

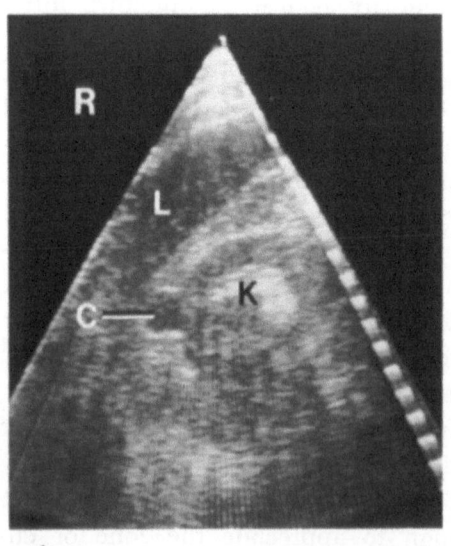

A'

Fig. 4.12. Scans in transverse planes. **A** and **A'** Via anterior abdominal wall or perpendicular to sagittal plane. **B** Via flank or perpendicular to coronal plane. Cyst (*C*) well defined in either approach. *L*, liver; *K*, kidney.

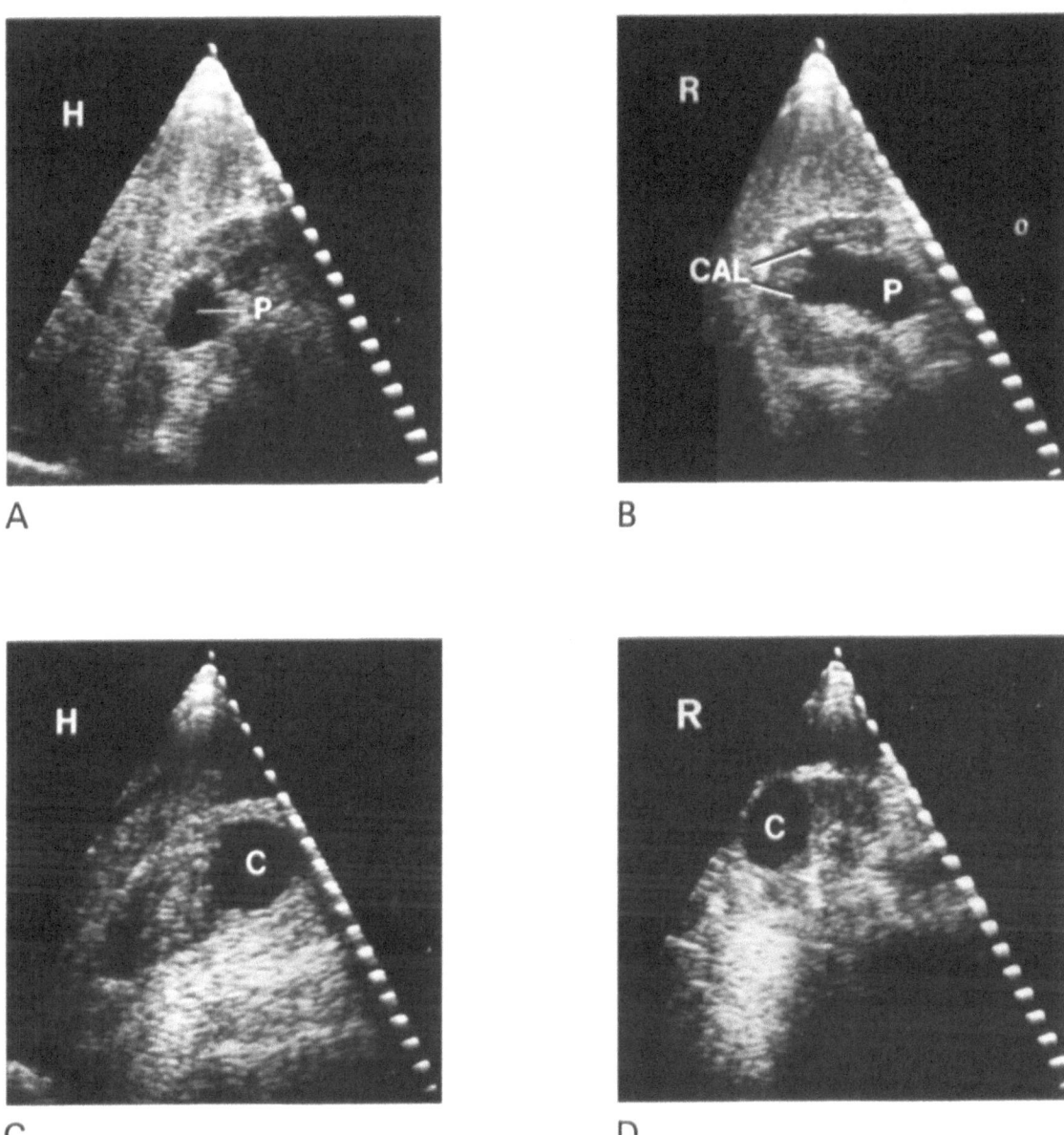

Fig. 4.13. Importance of obtaining views perpendicular to each other. **A** and **C** Sagittal views. Dilated pelvis (*P*) and peripelvic cyst (*C*) appear similar. **B** and **D** Transverse views. Dilated calyces (*CAL*) project from lateral margins of dilated pelvis (*P*) while cyst (*C*) maintains its circular appearance.

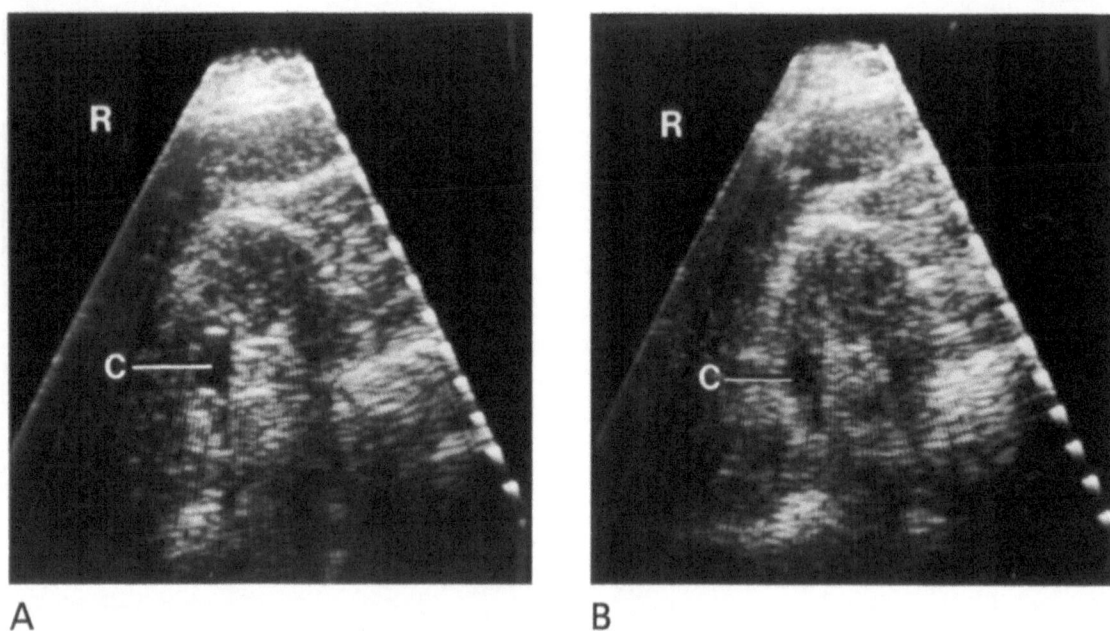

Fig. 4.14. A Beam width entirely within cyst. Typical appearance of cyst (*C*). **B** Beam partially through cyst and partially through adjacent solid tissue. Cyst contains faint echoes, walls not as strongly reflective, and zone of acoustic enhancement not present.

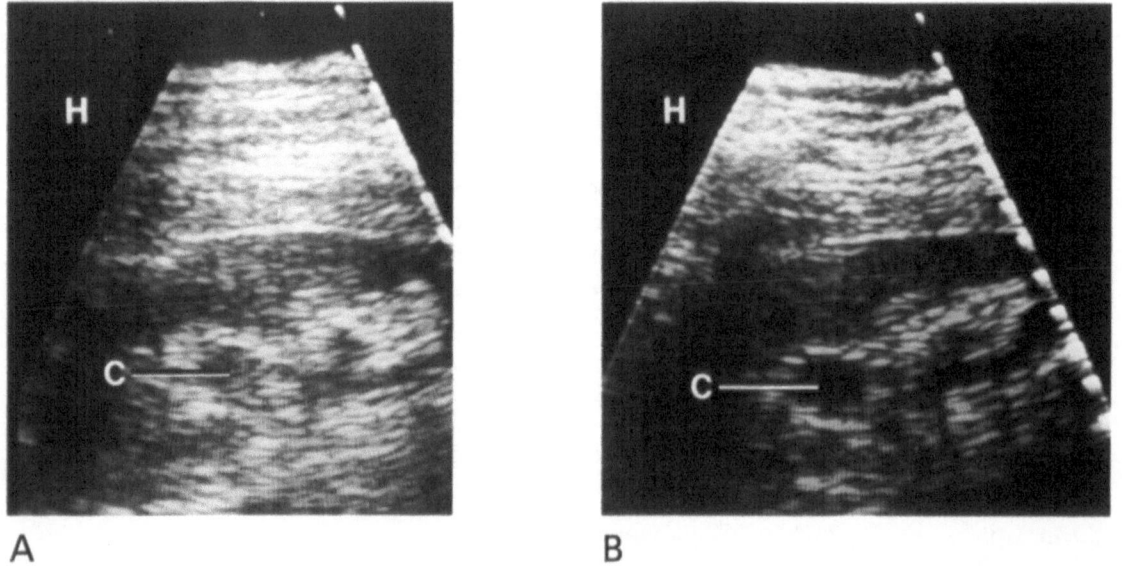

Fig. 4.15. Effect of gain on cyst identification. **A** Gain too high; echoes appear within cyst (*C*). **B** Correct gain level; cyst echo free.

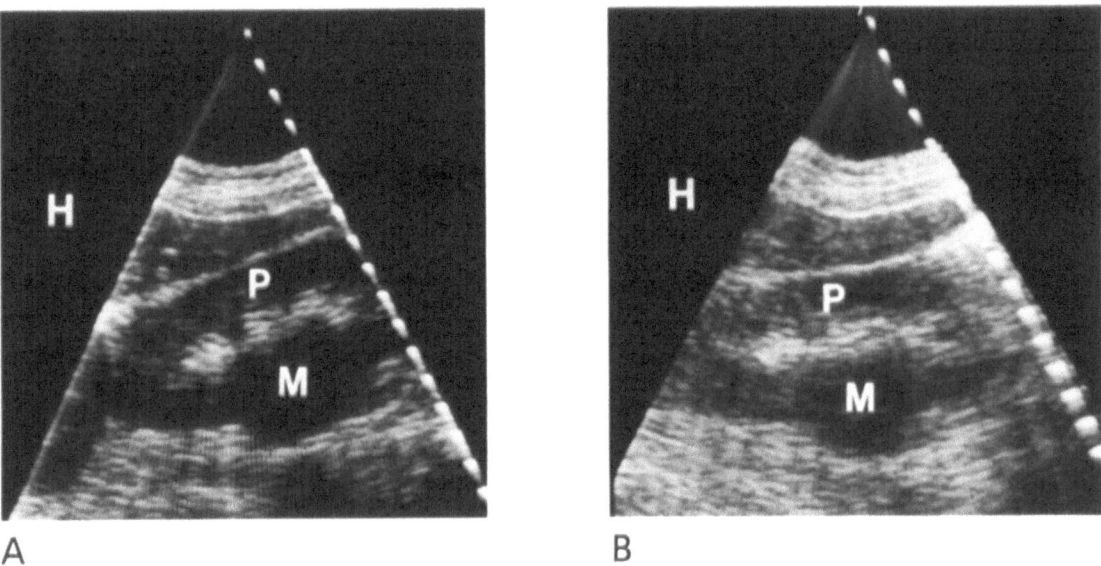

Fig. 4.16. Effect of gain on identification of solid mass. Carcinoma of lung metastatic to kidney. **A** Gain level too low. No echoes within mass (*M*) and few within normal renal parenchyma (*P*). **B** Correct gain level. Echoes produced from within both parenchyma and mass.

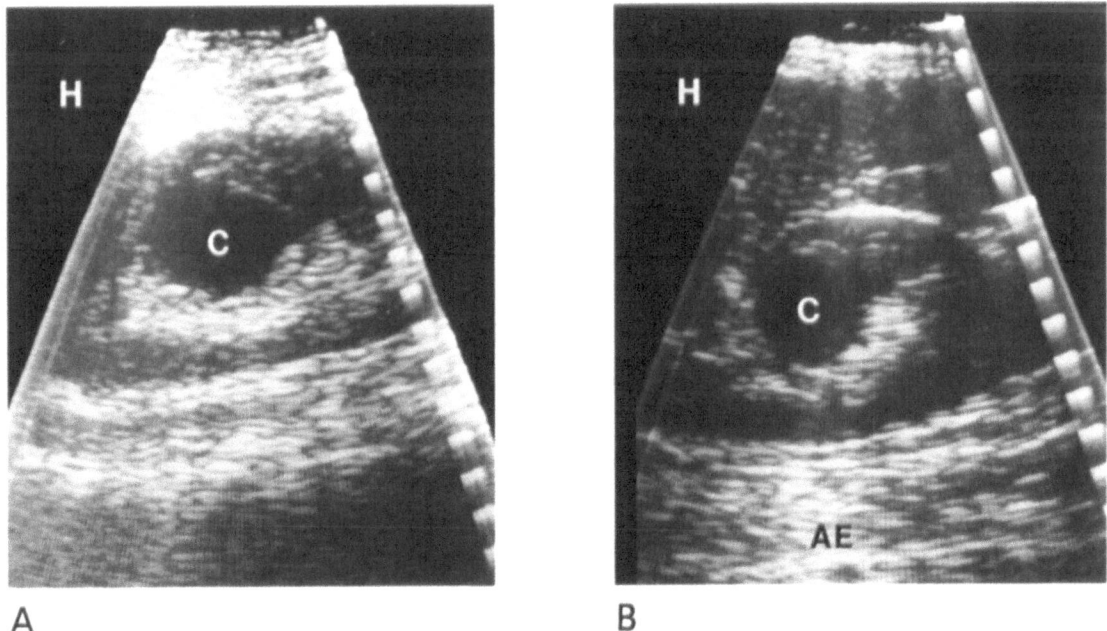

Fig. 4.17. Effect of gain level on detection of acoustic enhancement behind cyst. **A** Zone of acoustic enhancement behind cyst (*C*) is difficult to appreciate because of high level of all echoes behind kidney. **B** Lower gain level. Zone of enhancement (*AE*) becomes more distinct.

If the gain is reduced, then the zone of enhancement behind the cyst becomes more obvious (Fig. 4.17) because the echoes of the adjacent parenchyma become lower. However, if cysts are only studied at these lower gain levels, abscesses, hematomas, and necrotic tumors that can produce echoes in a fluid-filled cavity may be missed.

3. PATHOLOGY

A. Cysts

The diagnosis of a cyst depends upon three characteristics: (1) an echo-free mass with (2) smooth and sharply defined walls and (3) a zone of increased reflectivity in the tissues deep to the cyst produced by the reduced attenuation of the beam as it traverses through the cyst fluid (Figs. 4.12A, 4.13C and D, 4.14A, 4.15, 4.17, and 4.18) (4).

The spectrum of renal cysts is great. They range in size from less than 1 cm (Fig. 4.12A)

to many centimeters in diameter (Fig. 4.18). They can be located peripherally (Fig. 4.12A') or in the peripelvic region (Figs. 4.13C and D, 4.17, and 4.18) where they can be confused with a dilated renal pelvis. Two or more simple cysts can coexist in the same kidney. When this situation is suspected, the diagnosis can definitely be made by displaying the multiple cysts on one scan (Fig. 4.19). Multiple simple cysts should not be confused with polycystic disease (Fig. 4.20). In the latter condition both kidneys usually are similarly involved, and the cysts often show considerable variation in size (5). They are very numerous and diffusely involve the kidneys so that little or no normal renal tissue may be visible. By contrast, in kidneys with multiple simple cysts, the two kidneys are not symmetrically involved and a considerable amount of normal renal tissue remains.

B. Tumors

The criteria for designating a mass as solid are (1) the presence of echoes within the

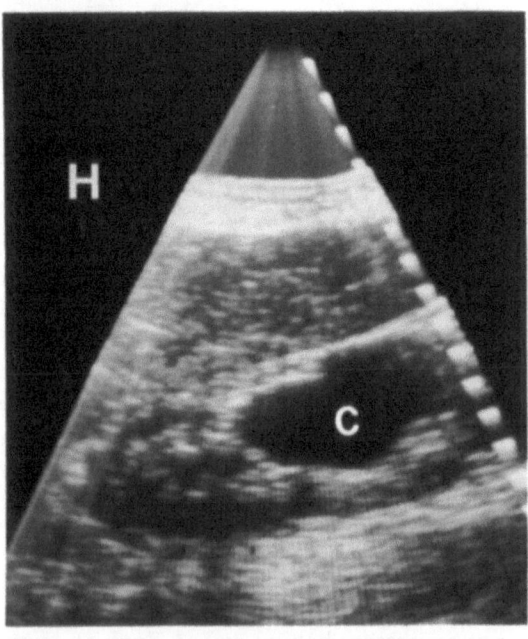

A

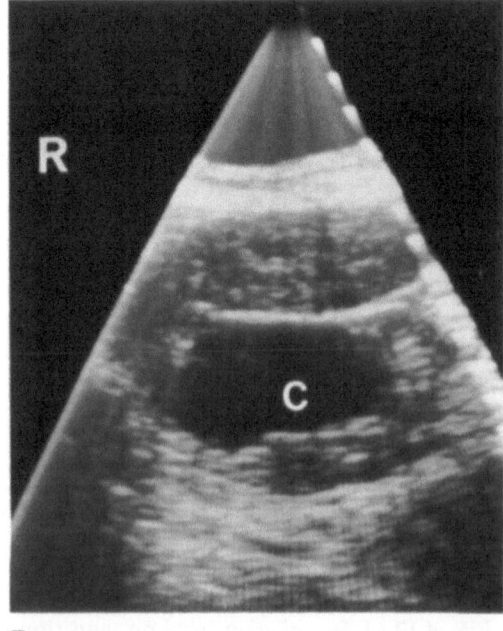

B

Fig. 4.18. Large cyst (*C*) entirely within confines of kidney. Sagittal (**A**) and transverse (**B**) planes.

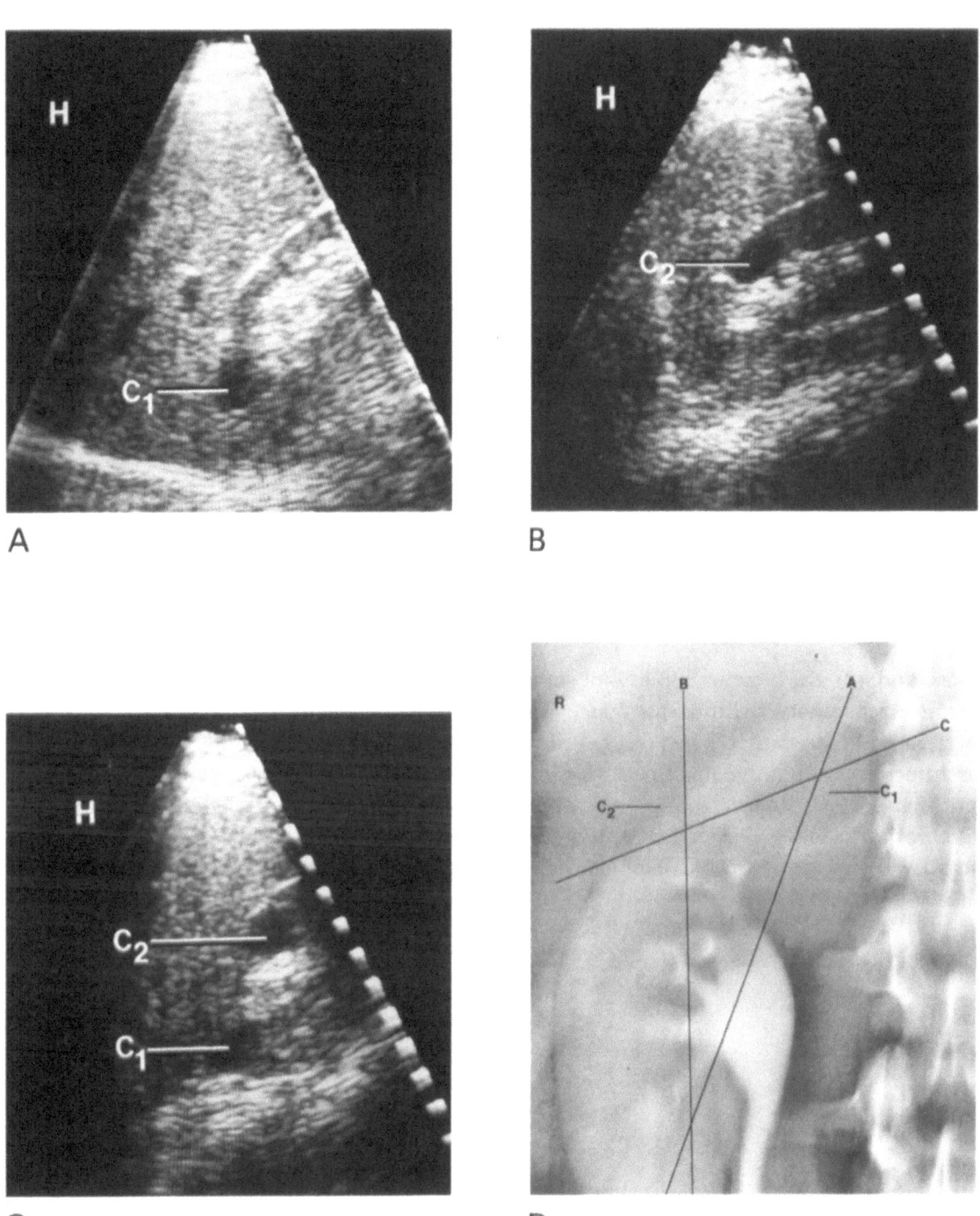

Fig. 4.19. Multiple cysts within right kidney. **A** Upper pole cyst (C_1); sagittal view. **B** Laterally located cyst (C_2); sagittal view. **C** Both cysts; diagonal view. **D** Intravenous pyelogram of kidney with planes of ultrasound scans superimposed.

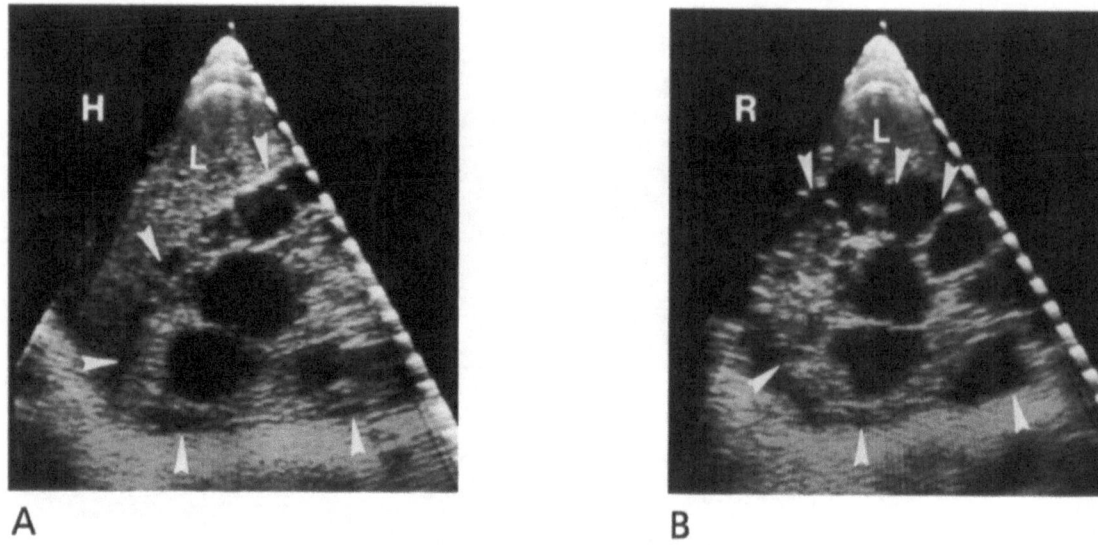

Fig. 4.20. Polycystic kidney (*arrowheads*). Sagittal (**A**) and transverse (**B**) planes. *L,* liver.

mass and (2) the absence of a zone of increased reflectivity behind the mass. However, a solid mass that has a very uniform architecture containing small cells that does not significantly reflect sound may appear as an echo-free mass. Nevertheless, there will usually be no zone of acoustic enhancement distal to the mass. Other masses may show a zone of decreased reflectivity behind if the attenuation of sound through the mass is greater than that through the adjacent normal renal tissue. Echoes within the mass can be increased (Fig. 4.21), be similar to the surrounding tissue (Fig. 4.22), or de-

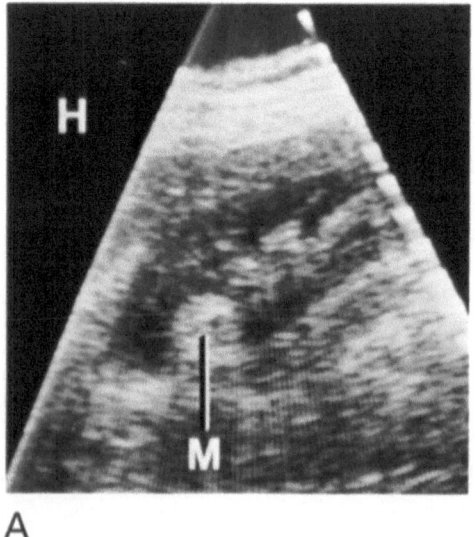 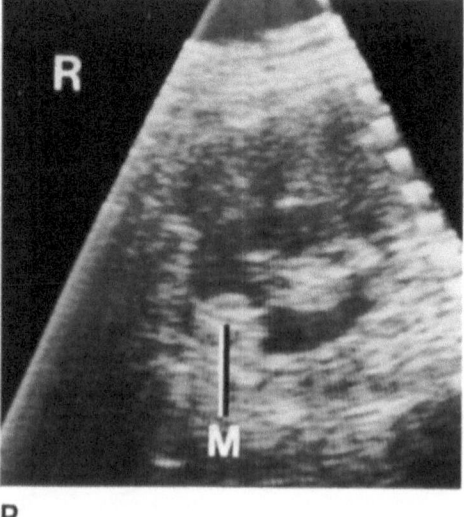

Fig. 4.21. Mass effect (*M*) produced by inserting perirenal fat into cavity from which a metastasis to the kidney was surgically shelled out. Similar type of focal highly reflective mass is typically seen in an angiomyolipoma. Sagittal (**A**) and transverse (**B**) views.

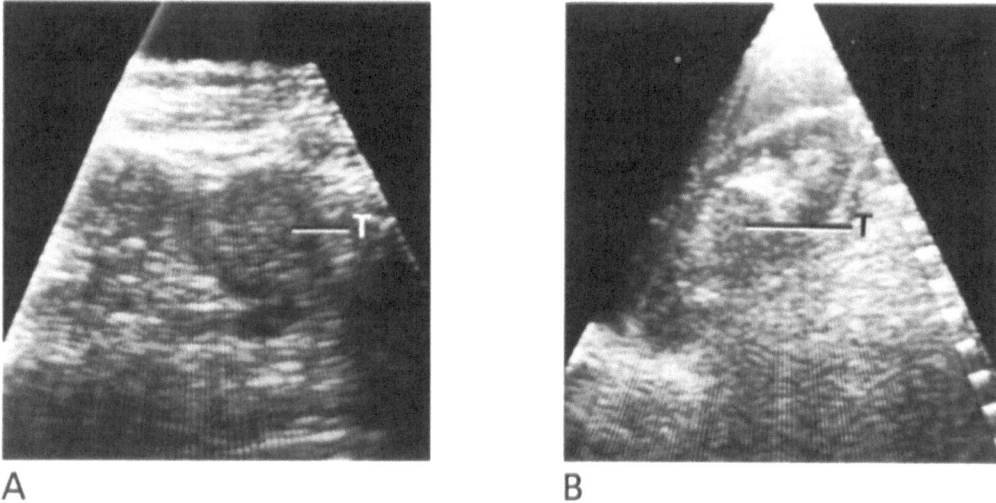

Fig. 4.22. Level of echoes from within tumor (*T*) similar to adjacent normal renal tissue. **A** Peripheral renal cell carcinoma. **B** Peripelvic metastasis from nasopharyngeal carcinoma.

creased (Fig. 4.23A). The most common appearance of a primary renal carcinoma is a mass with increased echoes which usually corresponds to a hypervascular mass on angiography (6). Occasionally renal carcinomas, although more often metastatic lesions, show

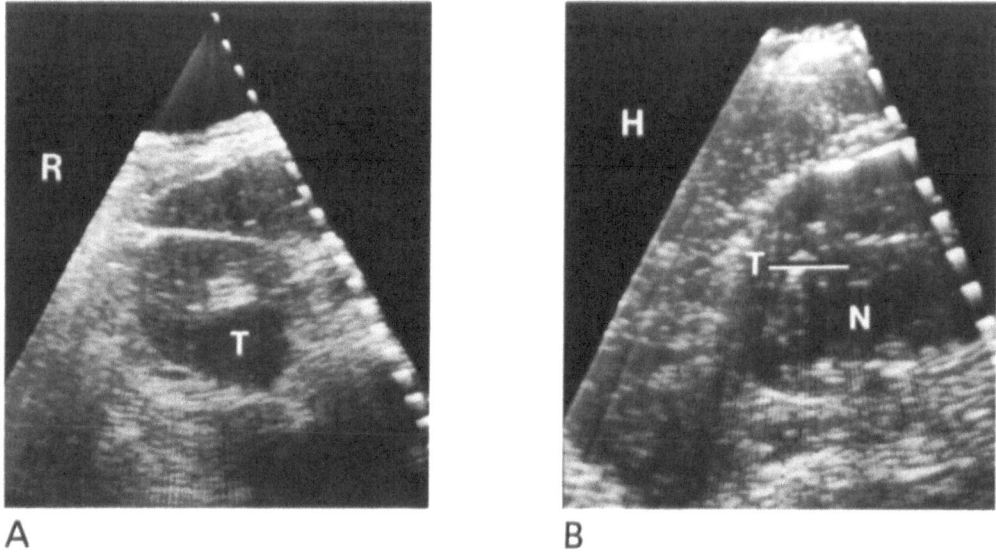

Fig. 4.23. Tumors with reduced echoes. **A** Carcinoma of the lung, metastatic to kidney. **B** Necrotic transitional cell carcinoma. *T*, solid peripheral part of tumor; *N*, central necrosis. Walls of necrotic area are irregular as compared to smooth walls of cyst and no zone of acoustic enhancement projects beyond necrotic area.

lower level echoes within the tumor than in surrounding normal tissue (6). When necrosis has occurred within the mass, a zone of absent or decreased echoes can be see (Fig. 4.23B).

A lesion that presents a characteristic ultrasonic appearance is an angiomyolipoma (7). It is a sharply circumscribed mass with uniform and intense internal echoes. We have also had one case in which a surgical effect mimicked the angiomyolipoma. This occurred in a patient in whom a nodule of metastatic renal carcinoma was shelled out of the kidney and the defect was filled with perinephric fat. The ultrasonic image of the fat packed in the cavity simulated an angiomyolipoma (Fig. 4.21).

When a renal carcinoma is detected by ultrasound, one should investigate the renal vein and the vena cava to see if there is ultravascular extension of tumor (Fig. 4.24) (8).

C. Intermediate Masses

Between the typical solid mass and typical cyst lies a spectrum of patterns that can represent an abscess, necrotic tumor, or a hematoma. These patterns are not completely specific but in conjunction with the clinical information can be strongly suggestive of a particular diagnosis.

Hematomas

The appearance of a hematoma, whether within the kidney or elsewhere in the abdomen (9), is quite variable depending upon whether it contains homogeneous fluid (either blood or serosanguineous fluid), clot, or a mixture of several fluids. Homogeneous blood attenuates sound in a manner similar to solid tissue, but internal echoes are not produced because individual red blood cells are too small to be identified as discrete structures by the ultrasound frequencies used for abdominal imaging. Clotted blood attenuates sound in a manner similar to nonclotted blood but, in addition, can produce internal echoes because of the grosser interfaces produced by the aggregates of blood cells and fibrin strands (10). If the mass contains mainly serosanguineous fluid, a fluid close to water density, a zone of increased transmission similar to that of a cyst may be seen behind the mass. Internal echoes

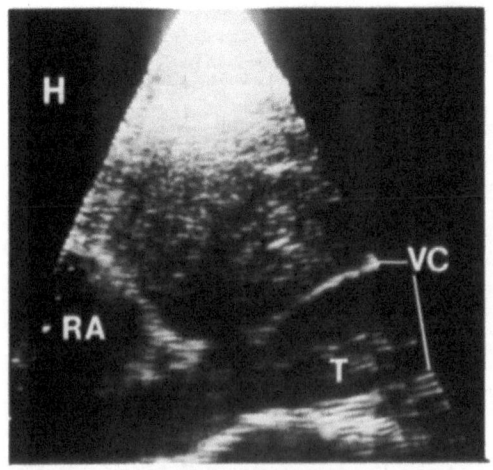

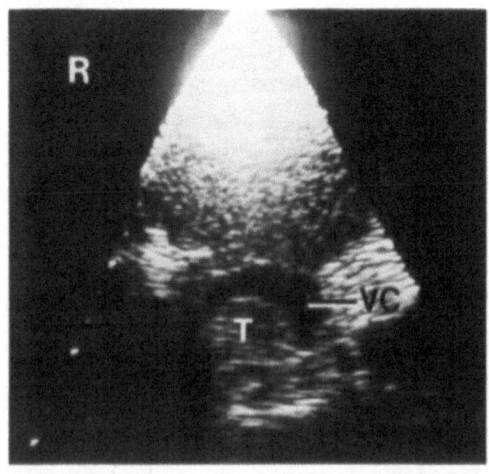

Fig. 4.24.

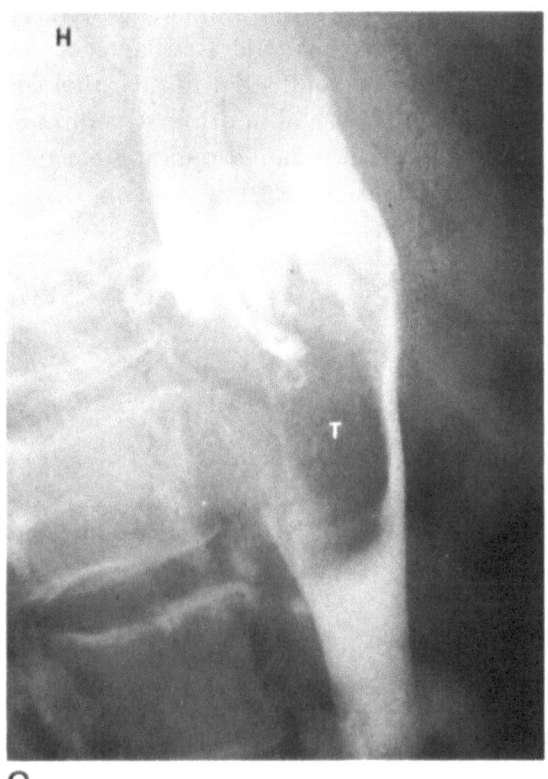

C

Fig. 4.24. Carcinoma of right kidney with tumor (T) extension into inferior vena cava (VC) to level of right atrium (RA). Sagittal (**A**) and transverse (**B**) views. **C** Inferior venocavogram confirming intraluminal tumor (T).

the protein content of the abscess fluid is high, it may absorb sound to the same degree as the surrounding tissue. Thus, the abscess may no longer have a zone of enhanced echoes deep to it and may be confused with a solid mass (11, 12). A focal region of cellulitis in which liquefaction has not yet occurred may also be indistinguishable from a solid mass.

Percutaneous fine needle aspiration of renal masses is a rapid and simple way of resolving diagnostic dilemmas. The technique will be discussed in detail in Chapter 10.

When a renal mass is identified, especially when tumor or inflammation is suspected, the degree of renal movement during respiration should also be evaluated. Reduced or absent movement suggests that the process has extended beyond the kidney and has fixed the kidney to the retroperitoneal tissues.

may or may not be seen depending upon whether or not the mass is homogeneous. The margins of a hematoma likewise can vary from smoothly circumscribed to somewhat irregular.

Abscesses

Abscesses can also present a spectrum of ultrasonic patterns. Depending upon the amount of tissue debris in the cavity, one may see many, few, or no internal echoes. The walls are usually irregular, but occasionally can be quite smooth. There is usually a zone of increased reflectivity behind the abscess since basically an abscess contains blood-free fluid mixed with a variable quantity of tissue debris (Fig. 4.25). However, if

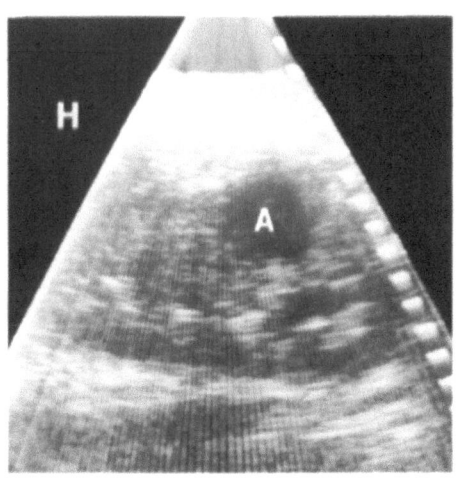

Fig. 4.25. Abscess (A) in lateral parenchymal region of left kidney. Sagittal view.

D. Normal Structures Simulating Masses

With the use of high resolution ultrasound scanners, the normal renal pyramids are frequently appreciated. These structures are conical zones of lower reflectivity (as compared to the renal cortex) arranged in a symmetric pattern around the central echo complex with the apex of the cone pointing toward the center of the kidney (Fig. 4.3) (1). When only one pyramid is seen on a section, it may be confused with a pathologic mass. The presence of multiple structures of similar appearance should indicate that they are not abnormal structures.

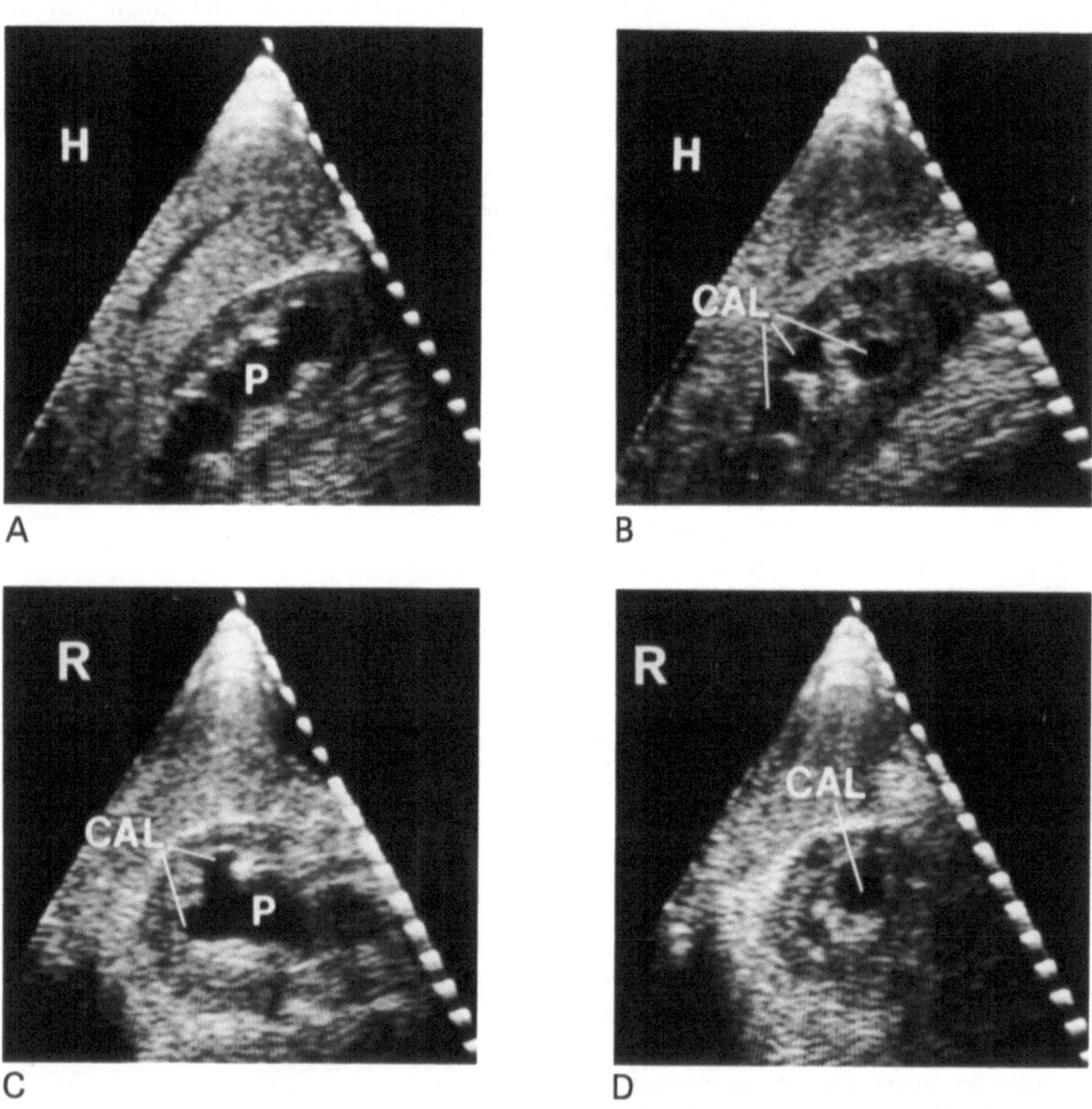

Fig. 4.26. Hydronephrosis; right kidney. **A** Sagittal plane through renal hilum. Dilated pelvis (*P*). **B** Sagittal plane lateral and parallel to plane **A** through dilated calyces (*CAL*). **C** Transverse plane through hilum. Dilated pelvis and calyces seen. **D** Transverse plane through dilated upper pole calyx (*CAL*). Dilated calyces in **B** and **D** can be confused with renal cysts if other views are not obtained.

E. Hydronephrosis

By this term we are referring to dilatation of the calyces, infundibula, and pelvis of the renal collecting system. If only one of these regions is dilated, then more specific terms such as calycectasis or dilatation of the renal pelvis should be used. To diagnosis hydronephrosis, dilatation of all three structures should be seen. The operator should examine the patient in suspended respiration and slowly sweep the transducer through the volume of the kidney in both the long and short axes (Fig. 4.26) so as to completely visualize the collecting system. A real-time scanner facilitates detection of mild degrees of hydronephrosis as compared to a static ultrasound imaging system because of its ability to continuously sweep the beam through the entire kidney. Although the diagnosis is frequently obvious on views made in one plane, views in the perpendicular scan should always be obtained to confirm the diagnosis.

The degree of hydronephrosis can vary considerably from minimal dilatation of infundibula and pelvis to such massive dilatation that the anatomy of the renal collecting system can no longer be identified (Fig. 4.27) (13). In the latter case, all that one may see is one or more fluid-filled saccular masses occupying almost the entire kidney volume. Short shelflike projections from the margins of these fluid structures representing the margins of the overdilated calyces (Fig. 4.27D) may be the only sign which indicates massive hydronephrosis and which differentiates this fluid-filled structure from a cystic renal mass.

One must be careful not to assume that a dilated renal pelvis means hydronephrosis. The pelvis may be extrarenal and thus have a large fluid capacity while the remainder of the collecting system is of normal caliber. Scans of the pelvis in transverse plane are best for making the distinction because this view shows the relationship of the pelvis to the renal parenchyma (Fig. 4.26C).

The state of the patient's urinary bladder can also affect the size of the renal collecting system. A very full bladder may temporarily produce distal ureteral obstruction which may show up as hydronephrosis (14). Therefore, it is important to reexamine kidneys demonstrating hydronephrosis after the patient has voided to see if the dilatation persists (Fig. 4.28). The bladder should also be examined after voiding to make sure it is empty. Examining the patient in the erect position can further clarify whether dilatation is secondary to obstruction and is unchanged in erect position or can indicate a capacious but nonobstructing system that drains when erect.

When the cause of hydronephrosis has not been determined from an intravenous pyelogram or retrograde study, then an ultrasonically guided percutaneous antegrade pyelogram can determine the site of obstruction and sometimes determine its cause by cytologic analysis of the aspirated urine. This procedure is discussed in Chapter 10.

F. Calculi

Stones within the kidney, whether calcified (15) or not (16), appear as focal areas of increased reflectivity with discrete acoustic shadows projecting behind them (Fig. 4.29). If the stones are within a dilated portion of the collecting system, the surrounding fluid can help define the size and shape of the stone (Fig. 4.30). One must also be sure that there are no gas bubbles in the renal pelvis from a recent retrograde pyelogram since gas can mimic a stone.

G. Intrapelvic Masses

A blood clot or a noncalcified tumor mass within a dilated renal pelvis may also appear by ultrasound as a reflective mass but will not cast an acoustic shadow behind it (17). Thus, when a noncalcified intrapelvic mass is identified by intravenous pyelography or retrograde pyelography, ultrasound can dis-

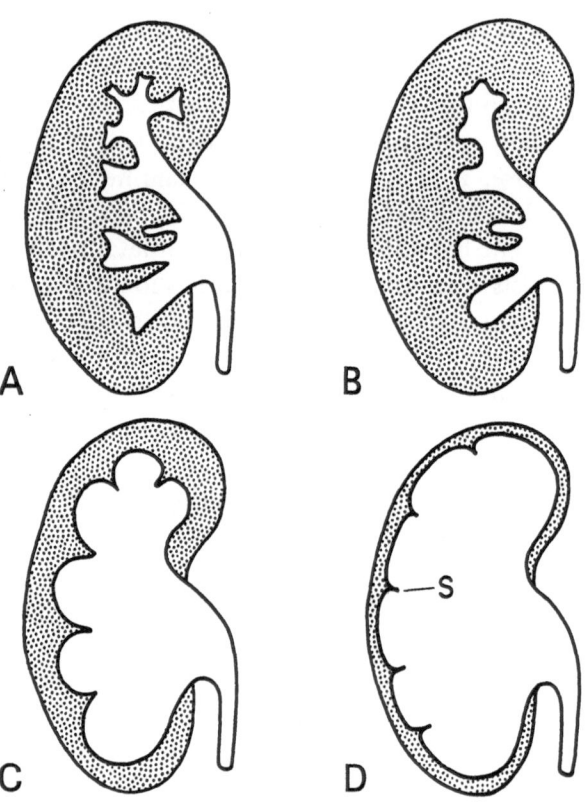

Fig. 4.27. Spectrum of hydronephrosis. **A** and **A′** Minimal dilatation of collecting system. Calyces (*CAL*) blunted but some pyramidal indentation remains. **B** and **B′** Moderate dilatation; calyces clubbed; no pyramidal indentation. **C** and **C′** Severe dilatation. Calyces still discretely defined and separate from each other. **D** and **D′** Extreme dilatation. Calyces so distented that they blend into one another except for residual margins that appear as thin septa (*S*).

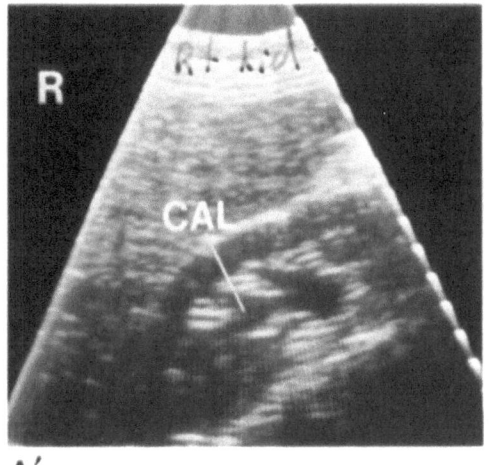

A′

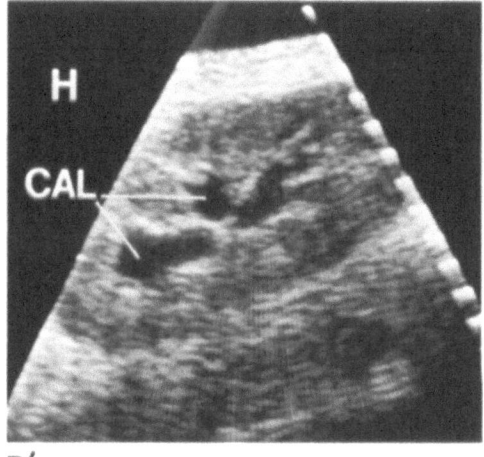

B′

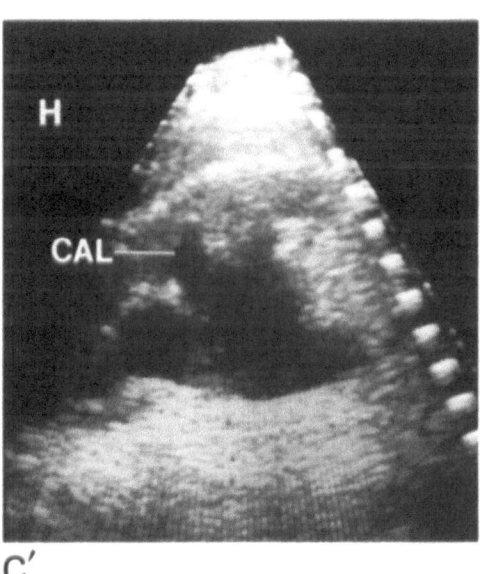

C′

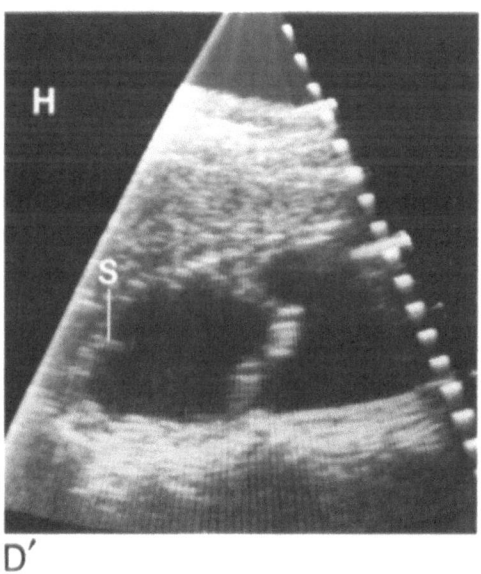

D′

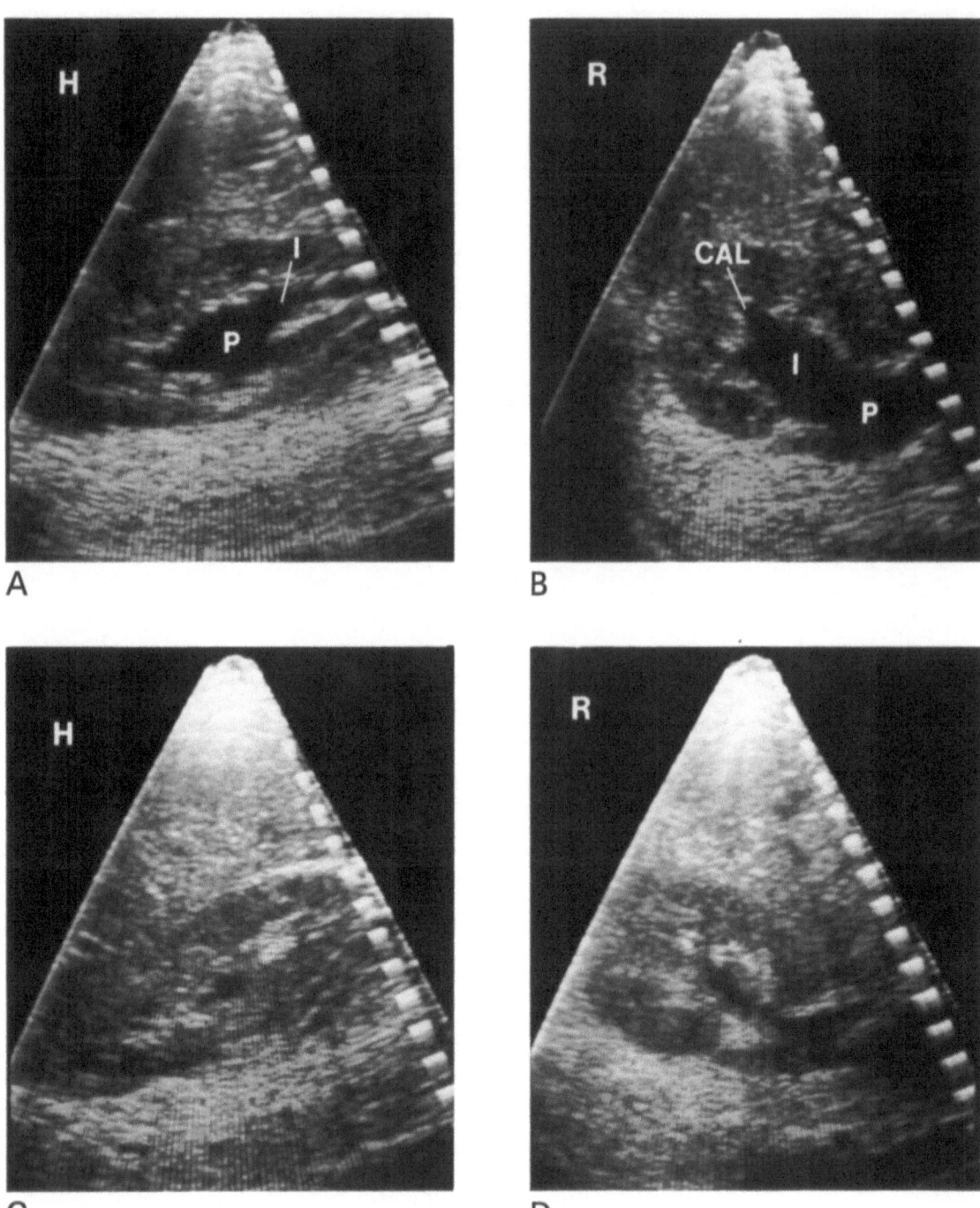

Fig. 4.28. Effect of urine volume within bladder upon degree of dilatation of renal collecting system. **A** and **B** Sagittal and transverse scans when bladder is full. Pelvis (*P*) and infundibula (*I*) are dilated but calyces (*CAL*) remain sharp. **C** and **D** Similar views postvoiding. Collecting system returns to normal size.

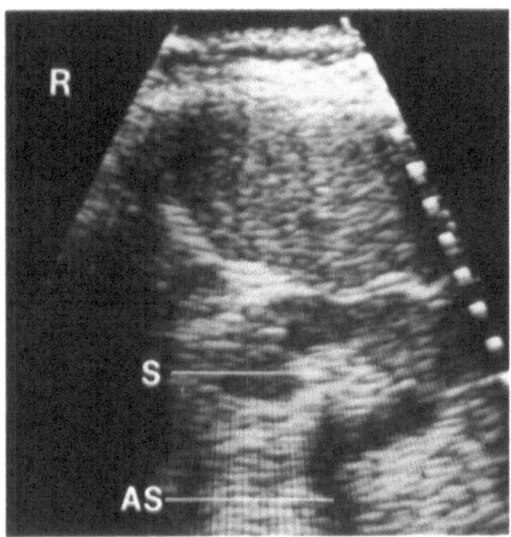

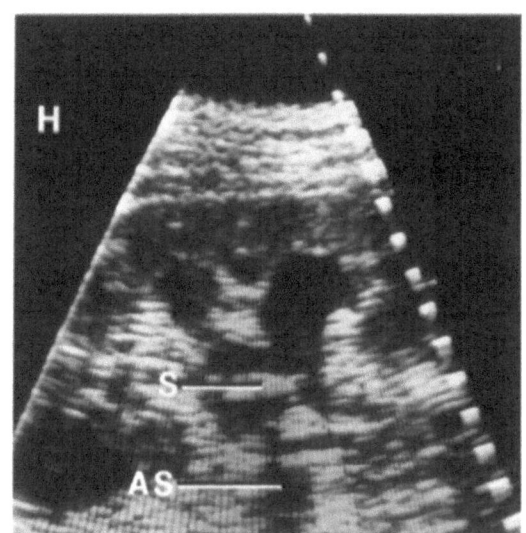

Fig. 4.29. Stone (*S*) within nondilated renal pelvis casting acoustic shadow (*AS*).

Fig. 4.30. Stone (*S*) obstructing and dilating renal collecting system. *AS,* acoustic shadow.

tinguish between stones on one hand and blood clot or tumor on the other. Ultrasound, however, cannot make the differential distinction between blood clot and tumor unless the mass is shown to be mobile when the patient changes position. Mobility supports the diagnosis of clot since tumor is usually fixed.

H. Transplants

Transplanted kidneys are usually placed laterally in either lower abdominal quadrant overlying the iliopsoas muscles. Although the kidneys are still anatomically in the retroperitoneal region, they are quite superficial, lying just below the abdominal musculature.

In this situation, a transducer with a larger-area near field, such as a linear array or a mechanical scanner producing a trapezoid format, is preferred to a sector scanner. Since the kidney is so close to the skin, only a small part of it can be seen with a sector field, whereas most or all of the kidney can fit into a trapezoid or rectangular field.

The major applications in which we have used ultrasound have been for the detection of hydronephrosis and perinephric fluid collections such as lymphoceles, hematomas, and abscesses.

Hydronephrosis in our experience is often caused by ureteral obstruction, either from edema or stenosis at the site of the ureteral anastomosis to the bladder or from an extrinsic mass compressing the ureter.

The most common extrinsic masses in our experience have been perinephric hematomas or lymphoceles following transplant surgery. The hematomas may be echo free if the blood is liquid. If the blood is clotted and the clot has fissures or fibrin strands, echoes may be seen within (Fig. 4.31). Lymphoceles (Fig. 4.32) typically have the characteristics of a cyst. However, since the normal urine-filled bladder may be confused with a lymphocele, one must be careful to distinguish between the two possibilities by scanning the patient with a full bladder and then after voiding. The fluid-filled mass that disappears or markedly decreases in size is the bladder. The lymphocele may change

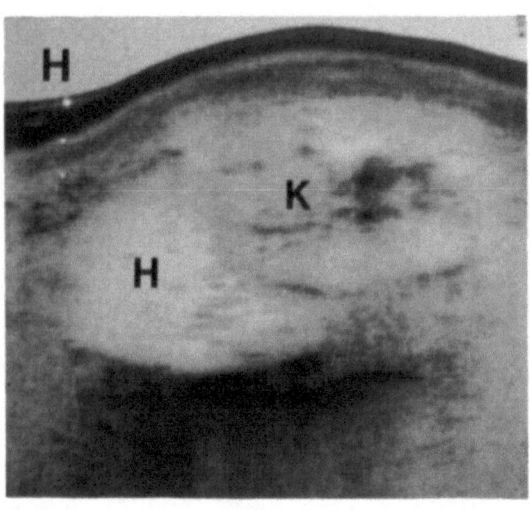
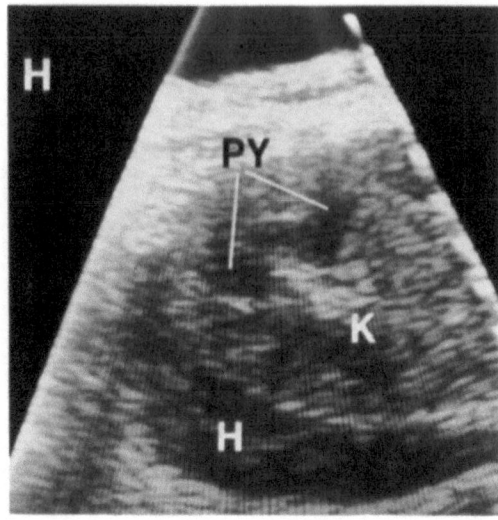

Fig. 4.31. Renal transplant in left iliac fossa. Large clotted hematoma (*H*) surrounds upper pole of kidney (*K*). *PY,* pyramids. Needle aspiration gave no blood or serum. Confirmation subsequently obtained surgically. Comparison of contact (**A**) and real-time (**B**) scanner images in sagittal plane. Although field of view is smaller with the trapezoid real-time than with the contact scanner, images of the trapezoid scanner are equally diagnostic.

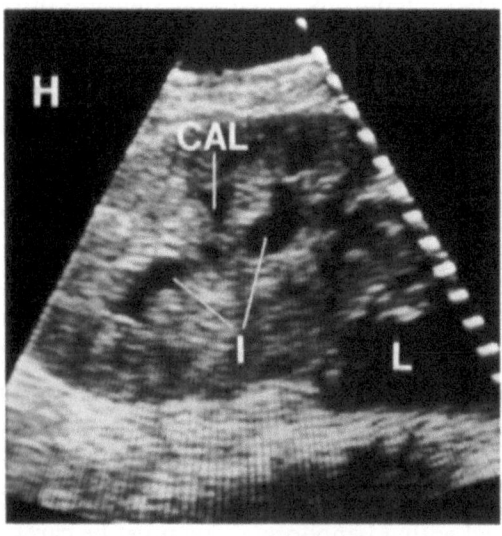
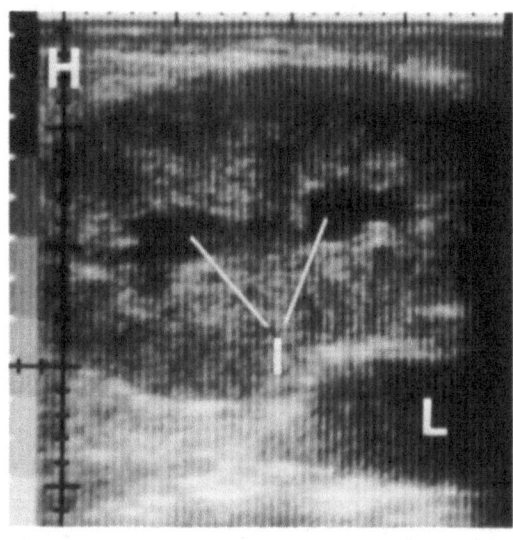

Fig. 4.32. Renal transplant. Lymphocele (*L*) obstructing ureter to produce dilatation of collecting system. *I,* infundibula; *CAL,* calyces. **A** and **B** Sagittal scans comparing trapezoid and linear array scanners. (Linear array scanner manufactured by Advanced Diagnostic Research Corp.)

shape and even enlarge after the bladder is emptied because of the disappearance of bladder pressure upon the lymphocele.

Both hematomas and lymphoceles can become infected. Usually the presence of infection cannot be detected just by their ultrasound appearance. Occasionally a previously echo-free lymphocele may develop internal echoes from clumps of inflammatory cells floating within.

Percutaneous aspiration and drainage of both lymphoceles and hematomas under ultrasonic guidance is a common practice at our institution (see Chapter 10). These studies are done when hydronephrosis is seen in the presence of a perinephric cystic-appearing mass to determine whether the mass is producing the obstruction.

Ultrasound can also detect rejection by the presence of swollen pyramids and patchy sonolucent areas within the cortex which may be regions of edema, hemorrhage, or infarction (18).

I. Abnormal Size and Shape

Uniformly enlarged kidneys are easily detected by real-time imaging. When the process is symmetric, lymphoma (19) (Fig. 4.33), amyloid, or other infiltrative processes should be considered. Symmetrically enlarged kidneys are also seen in diabetes. A unilaterally enlarged kidney is more likely to occur in renal vein thrombosis or in acute interstitial pyelonephritis.

Hypoplastic kidneys are more difficult to detect. The normal renal appearance of a highly reflective central echo cluster surrounded by a zone of lower echoes may no longer be evident because of severe cortical atrophy. The strong echoes from the collecting system and central vessels can appear similar to the echoes from the retroperitoneal fat surrounding the kidneys. It may be easier to first attempt to identify the kidneys in transverse plane (Fig. 4.34A) since the circular appearance on cross section is at times more readily appreciated than the fusiform appearance on long axis view. Once the kidney is found on cross section, the plane of the beam is rotated to define the long axis for measurement (Fig. 4.34B). When more of the cortex is preserved, identification is easier (Fig. 4.35).

Focal parenchymal atrophy such as occurs in chronic pyelonephritis (Fig. 4.36) can be appreciated as a localized zone of cortical thinning (20).

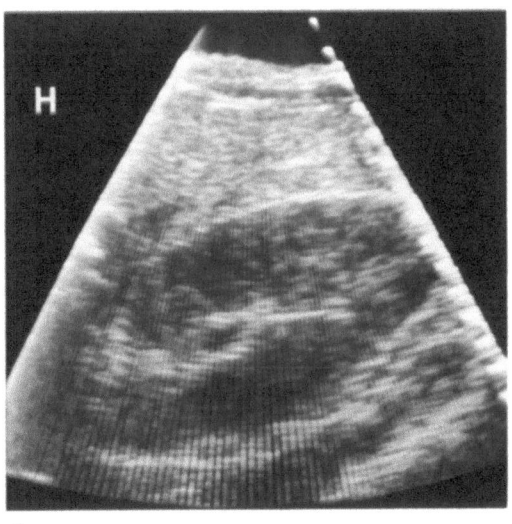

A

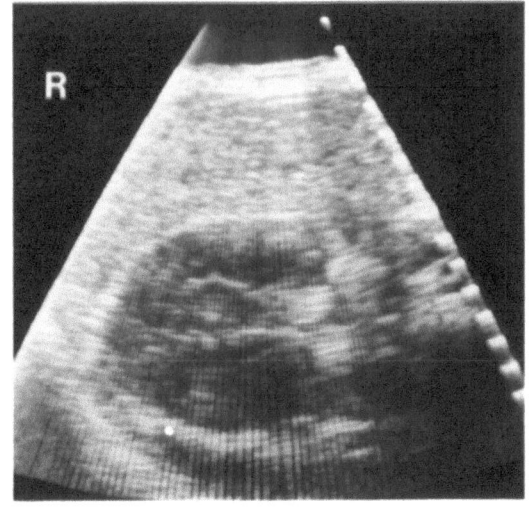

B

Fig. 4.33. Diffusely enlarged kidney; lymphoma. **A** Sagittal view. **B** Transverse view.

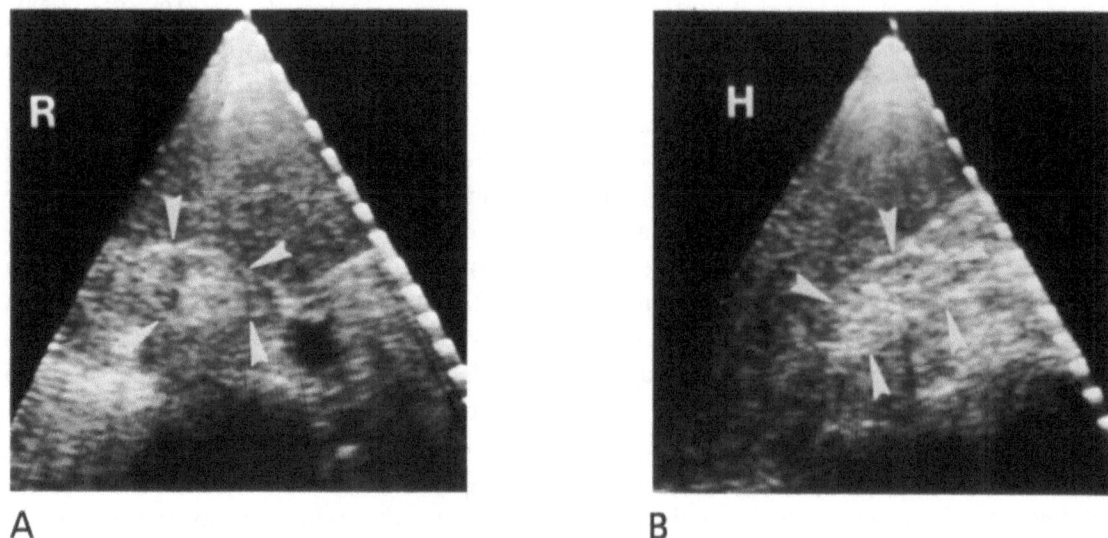

Fig. 4.34. Severe renal atrophy. No renal parenchyma. Renal capsule (*arrowheads*) better appreciated on transverse (**A**) than on sagittal (**B**) plane.

4. CHOICE OF INSTRUMENTATION

It would be ideal if each real-time instrument came with a variety of transducer configurations—bars, sector scanners, trapezoid scanners—so that the most appropriate instrument could be used for a specific patient.

Unfortunately, this possibility is usually not the case. Some instruments that use linear arrays provide arrays of different lengths usually representing different frequencies. Several of the manufacturers of sector scanners provide optional trapezoid standoff blocks so that a trapezoid type of image with a longer skin surface can be obtained, although similar results can be obtained by

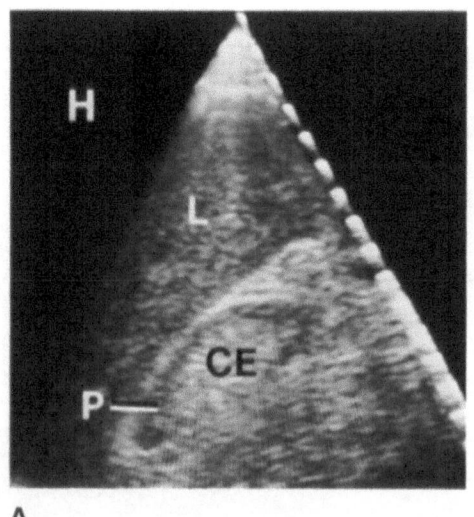

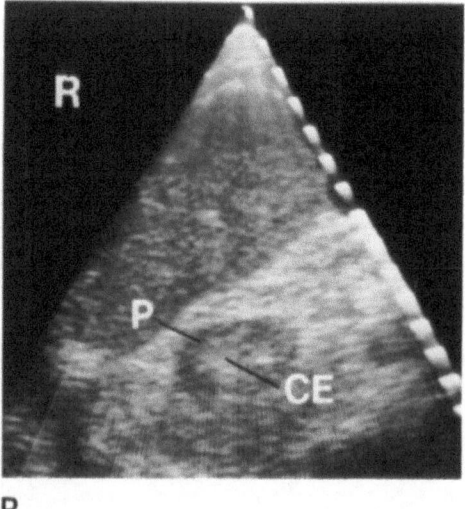

Fig. 4.35. Moderate renal atrophy. Thin rim of parenchyma (*P*) remains to separate capsule from central echo complex (*CE*). *L*, liver. Sagittal (**A**) and transverse (**B**) planes.

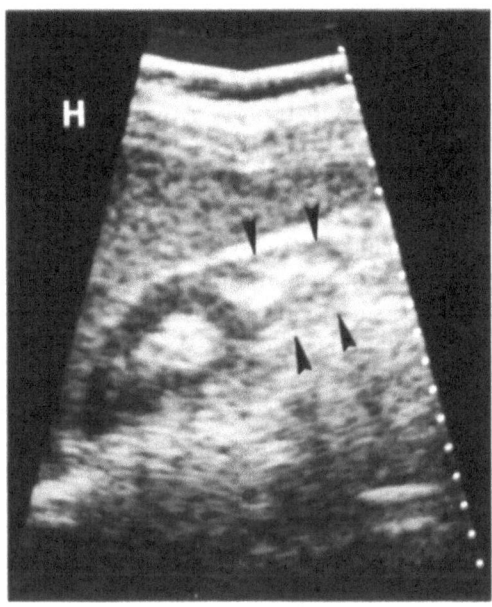

Fig. 4.36. Atrophic pyelonephritis producing localized parenchymal atrophy (*arrowheads*) in lower pole. (Xerox model 150 scanner.)

scanning through a water-filled bag placed between the skin and the transducer.[1] One manufacturer (Diasonics) can provide both sector and wide trapezoid images with the same transducer head, thereby combining advantages of either type of unit, while another manufacturer (Advanced Diagnostic Research Corporation) sells a system that incorporates both a linear array and mechanical sector scanner.

A. Linear Array

For long axis images of the kidneys, the linear array or its equivalent is ideal provided that the entire face of the transducer can make good contact with the patient's skin. This proviso is not as trivial as it seems. Not all patients possess a flat skin surface

overlying their kidneys. In patients in whom the skin has a concave configuration, the central part of the linear array may not touch the skin, whereas in those with a convex configuration, only the central portion of the transducer can make contact with the skin (Fig. 2.16). Often with some pressure the full length of the transducer can be made to contact the skin. Where complete skin contact cannot be made in one position, the array can still be effective if an alternate anatomic approach providing more uniform skin contact can be found. For example, one might not be able to obtain good images of the long axis of the right kidney using a sagittal approach with the patient supine but could do so with a flank, subcostal, or prone approach. Sometimes considerable care is required in positioning the patient to obtain a smooth and flat skin surface. This may entail the use of pillows or blankets to produce and maintain a desired position.

B. Sector Scanner

Since the sector scanner can fit within intercostal spaces and has a fan-shaped beam, one can image a kidney which lies below the rib cage without casting acoustic shadows into the field of view. Sometimes, however, the entire long axis of the kidney cannot be seen on one field of the sector scanner whereas it usually can be seen on one field of a linear array scanner. Therefore, with the sector scanner one may have to obtain separate long axis scans of the superior and inferior portions of the kidney. This extra effort usually does not significantly increase the examination time and does not lead to loss of information if one is careful to overlay portions of the kidney on both fields. The one disadvantage of not being able to encompass the entire kidney on one scan field is the situation where accurate measurements of renal length are desired. This limitation of the sector scan can be overcome at times if the patient is so positioned that the kidney is relatively far from the skin surface

---

[1] The prototype scanner designed by Dr. Terrance Matzuk that we have used extensively has a trapezoid head in which the transducer is displaced 5 cm from the face of the case (see Chapter 2).

so that the kidney projects within the wider portion of the transducer beam. Such positioning can best be achieved with the right kidney when scanning in the sagittal approach through the large mass of overlying liver. it is more difficult to obtain similar views of the left kidney because the spleen is usually less thick than the liver.

References

1. Cook JH, Rosenfield AT, Taylor KJW (1977) Ultrasonic demonstration of intrarenal anatomy. Am J Roentgenol 129:831–835

2. Rosenfield AT, Taylor KJW, Crade M, De-Graaf CS (1978) Anatomy and pathology of the kidney by gray scale ultrasound. Radiology 128:737–744

3. Green WM, King DL, Casarella WJ (1976) A reappraisal of sonolucent renal masses. Radiology 121:163–171

4. Pollack HM, Banner MC, Arger PH, Goldberg BB, Mulhern CB (1979) Comparison of computed tomography and ultrasound in the diagnosis of renal masses. In: Rosenfield AT (ed) Genitourinary radiology. Churchill Livingstone, New York

5. Rosenfield AT, Lipson MH, Wolf B, Taylor KJW, Rosenfield NS, Hendler E (1980) Ultrasonography and nephrotomography in the presymptomatic diagnosis of dominantly inherited (adult-onset) polycystic kidney disease. Radiology 135:423–427

6. Maklad NF, Chuang VP, Doust BD, Cho KJ, Curran JE (1977) Ultrasonic characterization of solid renal lesions: echographic, angiographic and pathologic correlation. Radiology 123:733–739

7. Lee TG, Henderson SC, Freeny PC, Raskin MM, Benson EP, Pearse HD (1978) Ultrasound findings of renal angiomyolipoma. J Clin Ultrasound 6:150–155

8. Goldstein HM, Green B, Weaver RM (1978) Ultrasonic detection of renal tumor extension into the inferior vena cava. Am J Roentgenol 130:1083–1085

9. Wicks JD, Silver TM, Bree RL (1978) Gray scale features of hematomas: an ultrasonic spectrum. Am J Roentgenol 131:977–980

10. Kay CJ, Rosenfield AT, Armm M (1980) Gray-scale ultrasonography in the evaluation of renal trauma. Radiology 134:461–466

11. Cunningham JJ (1976) In vitro gray scale echography of protein-lipid fluid collections in liver tissue. J Clin Ultrasound 4:255–258

12. Cunningham JJ, Wooten W, Cunningham MA (1976) Gray scale echography of soluble protein and protein aggregate fluid collections (in vitro study). J Clin Ultrasound 4:417–419

13. Ellenbogen PH, Scheible FW, Talner LB, Leopold GR (1978) Sensitivity of gray scale ultrasound in detecting urinary tract obstruction. Am J Roentgenol 130:731–733

14. Morin ME, Baker DA (1979) The influence of hydration and bladder distention on the sonographic diagnosis of hydronephrosis. J Clin Ultrasound 7:192–194

15. Edell S, Zegel H (1978) Ultrasonic evaluation of renal calculi. Am J Roentgenol 130:261–263

16. Pollack HM, Arger PH, Goldberg BB, Mulholland SG (1978) Ultrasonic detection of nonopaque renal calculi. Radiology 127:233–237

17. Arger PH, Mulhern CB, Pollack HM, Banner MP, Wein AJ (1979) Ultrasonic assessment of renal transitional cell carcinoma: preliminary report. Am J Roentgenol 132:407–411

18. Johnson MJ, Dunne MG, Watts B, Staples D (1978) Ultrasonography in renal transplantation. In: Rosenfield AT (ed) Genitourinary radiology. Churchill Livingstone, New York

19. Kaude JV, Lacy GD (1978) Ultrasonography in renal lymphoma. J Clin Ultrasound 6:295–382

20. Kay CJ, Rosenfield AT, Taylor KJW, Rosenberg MA (1979) Ultrasonic characteristics of chronic atrophic pyelonephritis. Am J Roentgenol 132:47–49

5
Liver and Spleen

The liver and spleen are difficult to image with ultrasound because the overlying ribs, by preventing the transmission of ultrasound, obscure portions of these organs. In addition, since regions of the liver and spleen are larger than the field of view of a real-time scanner, a cross section of either of these organs often cannot be included on a single image. However, real-time imaging of the liver has several advantages over contact scanning. Small intrahepatic lesions can be more readily identified by real-time imaging than by contact scanning because the entire volume of the liver is continuously imaged as the real-time transducer sweeps through it, whereas with contact scanning serial scans are obtained with discrete spaces between the scans. In addition, when a questionable mass is identified, it can be more readily characterized as cystic or solid by real-time than by contact scanning since the beam can be more easily manipulated perpendicular to the surface of the mass and swept through the mass from side to side so as to both define its margins and internal echo pattern.

1. SCANNING TECHNIQUES: LIVER

A. Sagittal

A systematic approach for imaging should be used. We begin with the patient supine. The first view is a midsagittal one of the liver and aorta. Then the transducer is moved to the left to obtain sequential parasagittal scans of the left lobe of the liver. The process is repeated on the right side to visualize the right lobe (Fig. 5.1A).

Since the abdominal wall curves as it extends laterally over the liver, the operator should maintain the scan plane perpendicular to the skin in order to maintain adequate contact with the skin. Thus, as one moves from more medial to more lateral planes through the liver, the plane of section changes from sagittal to coronal (Fig. 5.1A).

Since the right lobe is much larger than

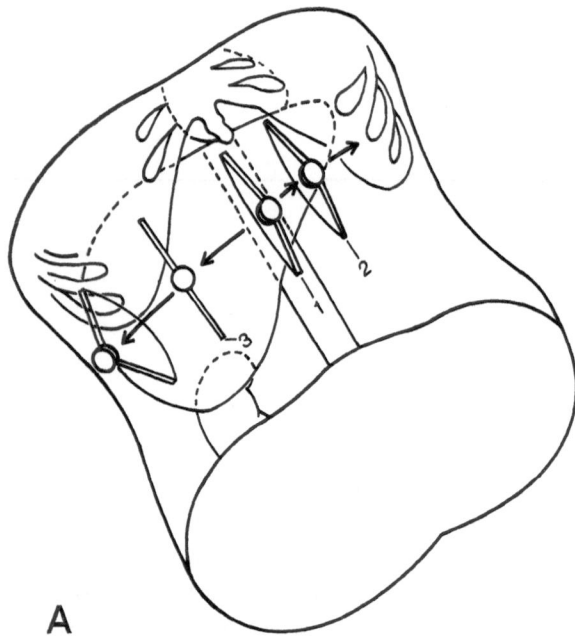

A

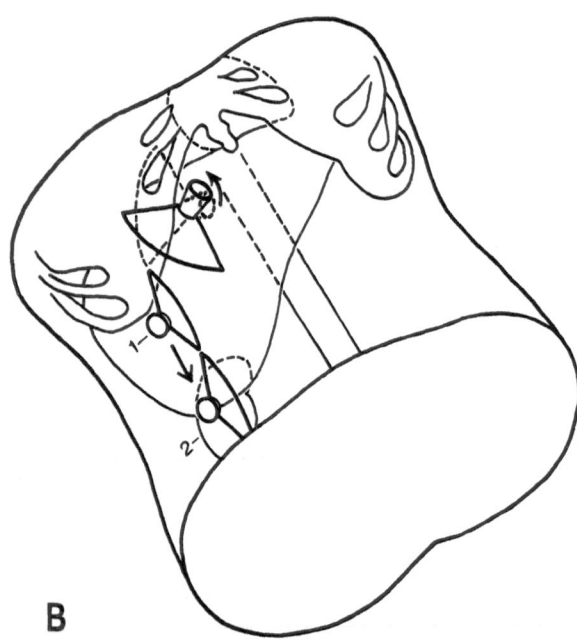

B

Fig. 5.1. A Examination of liver in sagittal planes. Transducer maintained perpendicular to skin (so as to be perpendicular to anterior liver capsule) as it is moved over liver. Scan plane changes from sagittal to coronal as transducer moves laterally over right lobe. Scanning begins in midsagittal plane and then sweeps over left lobe and back through right lobe. Representative parasagittal planes are as follows: **5.1A.1** Midline through left lobe (*LL*), aorta (*A*), hepatic vein (*HV*), right atrium (*RA*). **5.1A.2** Left lobe (*LL*), left ventricle (*LV*), stomach (*S*). **5.1A.3** Right lobe (*RL*), vena cava (*VC*), right atrium (*RA*). **B** Transducer moved or arced in superior-inferior direction along parasagittal plane when section of liver is too large to be encompassed within a single sector field. Representative superior (**5.1B.1**) and inferior (**5.1B.2**) images through parasagittal plane of right lobe (*RL*) and right kidney (*RK*). *D*, diaphragm.

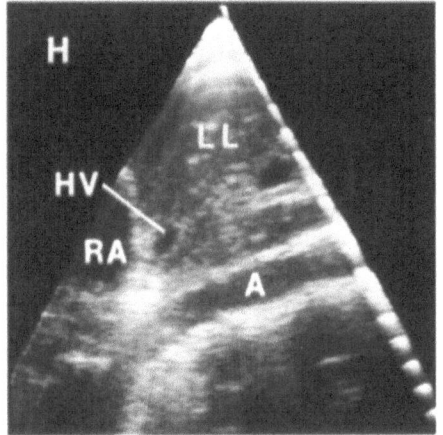

A1

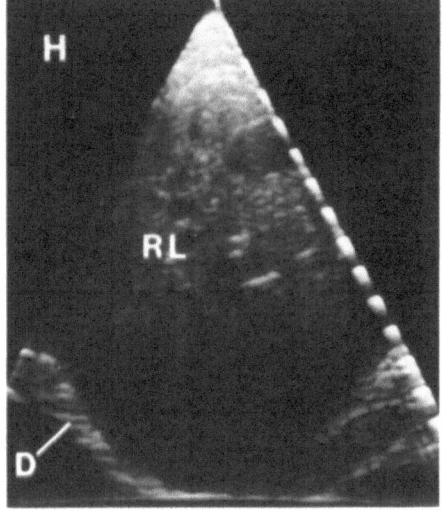

B1

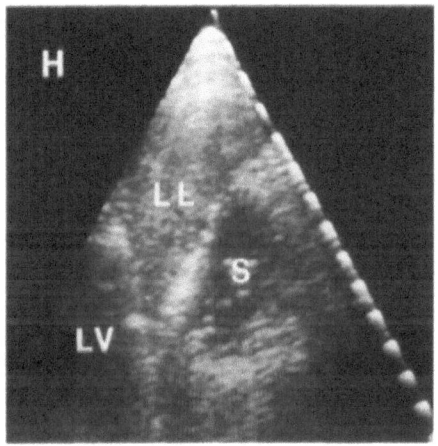

A2

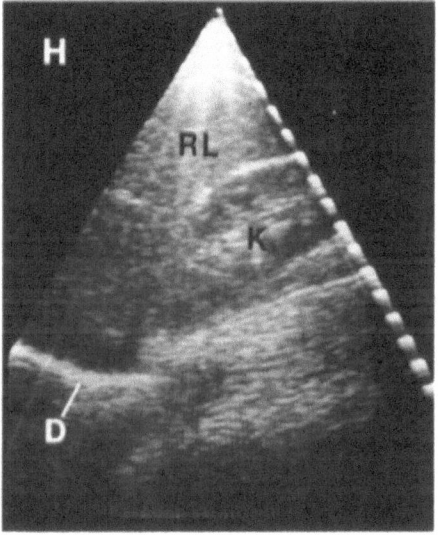

B2

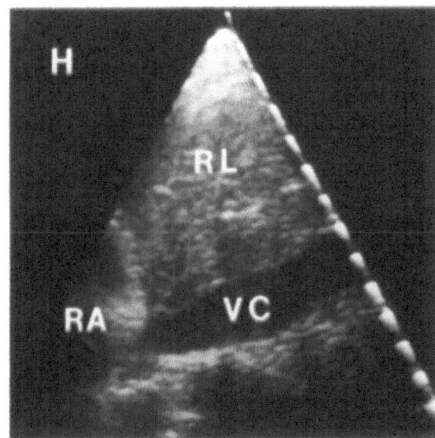

A3

the left lobe and is partially covered by ribs, a single real-time field of view often cannot encompass an entire parasagittal section. Therefore, to obtain complete parasagittal scans of the right lobe, the transducer must be moved through a series of superior-inferior sliding or arcing motions in each parasagittal scan plane (Fig. 5.1B). The operator mentally integrates partial images of each parasagittal liver section to obtain a complete image of that plane.

Because the ribs partially obscure the right lobe of the liver, several maneuvers are performed to image the liver free of the

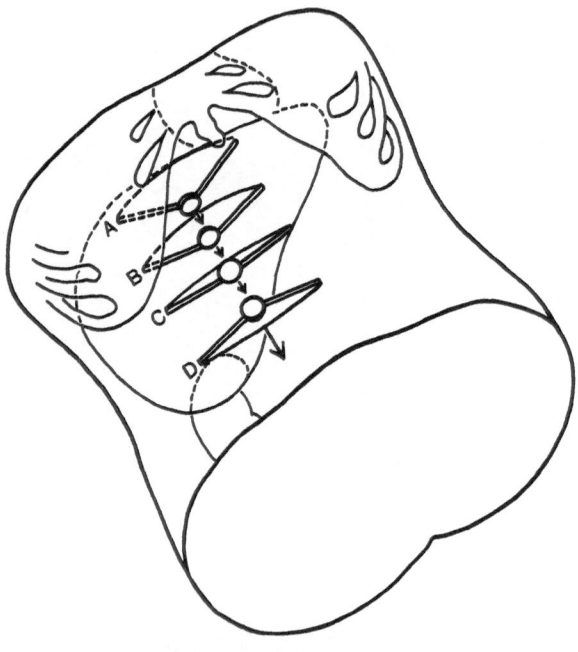

Fig. 5.2. Examination of liver in transverse planes. Transducer swept from superior to inferior direction. Representative planes are as follows: **A** Uppermost plane through liver and heart. **B** Through confluence of hepatic veins into vena cava. **C** Through central portion of liver. **D** Through left portal vein. *L*, liver; *RHV*, right hepatic vein; *LHV*, left hepatic vein; *A*, aorta; *VC*, vena cava; *LPV*, left portal vein *K*, right kidney.

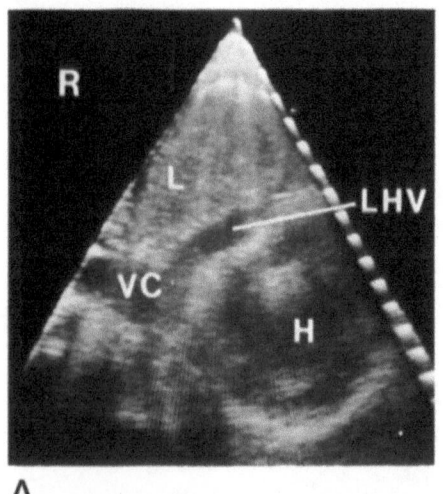

A

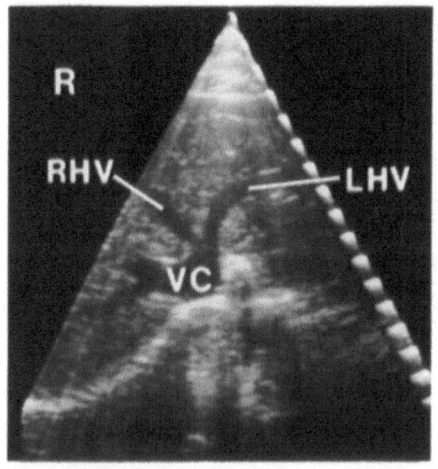

B

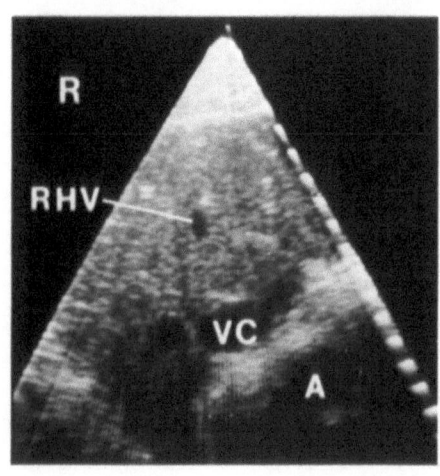

C

D

ribs. If a sector field transducer is used, the head can be placed in the interspace between each set of ribs, and with the patient in suspended respiration, the beam is swept in a superior to inferior direction to image the liver below the adjacent ribs. If a trapezoid or rectilinear transducer which extends over several ribs is used, then the transducer can be maintained in one position while the patient respires to expose adjacent regions of the liver to the ultrasound beam traveling through the interspaces (Fig. 3.16).

B. Transverse

The approach to transverse imaging of the liver is basically similar to sagittal imaging. The left lobe and medial portion of the right lobe are imaged by placing the transducer transversely high in the epigastric region and sweeping the beam from a superior to an inferior direction (Fig. 5.2). The same maneuver is used to image the more lateral portions of the right lobe except that multiple superior-inferior sweeps will be necessary in different sagittal planes since cross sections of the entire right lobe often cannot be encompassed by a single real-time field of view. The techniques used in sagittal planes to image between ribs are again repeated. It is important to angle the transducer quite superiorly at the beginning of the transverse scan to see the uppermost portion of the liver adjacent to the diaphragm. To ensure that this region of the liver is visualized, one should see portions of the heart (which lies just above the diaphragm) since the diaphragm itself is not often appreciated in transverse scans.

C. Modifications with Linear Array

Some modifications of the above scanning techniques may be necessary when a linear array is used with certain upper abdomen configurations. If the width of the subcostal space is narrower than the length of the array and the skin surface is concave, then in transverse scanning the ends of the array would rest upon the costal cartilages and not upon the anterior abdominal wall. Thus, no image would be obtained (Fig. 2.16A). If on the other hand the abdomen is convex anteriorly, then the skin may only make contact with the central portion of the transducer and a reduced width region would be imaged. Instead of true transverse scans, diagonal or subcostal images may be easier to obtain. The transducer is placed parallel to and below the costal margin and swept in an arcuate manner from the right shoulder to the left hip, thereby producing a series of diagonal slices through the right lobe of the liver (Fig. 2.17). In a like manner, the left lobe is imaged. The sagittal scans are performed in the usual manner as described above.

D. Respiratory Maneuvers

Any maneuver that exposes more of the liver below the ribs simplifies the imaging of that organ. Contrary to popular belief, instructing a patient to take a deep breath may actually expose less liver below the rib cage than occurs with a shallow breath. If the patient inspires by expanding the rib cage, the diaphragm can elevate and the liver moves further under the ribs. Therefore, we instruct the patient to bulge out his anterior abdominal wall by contracting his diaphragm. With this maneuver more of the liver descends below the ribs (Fig. 5.3). This maneuver also is useful for scanning the pancreas when it is obscured by overlying gas-filled bowel. The liver, when it descends, can displace the bowel inferiorly and interpose itself between the pancreas and anterior abdominal wall to provide a good acoustic window for pancreatic imaging.

As part of the examination of the liver, the extent of diaphragmatic motion should be evaluated. In order to document the degree of motion, a double exposure can be obtained in inspiration and expiration with

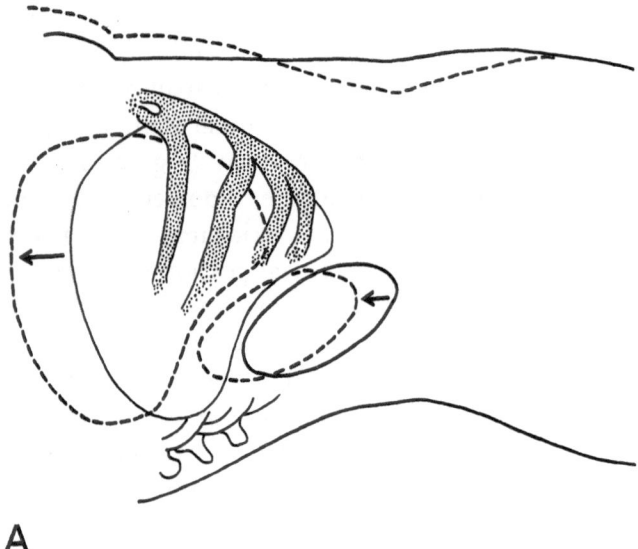

A

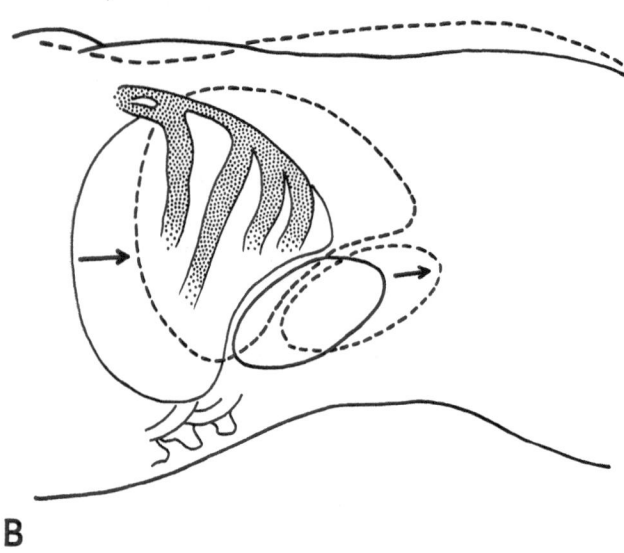

B

Fig. 5.3. Effects of respiration and diaphragm contraction on liver position. **A** Thoracic inspiration. Rib cage expands, diaphragm elevates, and liver moves superiorly under rib cage. ---, deep inspiration; ——, rest position. **B** Abdominal inspiration on "belly out" maneuver. Diaphragm contracts and liver descends below rib cage. ---, belly out; ——, rest position.

the operator holding the transducer fixed in position (Fig. 3.15). As an aid to obtaining a satisfactory photographic recording, one should close the iris of the camera by one or two stops, or reduce the gain by several decibels so as to prevent the diaphragm from being obscured by liver parenchyma.

If no pathology is seen, several representative views are photographed. When an abnormal region is observed, multiple views of the abnormality are obtained with slightly different transducer positions (in adjacent planes) to confirm that the abnormality is real. Since all the imaged portions of the liver are not recorded as still photographs, it is important to realize the considerable responsibility placed upon the operator for deciding what is normal and what is suspicious or pathologic.

E. Decubitus and Erect Positions

So far our discussion of liver scanning relates to the patient in the supine position. Any change in patient position that will project the liver further below the rib cage will improve the chances of fully imaging that organ. Two maneuvers will help: (1) Rotating the patient to the decubitus, left side down. In this position, the right lobe of the liver descends inferiorly and rotates medially, thereby exposing more of the upper portion of the right lobe. A repeat series of transverse and sagittal scans is then made. (2) Scanning the patient in erect position. This may be equally helpful in projecting the liver below the rib cage because of the effects of gravity. In the erect as in the decubitus position, further liver can be exposed by having the patient bulge out his anterior abdominal wall by contracting his diaphragm ("belly out" maneuver).

2. SCANNING TECHNIQUES: SPLEEN

The spleen, because it is also partially covered by ribs, gives rise to imaging problems similar to those of the liver. In addition, because the stomach (usually gas filled) normally lies anterior to the spleen, the anterior approach is not successful for imaging of the normal-sized spleen. Therefore, the spleen is usually imaged from the left flank using coronal and transverse planes (Fig. 5.4). The right lateral decubitus view can be used in a manner similar to the left lateral decubitus view for imaging the liver. This view causes the spleen to rotate anteriorly and inferiorly and projects more of the spleen below the rib cage than does the supine view.

3. NORMAL ANATOMY

Rather than simply sweeping the transducer throughout the liver, the operator should conscientiously seek to identify specific anatomic structures within and adjacent to the liver to ensure that a complete examination has been performed. In the midsagittal plane, the abdominal aorta and portal vein should be identified posteriorly to the liver (Fig. 5.1A.1). In a parasagittal scan slightly to the right of midline of inferior vena cava should be located and its continuity into the right atrium noted (Fig. 5.1A.3). In approximately the same plane, right hepatic veins can be seen entering the vena cava (Fig. 5.16). Unsuspected pericardial effusions can be found by demonstrating a fluid-filled space between the right atrium and the right hemidiaphragm during the routine examination of the liver (see Chapter 9). As one goes further to the right in the sagittal plane, the gallbladder and then right kidney should come into view (Fig. 5.5A).

In the transverse plane, the major landmarks are the confluence of the hepatic veins entering the vena cava just below the diaphragm (Fig. 5.2B), the left portal vein at a slightly lower level (Fig. 5.2D), and then the main portal vein branching into the right portal vein at a still lower level. As one continues inferiorly below the level of the main portal vein, the gallbladder comes into view as an echo-free space of increasing diameter, and the right kidney is seen posterolaterally to the liver (Fig. 5.5B).

The hepatic vein can be distinguished from the portal vein because (1) the wall surrounding the portal vein is thicker than that surrounding the hepatic vein and (2) portal veins become narrower as they go more superiorly in the liver and away from the porta hepatis, whereas hepatic veins become wider (Fig. 5.6) as they approach their junctures with the superior vena cava just below its penetration through the diaphragm (1). (Also see Fig. 2.9F)

The normal spleen is a crescent-shaped organ approximately the length and width of a normal kidney. The splenic architecture is uniform except for the echoes produced by branches of the splenic artery or vein. The splenic tissue contains an echo pattern more homogeneous but similar in intensity to that of the liver (Fig. 5.4).

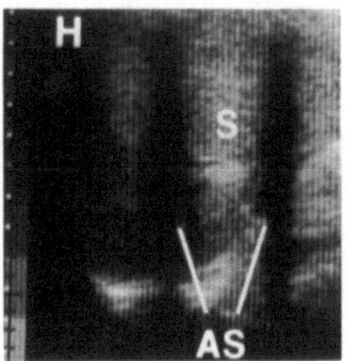

A1

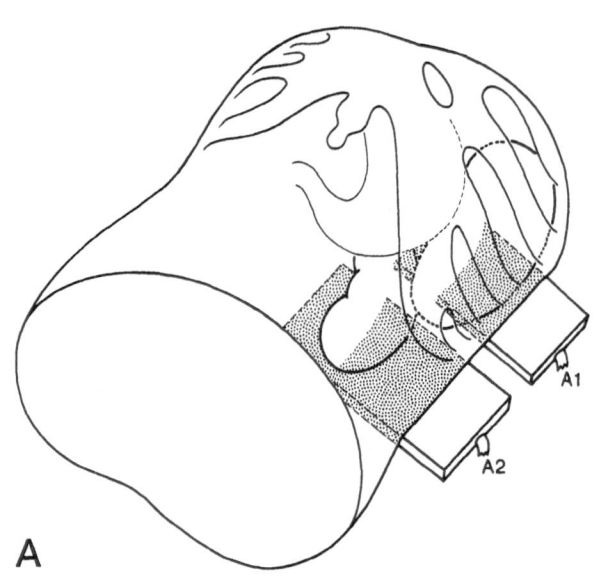

A

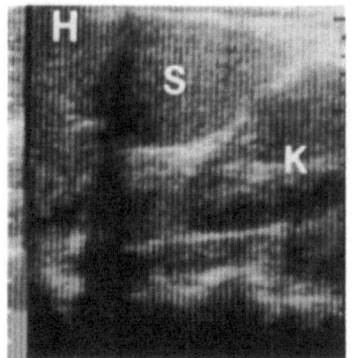

A2

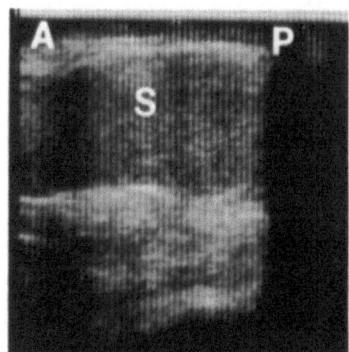

B1

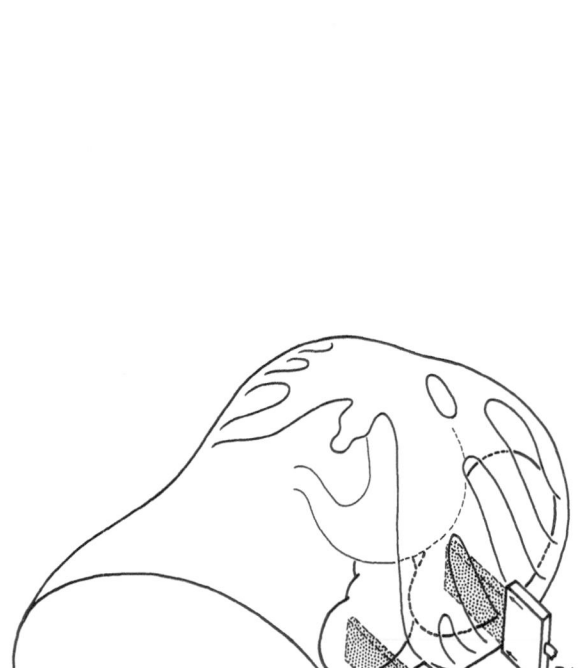

B

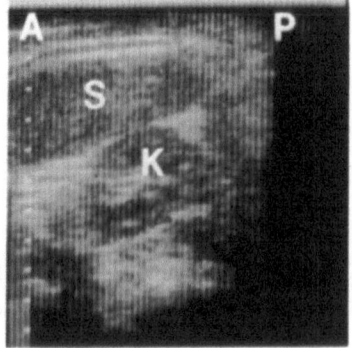

B2

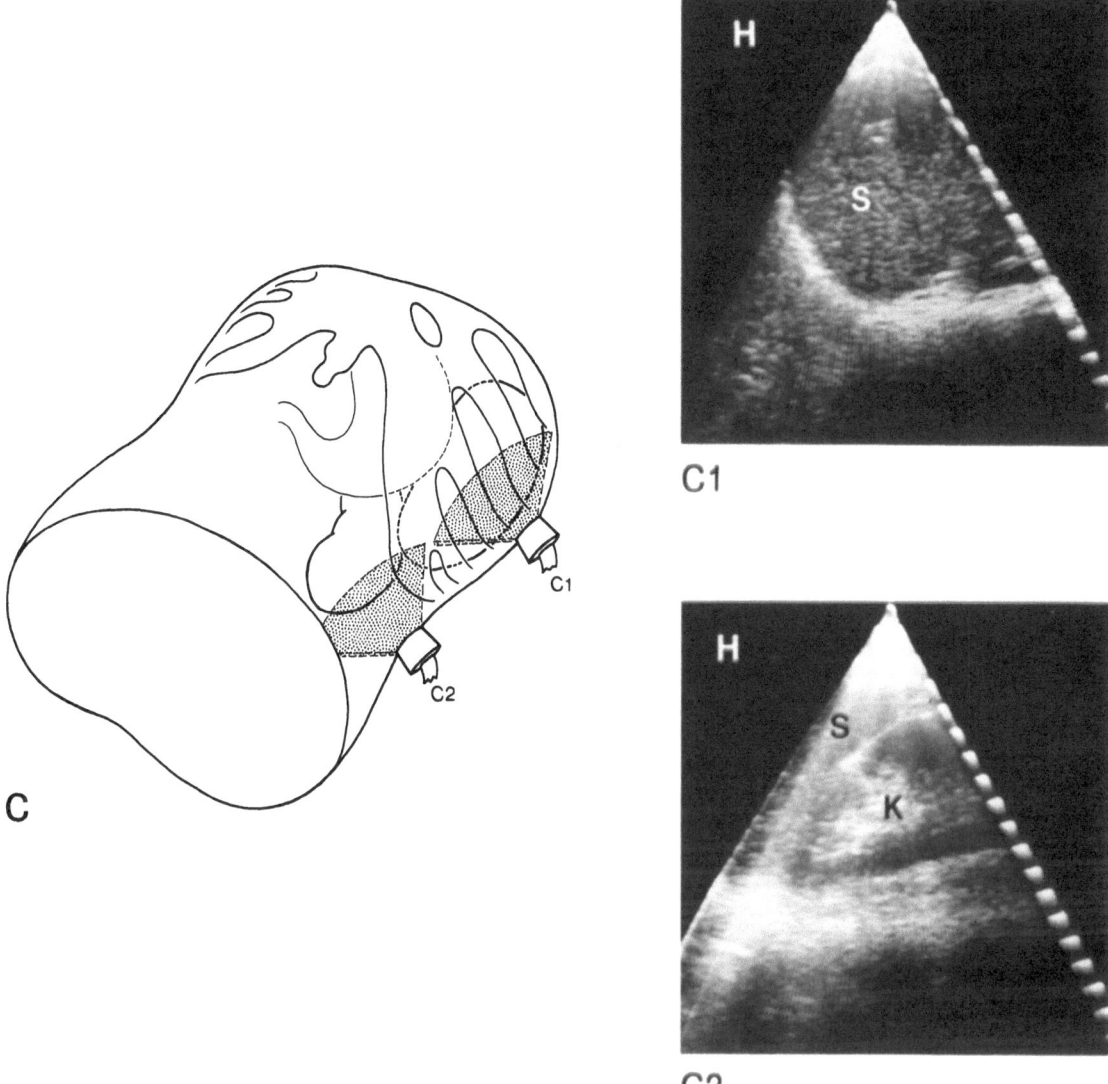

Fig. 5.4. Splenic imaging comparing linear array and sector scanner. Flank approach used because bowel obscures spleen from anterior approach. **A** and **B** Linear array; coronal and transverse planes. Superficial structures well seen but acoustic shadows cast by ribs obscure portions of spleen in coronal plane. In transverse planes length of image is shorter than in the coronal plane because part of linear array (*arrow*) does not make contact with skin. (Linear array manufactured by Advanced Diagnostic Research Corporation.) **C** and **D** Sector scanner; coronal and transverse planes. View of superficial regions more limited but scanner head conveniently fits within rib interspaces to readily image deeper structures. *S*, spleen; *K*, left kidney; *AS*, acoustic shadow; *H*, direction of head; *A*, toward anterior surface of abdomen; *P*, toward posterior surface of abdomen. (**D** on p. 100)

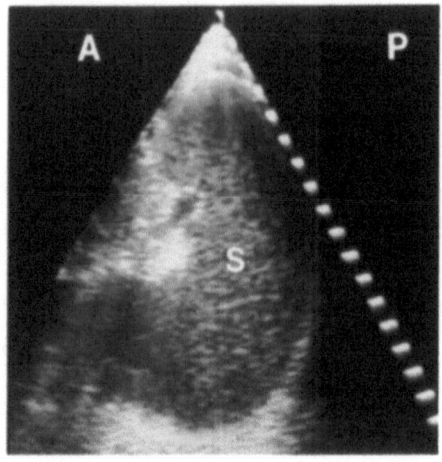

D1

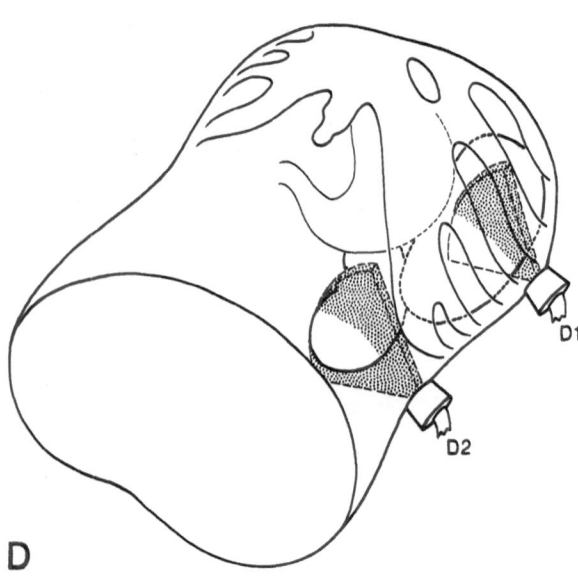

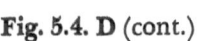

D

Fig. 5.4. D (cont.)

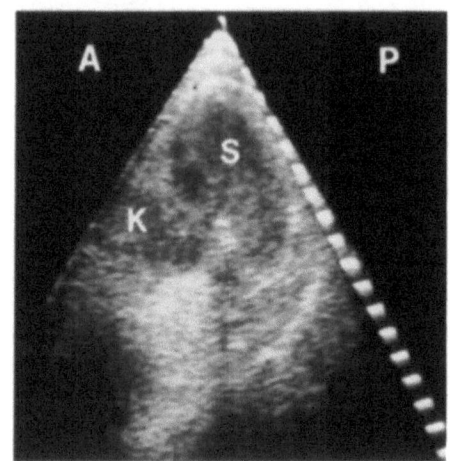

D2

4. PATHOLOGY: LIVER

In our experience the major applications of real-time scanners have been in the study of focal mass lesions—cysts, solid tumors, abscesses, and hematomas.

A. Cysts

Cysts can either be singular (Figs. 5.7 and 5.8) or multiple as in polycystic disease (Fig.

5.9). The typical cyst has a completely echo-free cavity with smooth and sharply delineated walls, and shows a zone of acoustic enhancement projecting behind it. Cysts may either be limited to the liver or be part of a spectrum of disease involving multiple organs. Therefore, when intrahepatic cysts are detected, it is important to examine the kidneys and pancreas (and ovaries in the female patient) for the presence of polycystic disease. When multiple septa or daughter cysts are seen within a larger hepatic cyst, the diagnosis of echinococcus disease should

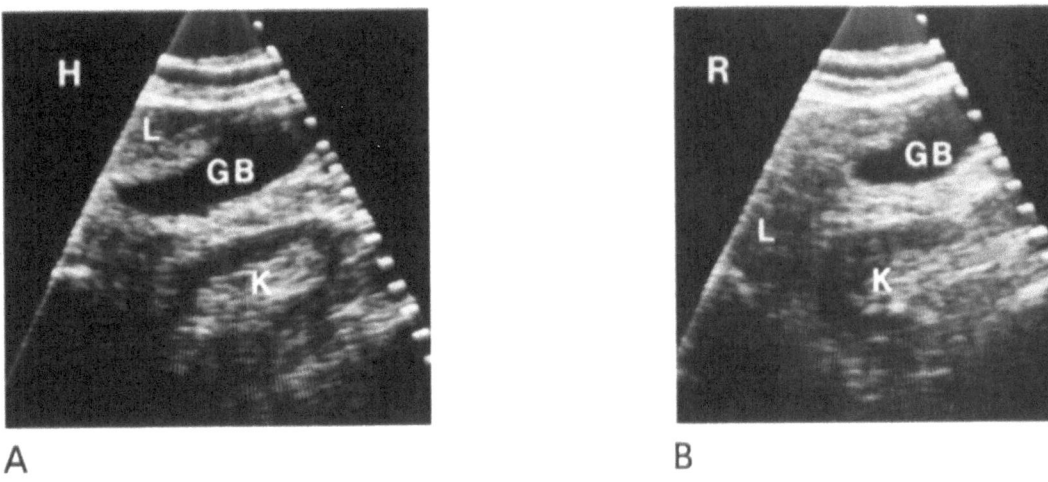

Fig. 5.5. Relationships of liver (*L*) to gallbladder (*GB*) and right kidney (*K*) in parasagittal (**A**) and transverse (**B**) scans.

be strongly entertained, and the cyst should not be percutaneously aspirated for fear of (1) causing an anaphylactic reaction from leakage of cyst fluid (1, 2) or (2) seeding the parasites along the needle track.

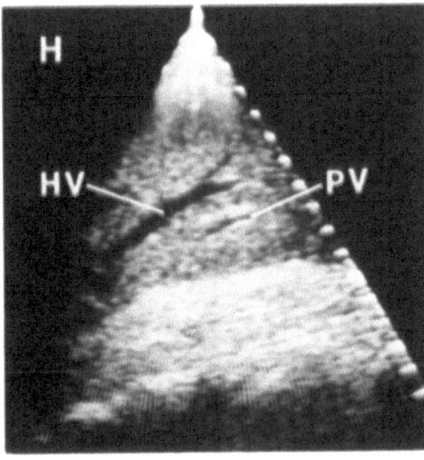

Fig. 5.6. Sagittal view; hepatic (*HV*) and portal (*PV*) veins. Walls of hepatic veins are thinner and less reflective than portal veins.

B. Tumors

Solid masses may represent either primary or metastatic tumors. These masses can either be homogeneous in their architectural pattern with echo levels weaker (Fig. 5.10) or stronger (Fig. 5.11) than the surrounding liver parenchyma, or may show a heterogeneous internal architecture indicative of either a tumor composed of several different types of tissue or a tumor containing areas of necrosis (3,4).

The necrotic zones will appear as regions of lower or absent echoes interspersed among the stronger echoes (representing the nonliquefied tumor) (Fig. 5.12). Zones of increased sound transmission as evidenced by greater reflectivity may be seen deep to necrotic areas if there is a significant amount of fluid in the necrotic area (5). The amount of sound absorbed by non–blood-containing fluid depends upon its composition and may depend on the size of particulate material within the fluid. According to in vitro studies reported by Cunningham et al. (6), protein microaggregates under 700 μm in water are indistinguishable from pure water and produce the typical appearance of a cyst.

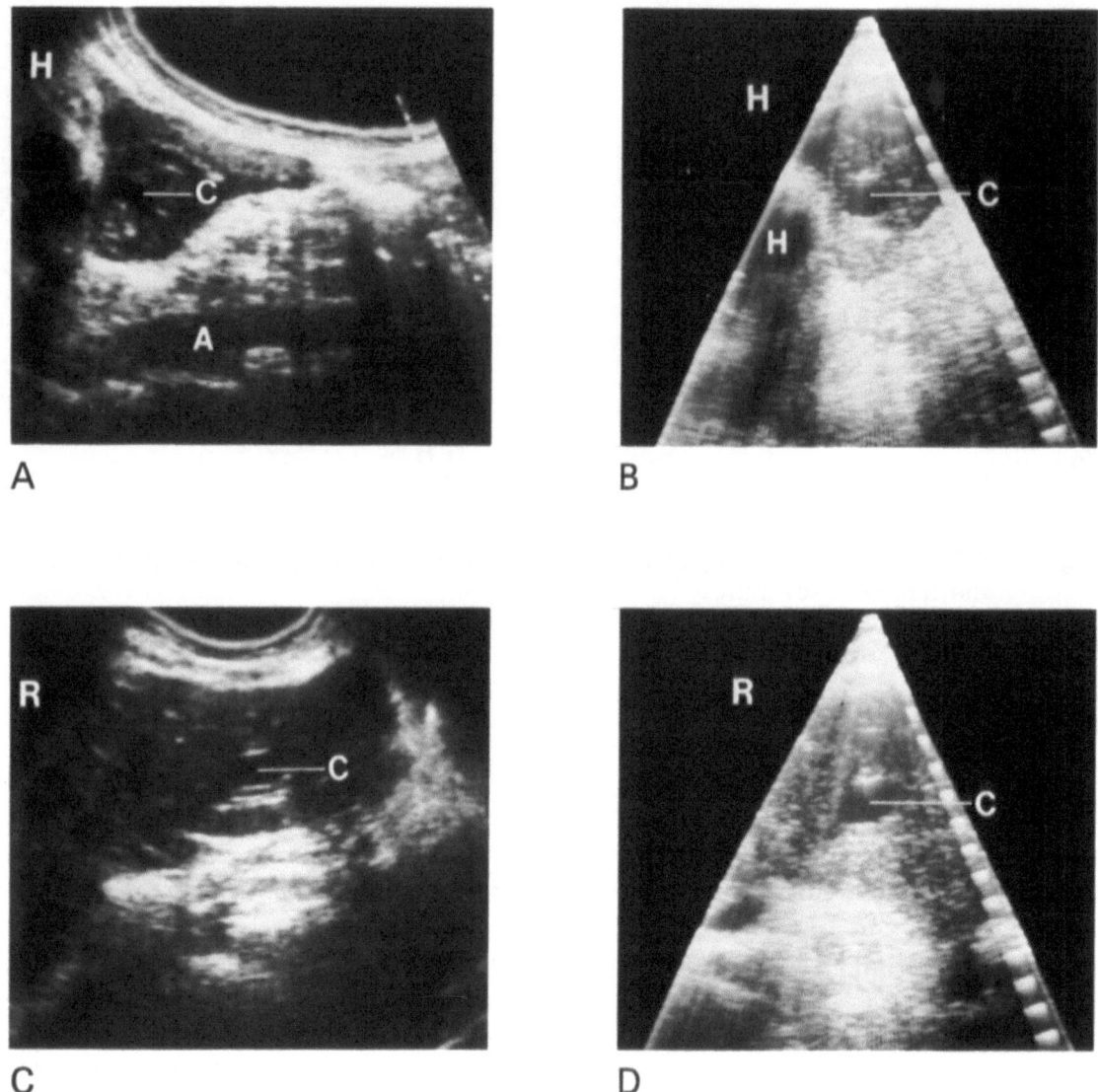

Fig. 5.7. Cyst; left lobe of liver. Comparison between contact scanner and sector scanner in sagittal (**A** and **B**) and transverse (**C** and **D**) planes. *C*, cyst; *A*, aorta; *H*, heart; *R*, right side of patient. Cyst equally well seen on real-time and on contact scanners.

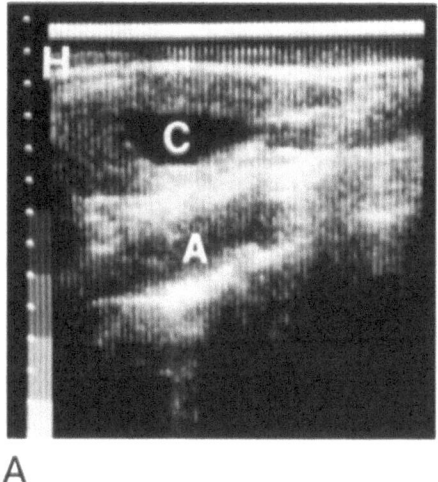 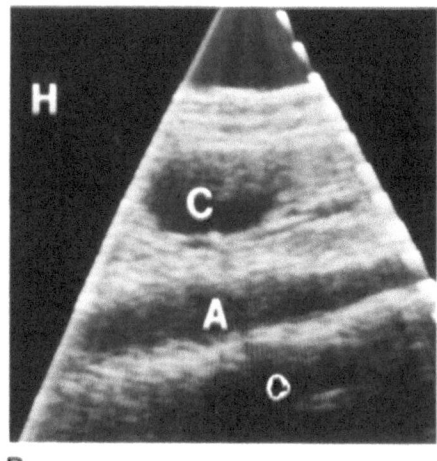

A   B

Fig. 5.8. Cyst left lobe of liver. Sagittal views. Comparison between linear array (**A**) and trapezoid scanner (**B**). *C*, cyst; *A*, aorta. (Linear array manufactured by Advanced Diagnostic Research Corporation.)

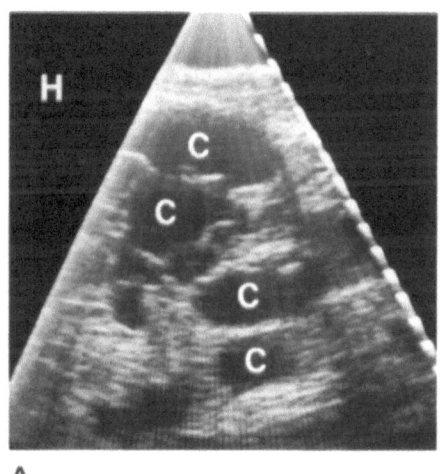 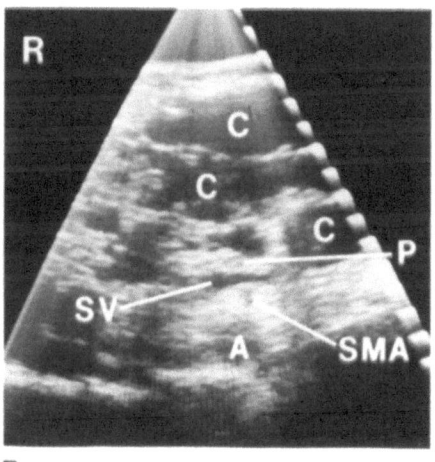

A   B

Fig. 5.9. Polycystic liver disease. Multiple cysts (*C*) of varying size. Midline sagittal view (**A**) and transverse view (**B**) of left lobe. *A*, aorta; *SMA*, superior mesenteric artery; *SV*, splenic vein; *P*, pancreas.

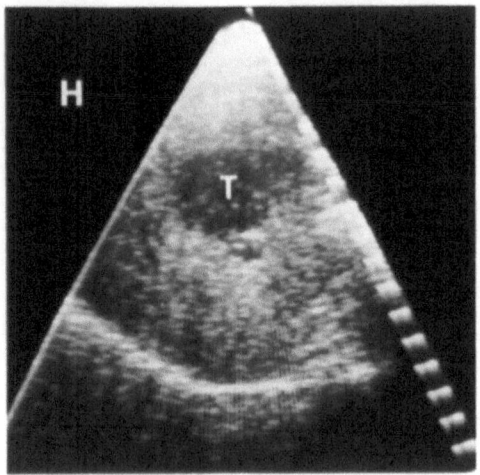

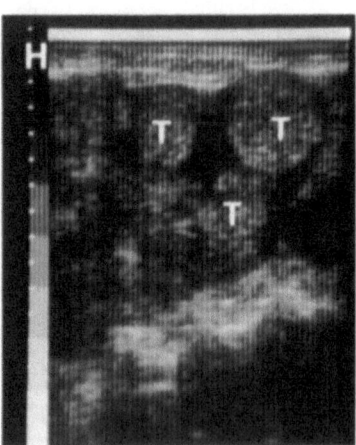

Fig. 5.10. Metastasis to liver; right parasagittal scan. Echo levels with tumor (*T*) lower than surrounding liver tissue.

Fig. 5.11. Hepatic metastasis (*T*) with echo levels greater than surrounding liver. Primary unknown. Right parasagittal scan. (Linear array manufactured by Advanced Diagnostic Research Corporation.)

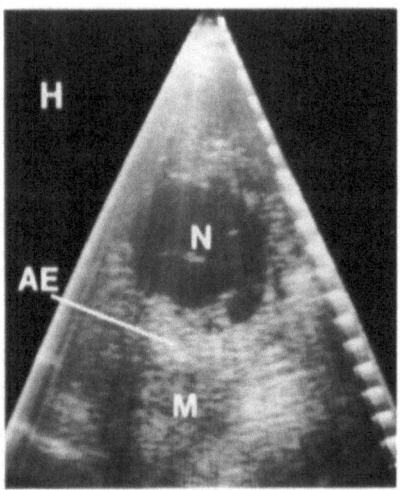

Fig. 5.12. Necrotic hepatic metastasis (*N*). Zone of acoustic enhancement (*AE*) deep to necrotic region. Another metastasis (*M*) is completely solid. Primary lesion is a dudodenal leiomyosarcoma.

When the particle size is between 1 and 3 mm, then the fluid containing these particles shows internal reflections and absorption of sound similar to that seen in a solid mass.

Thus, differentiation between a necrotic tumor and an abscess is often not possible on the basis of ultrasound alone (5). In such situations, the patient's clinical picture should also be considered.

When a tumor mass is large enough to occupy almost the entire field of view of the real-time scanner (and especially when using sector scanners), it may be difficult to appreciate the mass unless a portion of normal liver is included on that field for comparison (Fig. 5.13). The ability to identify the mass may become even more difficult when its boundaries form no distinct interface with normal liver.

The walls of solid intrahepatic masses may be smooth or irregular depending upon the gross architecture of the mass. The intensity of sound transmission behind the mass is either similar to the adjacent hepatic parenchyma or reduced if the absorption within the mass is greater than that of adjacent tissue.

The degree of reflectivity seen within a solid mass is usually related to its gross archi-

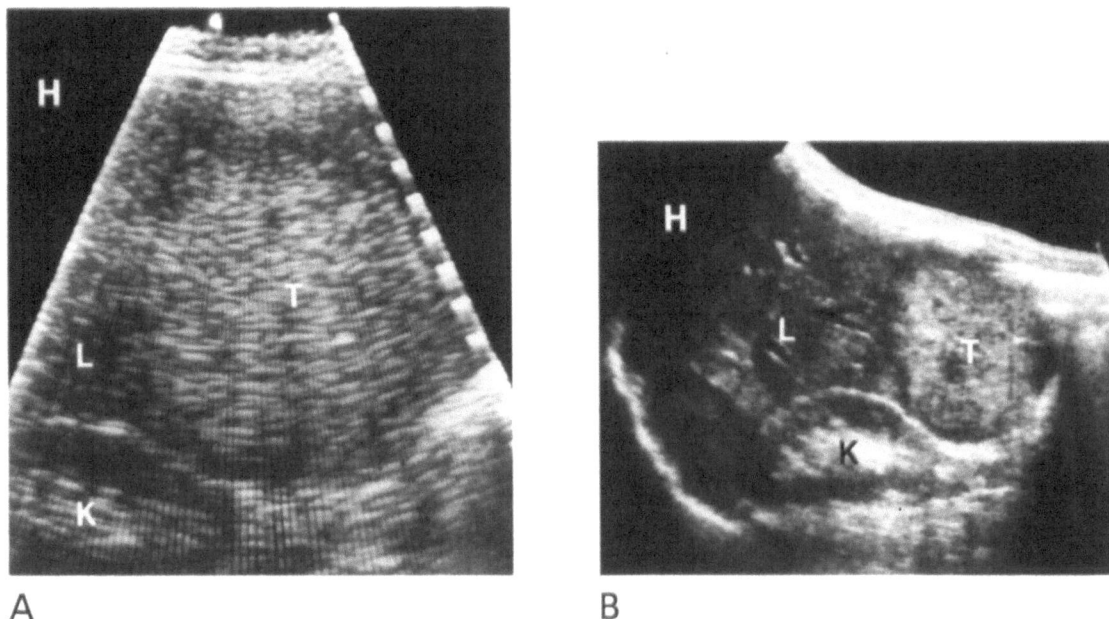

Fig. 5.13. Metastasis that occupies almost entire field of view may be difficult to detect with a real-time scanner because almost no normal liver is included for comparison. **A** Sagittal view, trapezoid scanner. *T*, tumor, metastatic from larynx; *L*, normal liver; *K*, right kidney. **B** Contact scan in similar plane. Tumor more readily distinguished from normal liver.

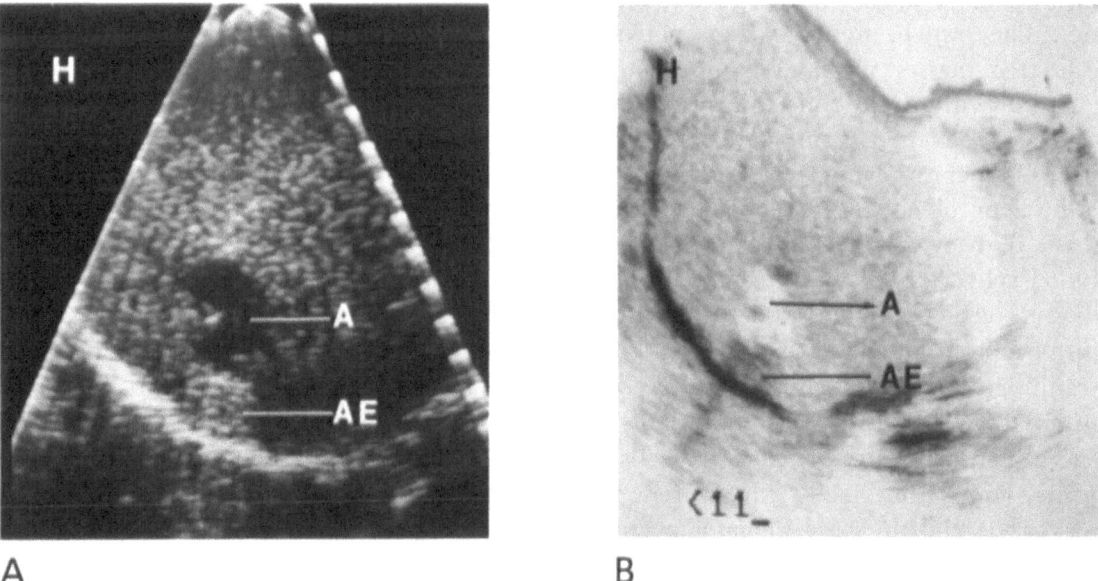

Fig. 5.14. Abscess (*A*) in lateral aspect of right lobe of liver. Confirmed by percutaneous aspiration and subsequent surgical drainage. Note zone of acoustic enhancement (*AE*) deep to abscess. **A** Right parasagittal view, sector scanner. **B** Similar plane, contact scanner. Both instruments are equally diagnostic.

tecture, although the specific type of tumor cannot be determined by the type of acoustic pattern produced by the mass. Both primary and metastatic tumors can produce either high or low level echoes (3, 4, 7). The effect of chemotherapy on the intensity of echoes within a tumor is not clear. Some investigators claim that echo levels can increase in hypoechoic masses (8), while others claim that no such change occurs (3, 9).

C. Abscesses

Abscesses often appear as mass lesions containing zones of increased transmission behind them. The mass may be echo free or may contain scattered internal echoes representing necrotic tissue. The walls of the mass can be smooth or irregular with the latter more common (Fig. 5.14) (10).

D. Hematomas

Hematomas may present diagnostic difficulties. They can be smoothly marginated and echo-free masses similar in appearance to cysts but without the zone of acoustic attenuation. Blood absorbs and attenuates sound in a manner similar to solid tissue so there is no zone of enhanced echoes deep to the mass. However, since the individual red blood cells are too small to be identified as discrete echo-producing structures with the ultrasound frequencies used for abdominal scanning, the hematoma usually produces no internal echoes. If a hematoma clots, the aggregated collection of red blood cells may form larger interfaces whose reflections may appear within the hematoma and resemble the echoes within a solid tumor mass (Fig. 5.15). Thus, when making the diagnosis of hematoma, the ultra sound images should be interpreted with knowledge of the patient's clinical findings.

The use of percutaneous fine needle as-

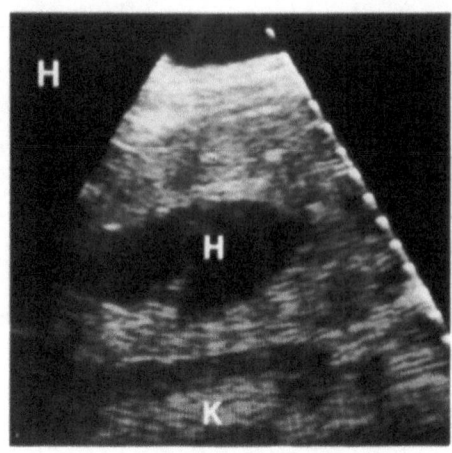

Fig. 5.15. Posttraumatic hematoma (*H*) within right lobe of liver. Faint echoes within hematoma probably represent interfaces produced by clotted blood. Sagittal view. *K*, right kidney.

piration under ultrasonic guidance is an excellent way of confirming the diagnosis of intrahepatic mass lesions. This technique will be discussed in Chapter 10.

E. Pseudomasses

A normal structure such as a hepatic vein may be confused with an echo-free and smoothly marginated mass when seen in only one plane. To avoid such mistakes, it is important for all suspected masses to be examined in multiple planes to see if their contours and internal architecture remain constant (indicative of a mass) or change to reveal a vessel or other normal structure. These multiple planes should include planes perpendicular to each other, serial closely spaced planes parallel to each other, and at times even a series of scans obtained by rotating the transducer over the suspected mass. Using these maneuvers, a true mass can be differentiated from a pseudomass (Fig. 5.16).

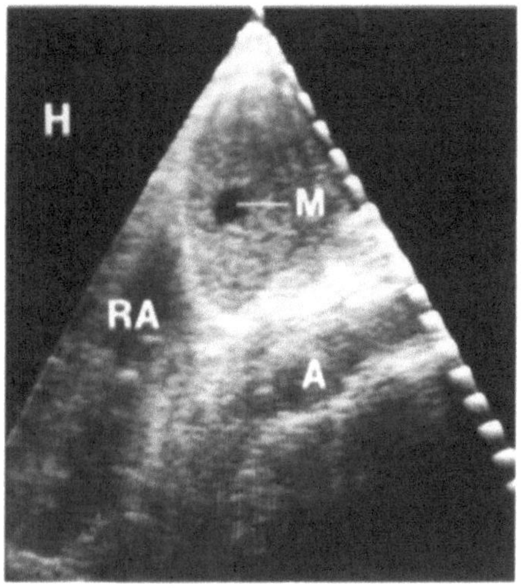

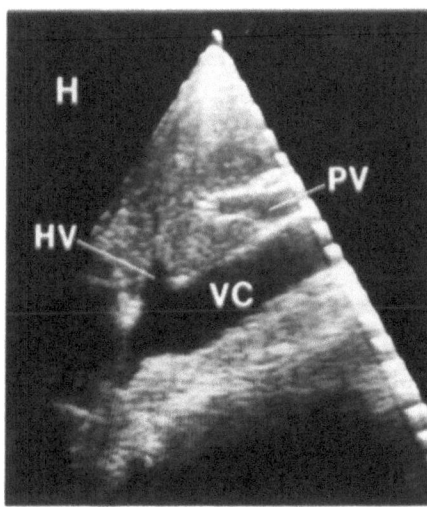

Fig. 5.16. Echo-free pseudomass produced by dilated hepatic vein seen in certain planes. Patient with congestive heart failure. **A** Sagittal view. *M*, "mass"; *A*, aorta; *RA*, right atrium. **B** Plane parallel and adjacent to **A**. "Mass" now identified as part of hepatic vein (*HV*). **C** Plane parallel and adjacent to **B**. Continuity of hepatic vein into dilated vena cava (*VC*) demonstrated. *PV*, portal vein. **D** Transverse plane. Hepatic vein has appearance of mass lesion (*M*) in cross section. **E** Plane parallel and adjacent to **D**. Continuity of "mass" with dilated hepatic veins and vena cava (*VC*) is shown.

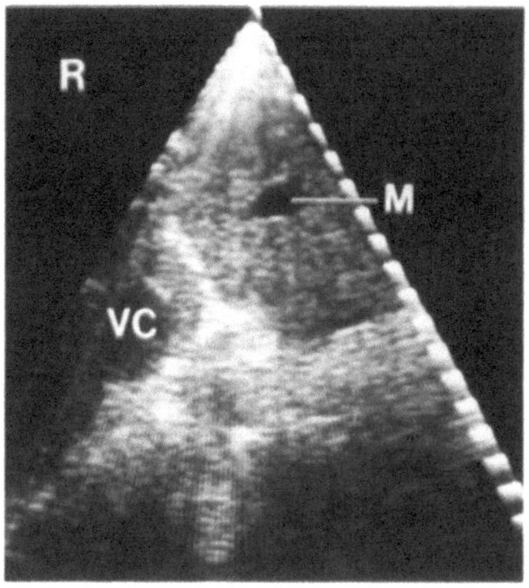

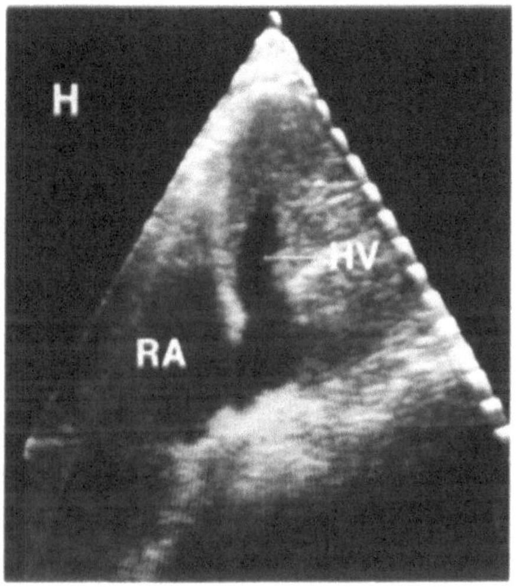

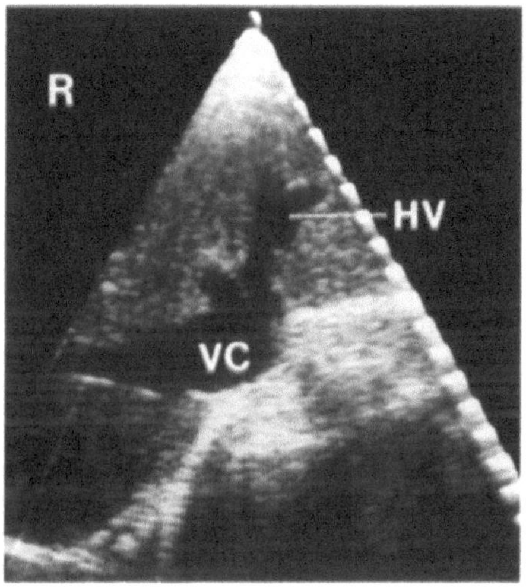

F. Vascular Abnormalities

The most common type of vascular abnormality is seen in patients with right heart failure. Because of the increased pressure in the right atrium, the hepatic veins become dilated (Fig. 5.16) and they fail to show the normal changes in caliber between inspiration and expiration. For the same reasons, the vena cava also is dilated and unchanging during respiration. Other lesions that impede the flow of blood into the right side of the heart (tricuspid atresia, tumors in the right atrium, constrictive pericarditis) can give a similar picture. By contrast in diseases such as hepatitis or cirrhosis the hepatic and portal veins may be reduced in caliber and difficult to see as a result of pressure of adjacent hepatic parenchyma.

Although thrombi within portal veins (11) have been reported in studies using contact scanning equipment, we have had no such personal experience with either contact or real-time scanners and have only identified them in the inferior vena cava and renal vein.

Abnormalities of the bile ducts will be discussed in the next chapter. However, one reason for identifying portal veins in both right and left hepatic lobes is to see if dilated bile ducts are present. Bile ducts, which lie adjacent to portal veins, are too small to identify when normal and are visualized only when dilated.

G. Diffuse Intrahepatic Disease

Because of the small field of view of real-time scanners, it has been our experience that detection of diffuse intrahepatic disease such as cirrhosis is more difficult with the real-time scanner than with the contact scanner and, therefore, a small-field-of-view real-time scanner is not recommended for such purposes. Nevertheless, one may suspect cirrhosis when much greater than usual gain

and time-gain compensation settings are required to obtain adequate penetration within the liver (8, 12).

5. PATHOLOGY: SPLEEN

In our experience focal intrasplenic masses are rare as compared to focal intrahepatic masses. An occasional splenic metastasis or calcification (with typical acoustic shadows) indicative of an old granuloma has been seen.

Our most common splenic lesion has been a subcapsular hematoma which is characterized as an echo-free mass in the subcapsular region (Fig. 5.17). Associated with the subcapsular hematoma there may be localized intrasplenic hematoma or infarcts which appear as focal zones of decreased reflectivity (Fig. 5.17) similar to some metastases.

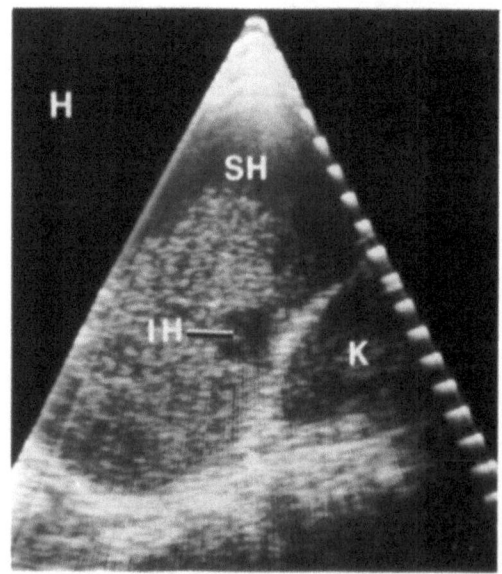

Fig. 5.17. Subcapsular hematoma (*SH*) within lateral aspect of spleen and small intrasplenic hematoma (*IH*) in patient who sustained flank trauma. *K*, Left kidney.

Splenomegaly is easy to appreciate with real-time instruments as the patient is being scanned, but more difficult to demonstrate from photographs of ultrasound images. The operator can readily determine gross splenic size as the transducer is swept over the left upper quadrant, but since the spleen usually has a larger area than can be encompassed by the field of a real-time scanner, accurate size is difficult to determine. For this purpose, the contact scanner is the more appropriate instrument.

Normally the spleen and left kidney are not imaged from the anterior surface because gas in the stomach obscured these deeper lying organs. As the spleen enlarges, it both displaces the stomach medially and extends over the left kidney. Thus, when the spleen and left kidney can be imaged from the anterior approach, the organ is probably enlarged. A rough approximation of splenic size can also be obtained by comparing splenic size to renal size (assuming normal kidneys) when imaging both the spleen and left kidney via the left flank approach.

References

1. Marks WM, Filly RA, Callen PW (1979) Ultrasonic anatomy of the liver: a review with new applications. J Clin Ultrasound 7:137–146
2. Babcock DS, Kaufman L, Cosnow I (1978) Ultrasound diagnosis of hydatid disease (echinococcosis) in two cases. Am J Roentgenol 131:895–897
3. Green B, Bree RL, Goldstein HM, Stanley C (1977) Gray scale ultrasound evaluation of hepatic neoplasms: patterns and correlations. Radiology 124:203–208
4. Scheible W, Gosink BB, Leopold GR (1977) Gray scale echographic patterns of hepatic metastatic disease. Am J Roentgenol 129:983–987
5. Wooten WB, Green B, Goldstein HM (1978) Ultrasonography of necrotic hepatic metastases. Radiology 128:447–450
6. Cunningham JJ, Wooten W, Cunningham MA (1976) Gray scale echography of soluble protein and protein aggregate fluid collections (in vitro study). J Clin Ultrasound 4:417–419
7. Broderick TW, Gosink B, Menuck L, Harris R, Wilcox J (1980) Echographic and radionuclide detection of hepatoma. Radiology 135:149–151
8. Taylor KJW, Carpenter DA, Hill CR, McCready VR (1976) Gray scale ultrasound imaging. Radiology 119:415–423
9. Bernardino ME, Green B (1979) Ultrasonographic evaluation of chemotherapeutic response in hepatic metastases. Radiology 133:437–441
10. Sukov RJ, Cohen LJ, Sample WF (1980) Sonography of hepatic amebic abscesses. Am J Roentgenol 134:911–915
11. Merritt CRB (1979) Ultrasonographic demonstration of portal vein thrombosis. Radiology 133:425–427
12. Gosink BB, Lemon SK, Scheible W, Leopold GR (1979) Accuracy of ultrasonography in diagnosis of hepatocellular disease. Am J Roentgenol 133:19–23

6
Biliary System

In our experience, the examination of the gallbladder lends itself more readily to real-time studies than to static imaging with an articulated arm contact scanner. Since there can be considerable variation in position of the gallbladder in the right upper quadrant, its visualization is more rapidly and easily obtained with real-time instrumentation. In addition, since a major purpose of the gallbladder examination is for the detection of stones, real-time scanning is preferable to contact scanning because real-time scanners can sweep through the entire volume of the organ in a variety of planes so as to better document the presence and movement of stones.

1. ANATOMIC CONSIDERATIONS

The gallbladder is located in the right upper abdomen along the inferior surface of the right lobe of the liver. Depending upon the size of the liver and the patient's habitus, the position of the gallbladder can range anywhere from the midline to the extreme lateral portion of the right upper abdomen. The gallbladder can be subcostal or supercostal in location. Although the gallbladder usually lies with its long axis roughly parallel to the long axis of the body, considerable variation in gallbladder position occurs. The organ varies in size depending upon whether the patient has fasted or has recently eaten. The configuration is usually oblong. Gallbladder size is usually not indicative of the presence or absence of obstruction per se. In the patient who has been fasting for several days (usually on intravenous fluids), the gallbladder can reach sizes as great as 10 cm in length without having cystic duct obstruction.

The lumen of the gallbladder may be completely echo free in the normal state (Fig. 6.1) or may reveal septa partially projecting from the walls (Fig. 6.2). In addition, near the neck of the gallbladder one may occasionally identify portions of the spiral valve that project as small shelves into the lumen. Sometimes portions of these shelves can be confused with gallstones depending upon how the gallbladder is ultrasonically imaged (Fig. 6.3).

In the normal subject, the common bile duct can often be identified in the right parasagittal plane as a longitudinally oriented tubular structure that courses anterior to the portal vein (Fig. 6.4) and then continues inferiorly into the head of the pan-

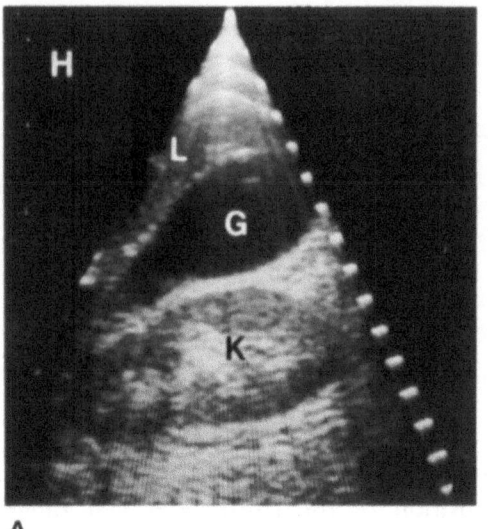

A

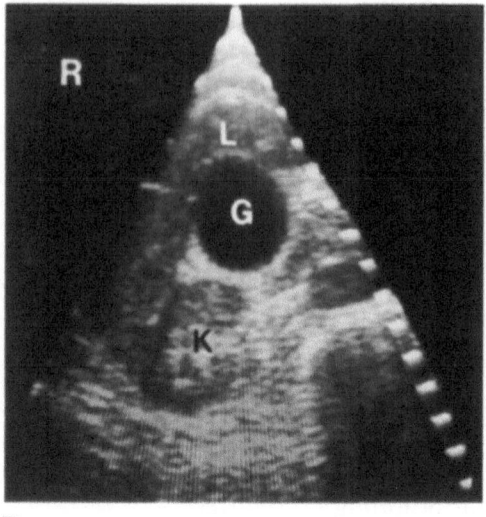

B

Fig. 6.1. Normal gallbladder (*G*) in sagittal (**A**) and transverse (**B**) scans. *L*, liver; *K*, right kidney.

creas (Fig. 6.5A and B). The maximum normal diameter of the common duct when measured where it crosses anterior to the portal vein ranges from 5 to 8 mm (1, 2, 3, 4) with the smallest diameter being reported using a real-time scanner (1). In asymptomatic post-cholecystectomy patients, the upper limits of the common duct have been reported as 10 mm, though in the majority of these patients the duct is still at or below

4 mm (5). In transverse scans the common duct is seen in cross section anterior to the portal vein (Fig. 6.4B) and in the posterior portion of the pancreatic head (Fig. 6.5C and D). One should be careful to distinguish between the superior mesenteric vein and the common duct. Although they both are longitudinally oriented, the former lies more medially and runs anteroinferiorly, going anteriorly to the uncinate process of the pancreas and terminating in the portal vein, whereas the latter lies more laterally and runs posteroinferiorly, going anteriorly over the portal vein and terminating in the posterior part of the pancreatic head (Fig. 6.6).

The normal caliber intrahepatic bile ducts are usually not seen, although Zemen et al. have reported that intrahepatic bile ducts under 2 mm can be seen and are considered of normal size (6). However, when they dilate, they can be easily identified as tubular structures running parallel to branches of the portal vein (Fig. 6.25).

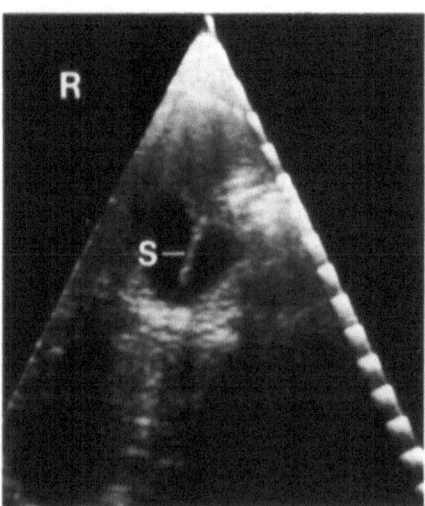

Fig. 6.2. Septum (*S*) projecting from one wall of gallbladder. Transverse scan.

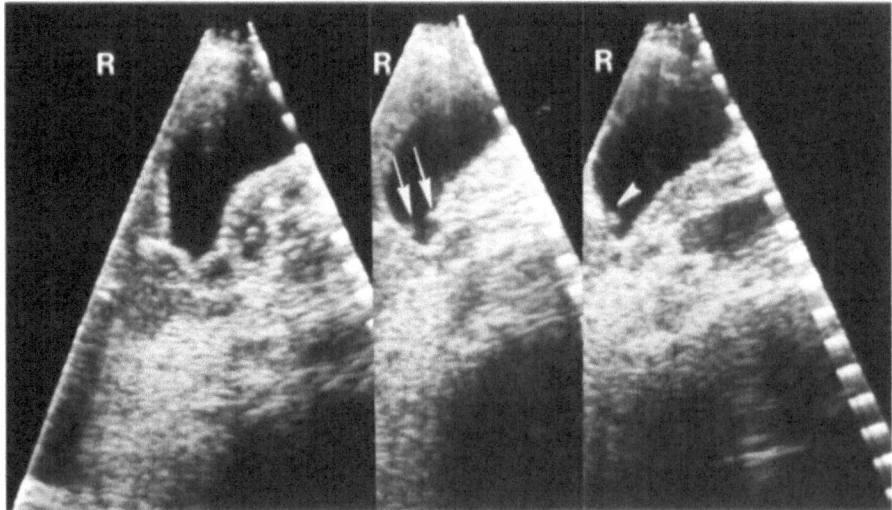

Fig. 6.3. Three adjacent transverse scans through gallbladder including spiral valve. Although portions of valve can be confused with polyp or small stone on single image (*arrowhead*), symmetric appearance of similar tissue projections (*arrows*) on adjacent images is indicative of normal valve.

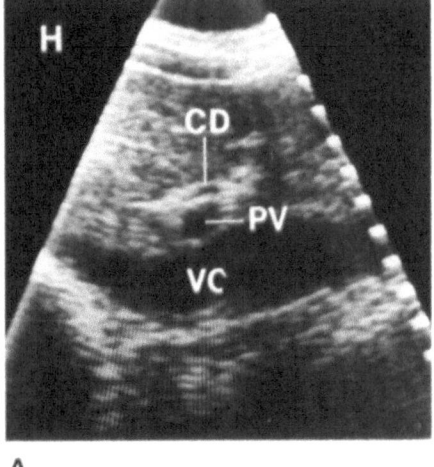

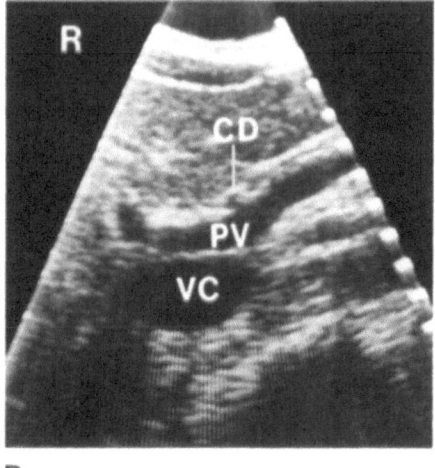

Fig. 6.4. Normal common duct (*CD*) as it crosses anterior to portal vein (*PV*) in sagittal (**A**) and transverse (**B**) planes. *VC,* vena cava.

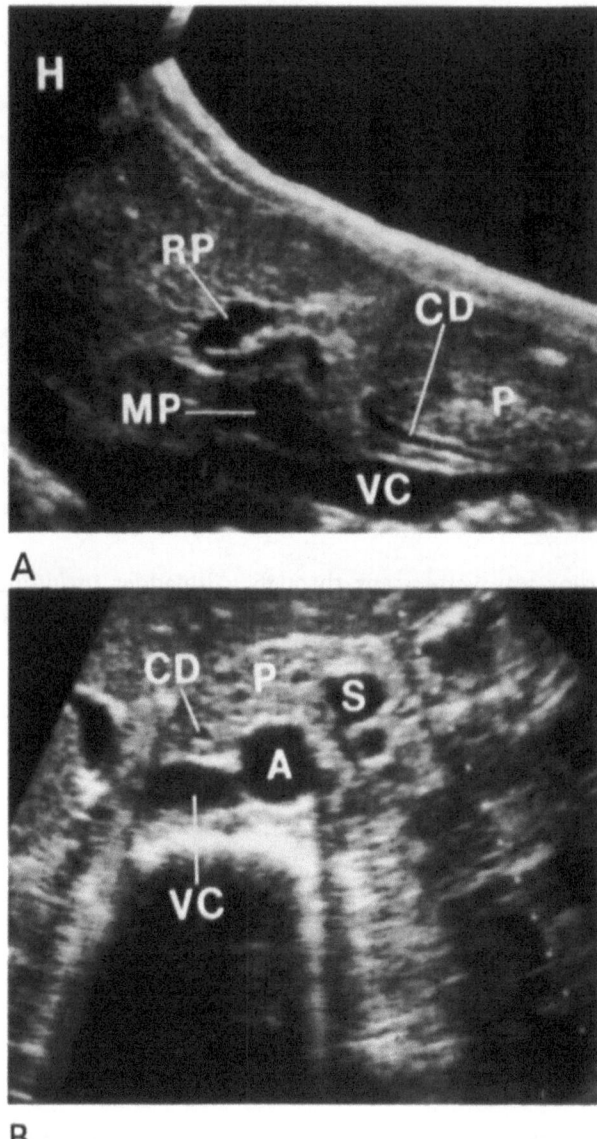

A

B

Fig. 6.5. Normal common duct (*CD*) within head of pancreas (*P*). Images in sagittal (**A** and **A′**) and transverse (**B** and **B′**) planes comparing contact and real-time mechanical sector scanners. *A*, aorta; *VC*, vena cava; *S*, splenic vein; *MP*, main portal vein; *RP*, right portal vein.

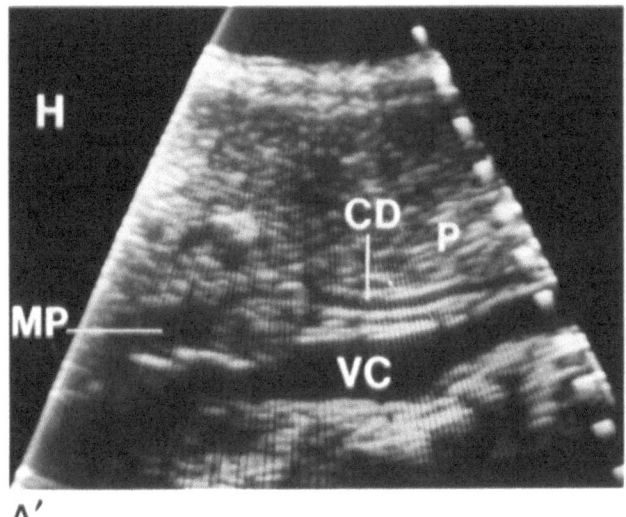

A'

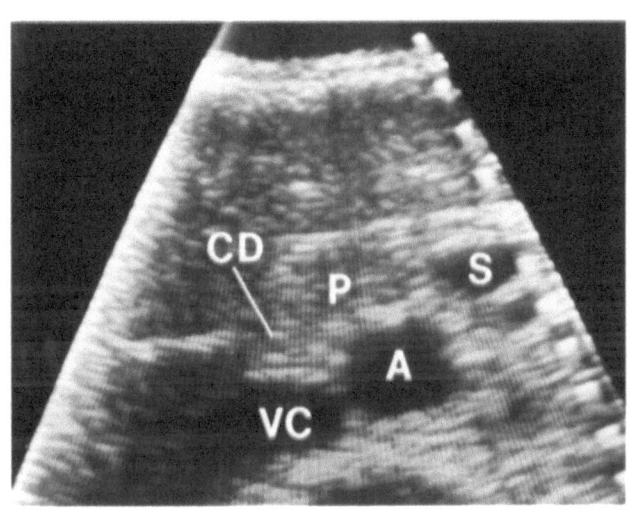

B'

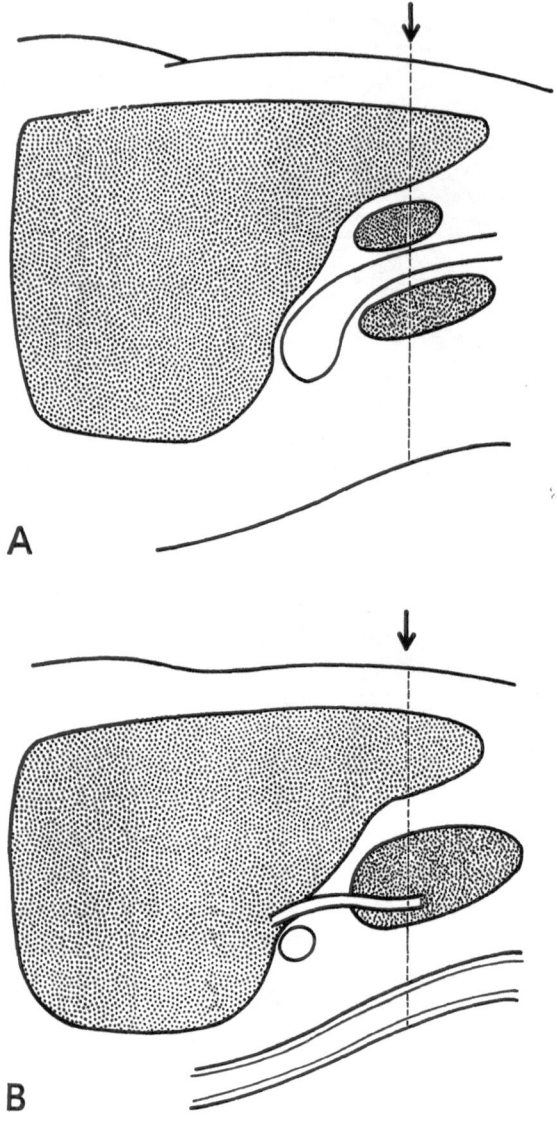

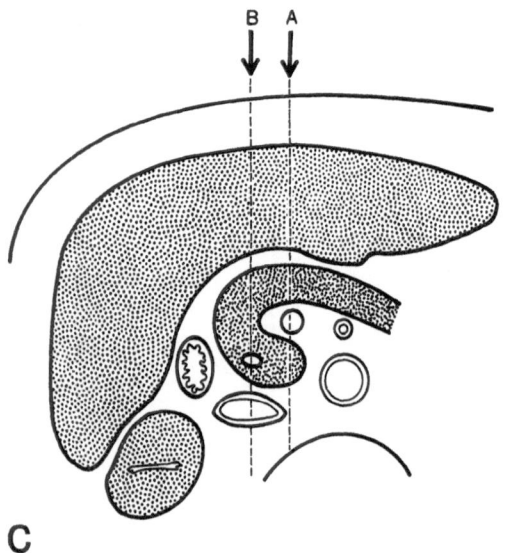

Fig. 6.6. Course and position of common duct versus superior mesenteric vein (SMV). **A** and **A'** Sagittal plane through SMV. **B** and **B'** sagittal plane through common duct (*CD*). **C** Transverse plane through pancreas (*P*) relating position of SMV to common duct. SMV is medial to common duct and courses anteroinferiorly while common duct courses posteroinferiorly. *L,* liver; *PV,* portal vein; *IVC,* inferior vena cava; *A,* aorta; *SMA,* superior mesenteric artery; *HA,* hepatic artery.

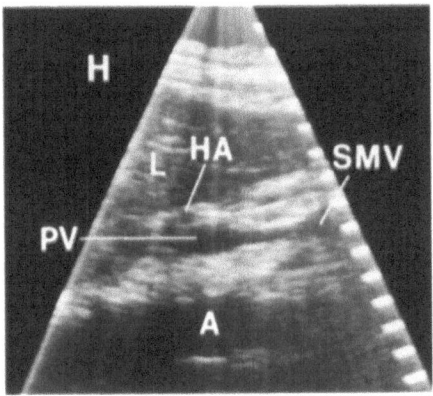

Fig. 6.6.A′

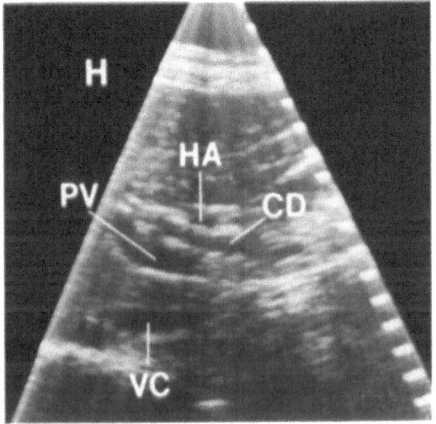

Fig. 6.6.B′

2. STRUCTURES CONFUSED WITH THE GALLBLADDER

Adequate history is vital for the satisfactory performance and correct interpretation of any imaging study. It is especially important for the ultrasound study of the gallbladder to know whether the gallbladder has been removed and whether other types of surgery have been performed in the area, since other structures in the right upper quadrant can be confused with the gallbladder. A

fusiform fluid-containing structure mimicking the gallbladder in shape and location can occur in patients following cholecystectomy which represents a postoperative hematoma or bile collection in the gallbladder bed (7). A loop of small bowel that has been anastomosed to the proximal common duct or common hepatic duct as part of the reconstructive procedure following resection of a carcinoma of the pancreatic head can resemble a gallbladder when the bowel is fluid filled. If food particles float within the fluid, they can be confused with stones (Fig. 6.7).

On occasion the fluid- and food-filled duodenum, especially in transverse view, can be confused with a gallbladder containing stones (Fig. 6.8). Continuous observation for several seconds usually will reveal that the intraluminal particles change in position and number, thus clearly distinguishing them from gallstones. If the duodenal contents do

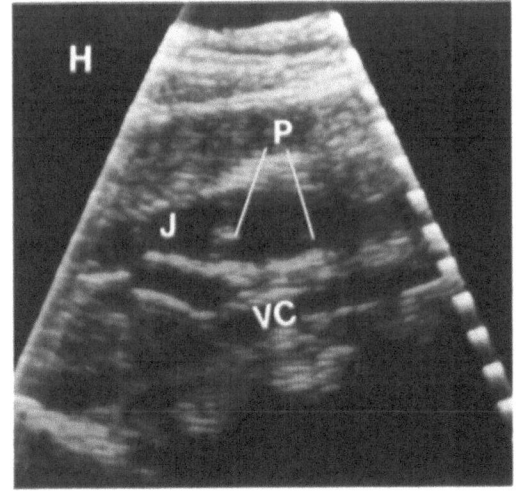

Fig. 6.7. Choledochojejunostomy. Jejunum (*J*) filled with fluid and food particles (*P*) can be confused with stones in gallbladder unless patient's history is known. Sagittal view. *VC*, vena cava.

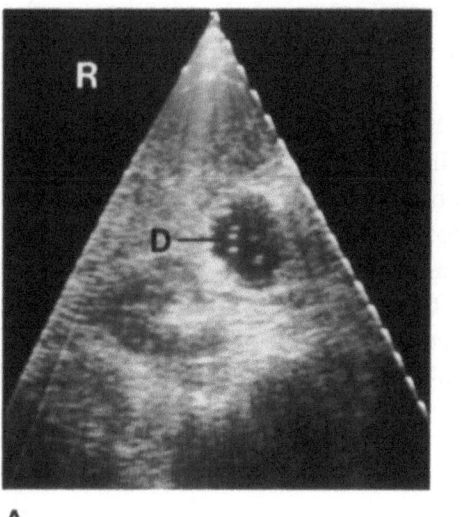

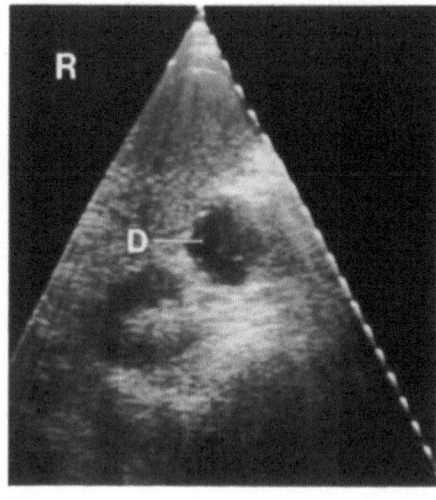

Fig. 6.8. **A** Fluid- and food-filled duodenum (*D*) can be confused with small stones within gall-bladder on single image. **B** Changing number and position of particles within the fluid indicates that structure is duodenum and not gallbladder. Transverse scans.

not move, the patient can be given a drink of water and a rapid change in duodenal contents will be observed.

3. SCANNING PROCEDURES

Before examining the gallbladder, the patient should fast preferably for at least eight hours so as to allow the organ to distend and, therefore, to be more readily detected. In addition, the larger amount of fluid within a fasting gallbladder helps visualize stones because the posterior wall becomes smoother from increased fluid volume and small stones can be more readily appreciated as slight irregularities lying against the wall.

Since the gallbladder lies quite close to the right kidney and since pain caused by gallbladder disease may at times be confused with symptoms caused by renal disease, the examiner should routinely examine the right kidney as well, especially when the gallbladder is normal. Two examples illus-

trate this point. In one patient for whom a gallbladder study was requested because of right upper quadrant pain suggestive of gall-stones, hydronephrosis was detected and an intravenous pyelogram showed that a ureteral calculus was the cause of this patient's pain (Fig. 6.9A). In another patient with vague right upper quadrant pain for whom a gallbladder study was requested, a small carcinoma of the right kidney was found (Fig. 6.9B) which may or may not have caused the patient's discomfort.

A. Supine Position

This is the usual starting position for the examination of the gallbladder and biliary tree. The real-time transducer is placed in the subcostal region in a sagittal orientation. The transducer is moved in the sagittal plane until the lower edge of the right lobe of the liver is identified. If the gallbladder is not immediately seen, the transducer is then moved medially or laterally while maintaining sagittal orientation until the gallbladder

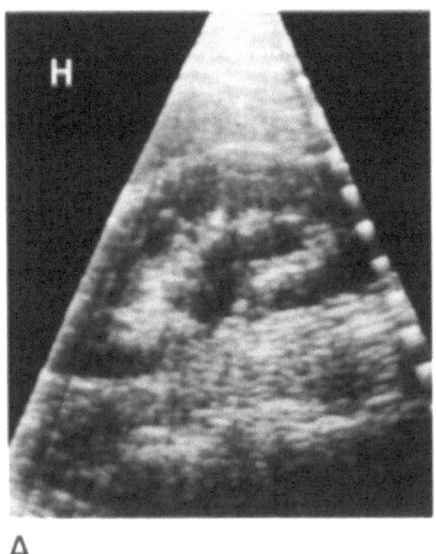

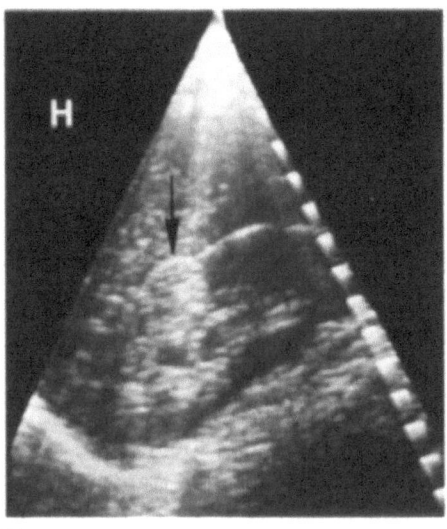

Fig. 6.9. Detection of unsuspected renal lesions because right kidney is routinely included in the examination of the gallbladder. **A** Hydronephrosis caused by distal ureteral calculus. **B** Two-centimeter carcinoma *(arrow)* in anterior parenchymal region.

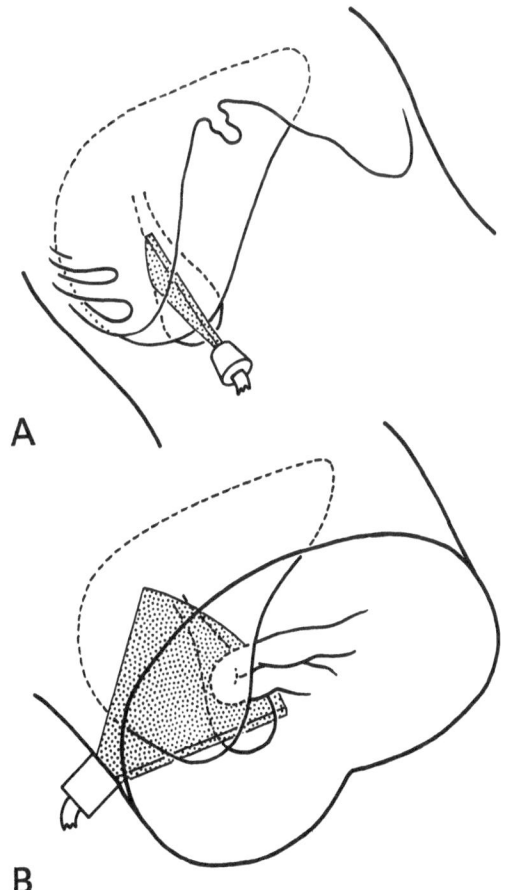

Fig. 6.10. Transducer positions for imaging gallbladder. **A** Sagittal plane. Transducer subcostal with beam angled superiorly under rib cage. **B** Coronal plane. Transducer within intercostal space in region of anterior or middle axillary line. This view is best when gallbladder is under rib cage or when bowel (B) is interposed between gallbladder and liver.

is identified. During this examination, the patient should either perform the "belly out" maneuver (Fig. 5.3) or maintain deep inspiration in order to project the liver and gallbladder below the costal margin (Fig. 6.10A). If one cannot identify the gallbladder using this approach, it is usually because the gallbladder is obscured by overlying gas-filled bowel or because it is located under the ribs in either a more superior or more lateral position. Therefore, the transducer should then be placed in one of the lower right intercostal spaces along the anterior or midaxillary line with the beam coronally oriented (Fig. 6.10B). In each interspace in which the transducer is placed, it should be swept through a large arc in an attempt to detect the gallbladder. When the right kidney is identified in one of these sweeps, the examiner knows that the beam is angled too posteriorly. It may be necessary to perform this maneuver in multiple intercostal spaces and in several positions within each intercostal space, first more an-

teriorly and then more laterally toward the axillary region, until the gallbladder is detected.

Once the gallbladder is detected in the sagittal or coronal plane, then the operator rotates the transducer in order to image the long axis of the gallbladder (Fig. 6.11A) since the organ, when initially detected, may be seen in a diagnonal plane rather than in the true long axis. After the long axis is identified, the transducer is swept in an arcuate manner from one side of the gallbladder through the true long axis to the other side with the patient in suspended respiration (Fig. 6.11B). This sweeping maneuver allows the entire organ to be scanned. At the completion of the maneuver, the transducer is rotated 90° in order to image the gallbladder along its true short axis. Then, with the patient again in suspended respiration, the transducer either is arced in a superior-to-inferior direction at one location on the skin so as to sweep the beam through the gallbladder from the neck to the fundus

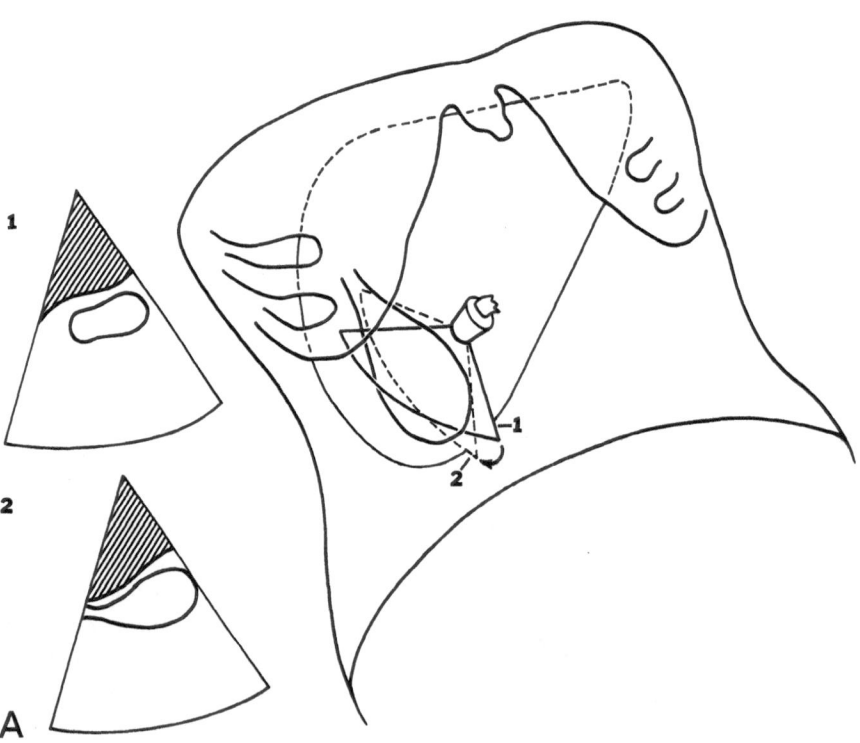

Fig. 6.11.

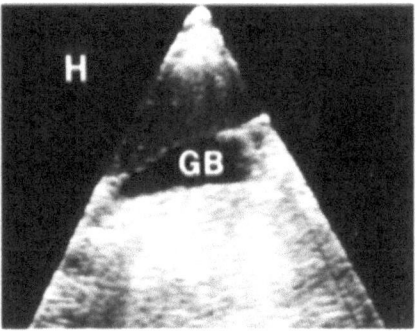

B1

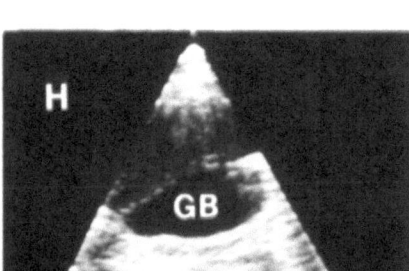

B2

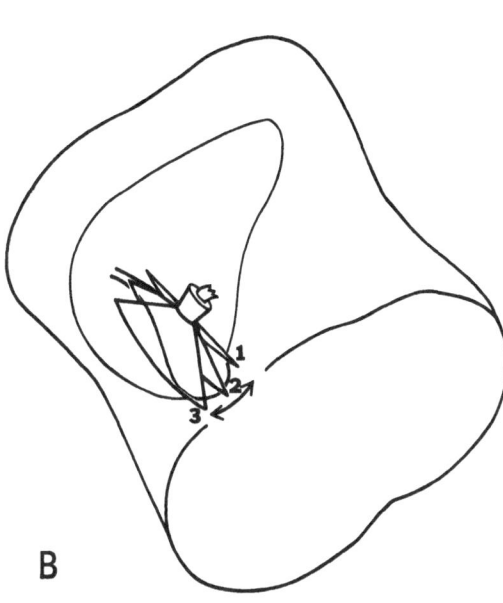

B

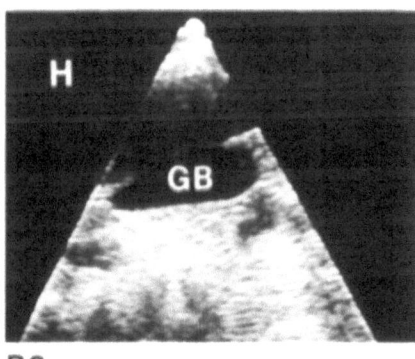

B3

Fig. 6.11. **A** Finding true long axis. Transducer rotated over gallbladder (*GB*) from initial position (*1*) in either direction until image showing greatest length of gallbladder is displayed (*2*). **B** Arcing transducer from side to side in plane of long axis to sweep beam through entire volume of gallbladder. *1,* median section; *2,* central section; *3,* lateral section.

(Fig. 6.12) or is slid over the skin in the same manner. The sliding maneuver is used when the gallbladder is relatively long (Fig. 3.3) and the arcuate one when the gallbladder is relatively short. Sometimes a combination of both maneuvers is used.

Longitudinal views in the sagittal plane (vertically oriented beam entering from the anterior abdominal wall) readily identify stones since the beam is perpendicular to the posterior wall, the most dependent part of the gallbladder. However, when the longitudinal view of the gallbladder is obtained in the coronal plane (beam entering through

flank), the beam is horizontal and perpendicular to the lateral and medial walls. In this orientation stones may not be visualized (Fig. 6.13).

The transverse view provides a better chance of detecting stones than the longitudinal view since stones will be seen in transverse view regardless of whether the beam enters the body from the anterior abdominal surface or through the flank. The only difference will be the direction of the acoustic shadow cast by the stone. The shadow will be vertical when the beam enters from the anterior abdominal wall and

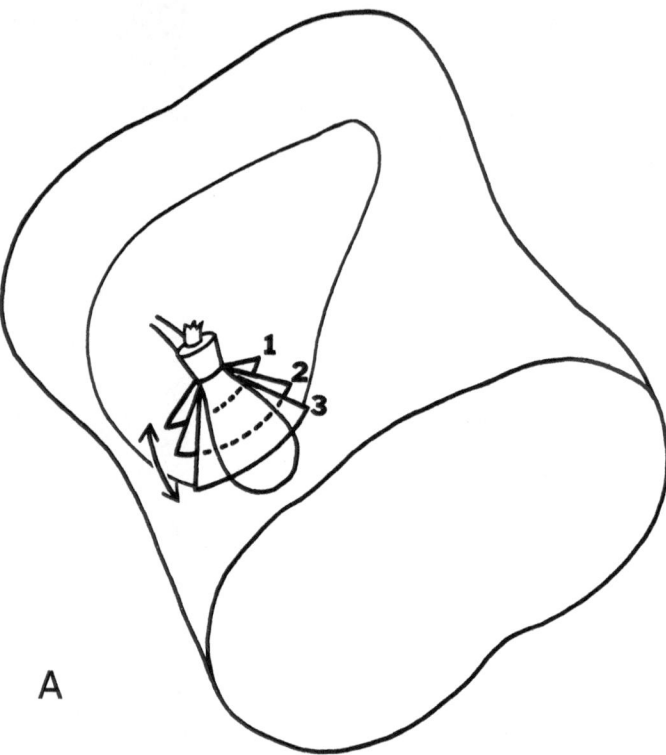

Fig. 6.12. A Short axis scanning through gallbladder by arcing transducer superiorly and inferiorly. Serial transverse scans. **A** *1*, superior section; **A** *2*, middle section; **A** *3*, inferior section.

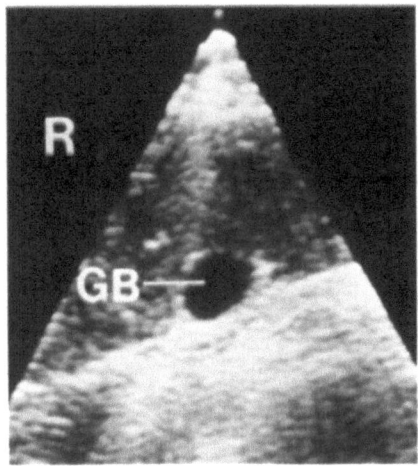

A1

Fig. 6.12. (cont.)

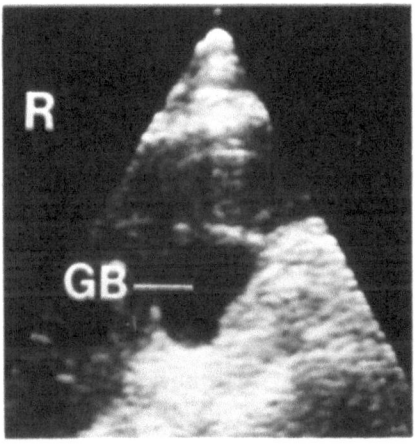

A2

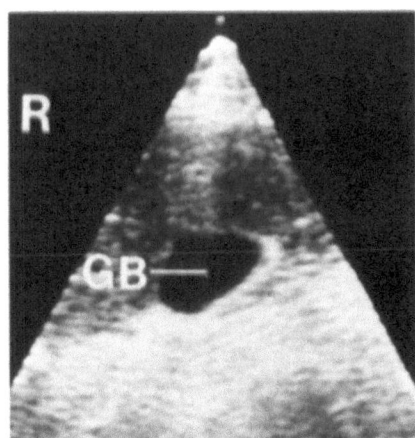

A3

horizontal when the beam enters from the flank (Fig. 6.14).

After the gallbladder is examined with the patient supine, then the region of the common duct is examined to see if this structure is dilated and if so whether it contains intraluminal stones. Lastly, the liver is briefly scanned to visualize branches of the portal system and to determine whether dilated bile ducts lie adjacent to them.

If dilated intrahepatic biliary ducts or a dilated common duct are detected, the region of examination should be enlarged to include the head of the pancreas, in the hope of detecting a mass lesion which may be the cause of biliary obstruction, and the porta hepatis and the liver to see if there are any focal masses suggestive of primary or metastatic tumor. In the examination of the pancreas, besides examining the head carefully for a mass lesion, the body and tail should be examined to see if evidence of pancreatic duct dilatation can be detected. Duct dilatation will further support the diagnosis of a mass lesion in the region of the head of the pancreas even if the mass lesion itself cannot be detected by ultrasound, since sometimes the lesion can be at the ampulla of Vater and be too small for ultrasonic detection.

B. Decubitus and Erect Positions

Whenever possible the gallbladder should be examined in the erect or decubitus view in addition to the supine one in order to demonstrate motion of the stones even if an apparently typical pattern of gallstones is seen in the supine view. Occasionally structures such as a portion of the spiral valve will mimic the appearance of stones in the gallbladder in supine position but will show no movement when the patient shifts position.

In the decubitus position the transverse view is again the crucial view for the same reason as was described for the supine position. To identify moving gallstones in this

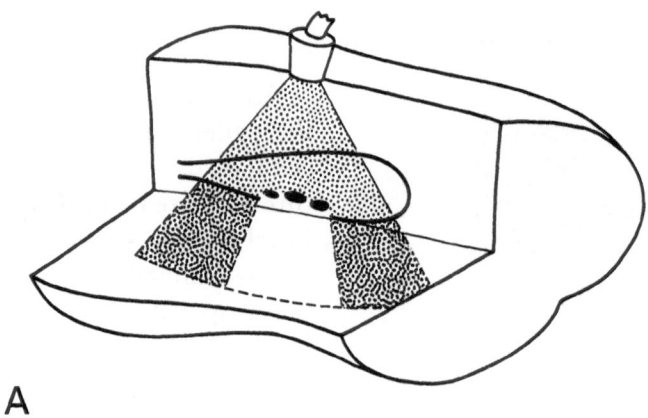

A

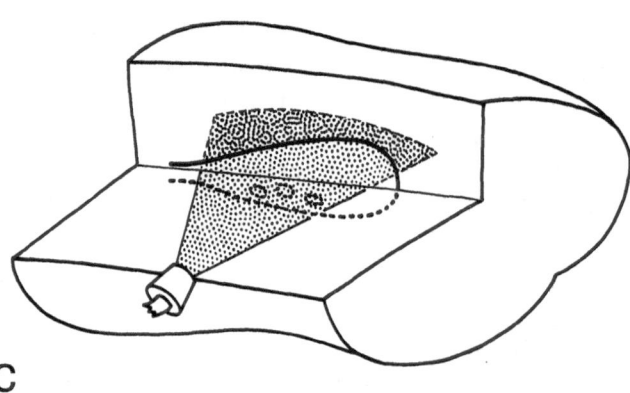

C

Fig. 6.13. Effect of sagittal versus coronal scans in detecting gallstones in supine patient. **A,B** Sagittal scans. Anterior (*A*) and posterior (*P*) walls of gallbladder visualized. Stones (*S*) lying on posterior wall are identified. **C,D** Coronal scans. Medial (*M*) and lateral (*L*) walls are visualized. Stones are not seen.

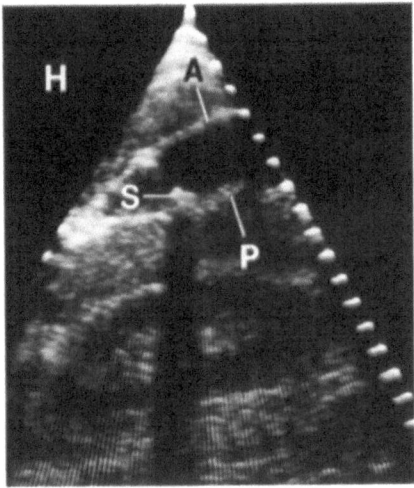

B

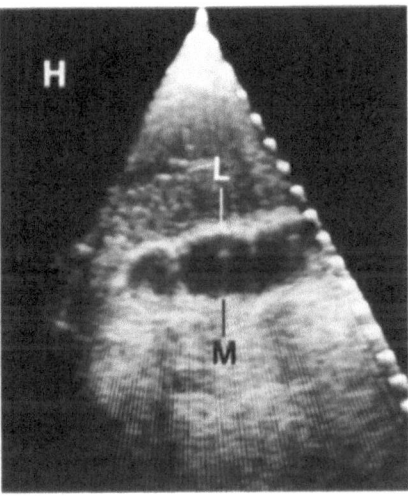

D

Fig. 6.13. (cont.)

view one must demonstrate that the position of the gallstones changes from resting on the posterior wall (in supine position) to resting on the left lateral wall (in decubitus position) (Fig. 6.15). Sagittal views are much less useful in the decubitus position because for this view the transducer is still placed over the anterior abdominal wall with the beam directed perpendicular to the anterior wall. In such orientation, the ultrasound beam traverses the anterior and posterior walls of the gallbladder, neither of which are the dependent walls in decubitus position (Fig. 6.16A). To obtain a meaningful long axis view of the gallbladder for stone detection in the decubitus view, the ultrasound beam should be oriented along the coronal plane (Fig. 6.16B). However, in practice it is difficult with the patient in decubitus position to see the gallbladder in the coronal plane since in this plane the gallbladder is quite far from the flank and sometimes obscured by intervening gas-filled bowel.

When the patient is examined in the decubitus position, often the gallbladder changes its long axis from one that is roughly parallel to the long axis of the body to one that is roughly parallel to the transverse axis of the body. When the gallbladder shifts its long axis between supine and decubitus positions, it is more difficult to determine whether the stones have moved than when the gallbladder maintains roughly the same axis in the two views.

In the erect position the gallstones fall to the fundus of the gallbladder and are best seen with the sagittal view. It is important to fully visualize the fundus so as not to miss small stones. At times the erect position may be the only position in which stones can be visualized (Fig. 6.17). One difficulty that can occur in both the supine and the erect position is that gas in the hepatic flexure of the colon may produce an acoustic shadow just beneath the gallbladder wall that could be confused with the shadow of gallstones. The key differential point is that with gallstones, one should see localized reflective structures lying inside of and against the wall of the gallbladder, whereas with gas in the bowel the inferior wall of the gallbladder is completely smooth on its intraluminal surface and the acoustic shadow begins below the wall of the gallbladder (Fig. 6.18). On rare occasions loops of the bowel may indent the gallbladder wall, mimicking intraluminal stones; but the relationship of these indentations to the gallbladder changes as the patient breathes

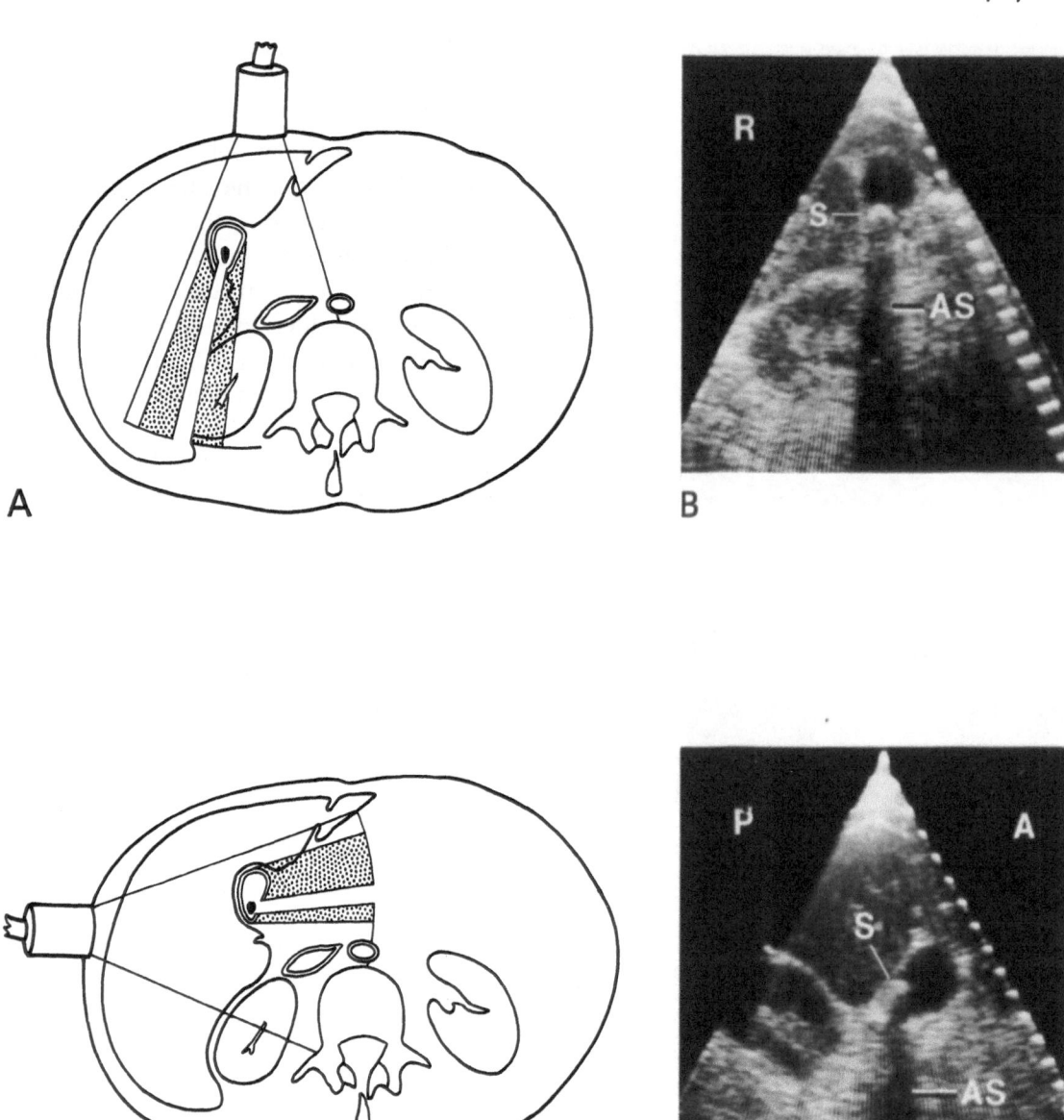

Fig. 6.14. Transverse scans of gallstone (*S*). Direction of acoustic shadow related to position of transducer. Patient is supine. **A,B** Transducer on anterior abdominal wall. Acoustic shadow (*AS*) is vertical. **C,D** Transducer on lateral abdominal wall (*L*). Acoustic shadow is horizontal. *A,* anterior direction; *P,* posterior direction.

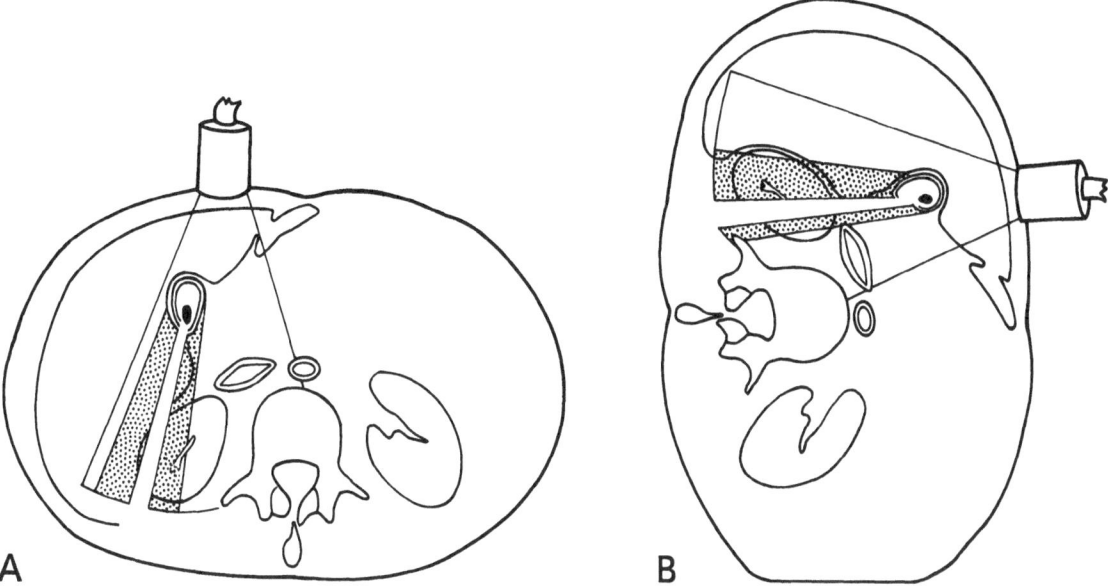

Fig. 6.15. Scans in transverse plane demonstrate movement of gallstones as patient shifts from supine (**A**) to decubitus (**B**) position, left side down.

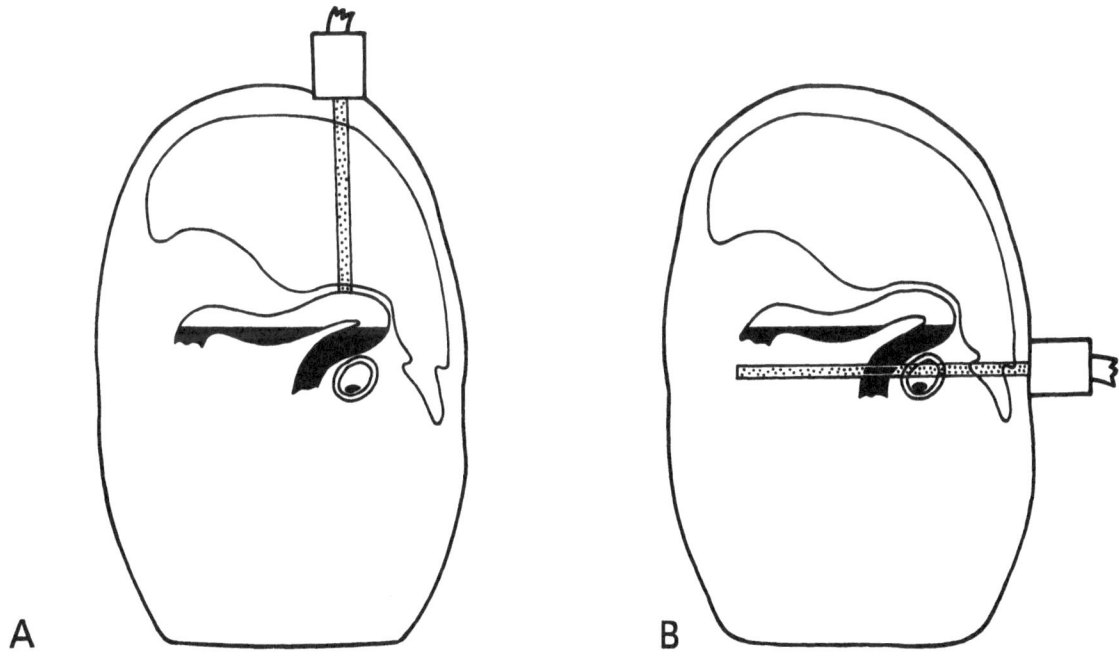

Fig. 6.16. Limitations of sagittal and coronal planes for detecting gallstones when patient lies in decubitus position. **A** Sagittal plane. Beam does not pass through plane of stones. **B** Coronal plane. Beam passes through plane of stones, but gas-filled bowel can be interposed between liver and gallbladder, blocking the passage of sound.

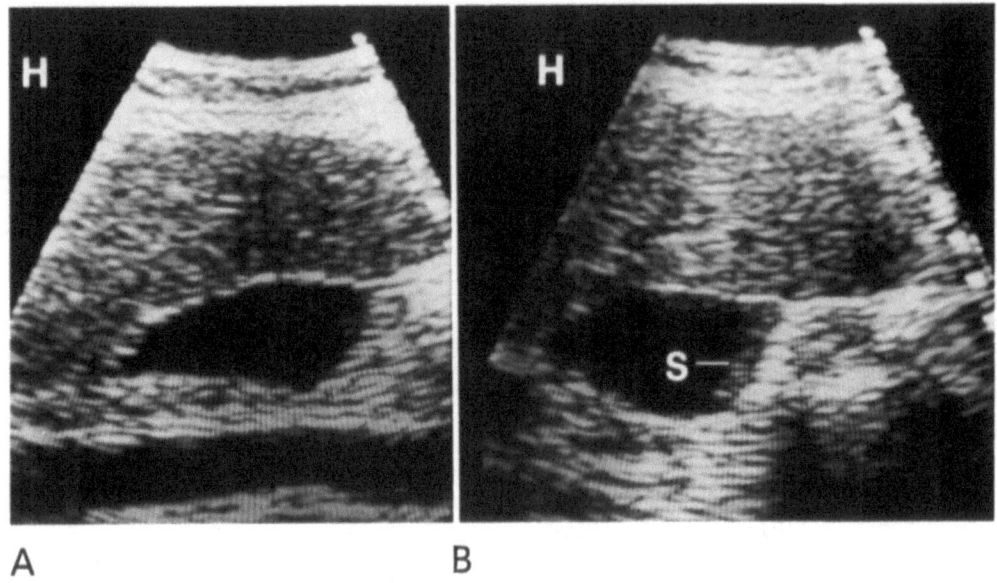

Fig. 6.17. Small gallstones (*S*) seen only with the patient erect. **A** Supine sagittal view; no stones seen. **B** Erect sagittal view. Layer of stones lying above inferior wall.

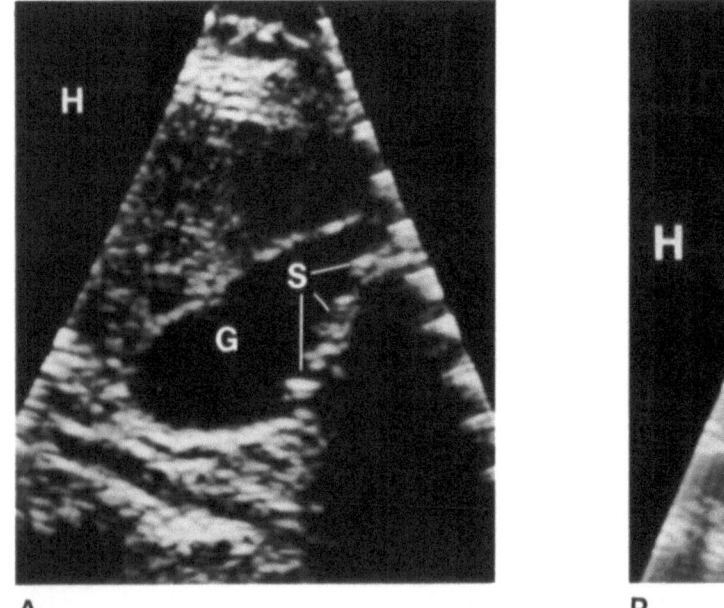

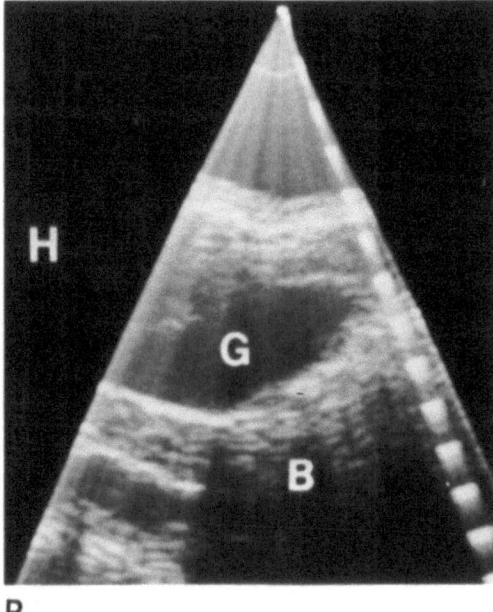

Fig. 6.18. Differentiating gallstones from a loop of bowel adjacent to inferior wall of gallbladder (*G*). Patient is erect. **A** Stones (*S*) present. Inferior surface of dependent wall of gallbladder is irregular. **B** Bowel loop (*B*) adjacent to gallbladder. Inferior surface of gallbladder wall is smooth.

because the gallbladder slides over the bowel (8).

The approach to erect gallbladder scanning is similar to that with the patient supine. The initial examination is conducted in the right parasagittal plane and the lower edge of the liver is used as a reference point. However, since the liver and gallbladder may descend a considerable amount as compared to their position when the patient is supine, if the gallbladder is not found in the right upper quadrant, it should be looked for in the right lower quadrant.

Of the two views, we prefer the erect position because the stones have a greater distance through which to move and, therefore, change in stone position is more readily appreciated. The key view in the erect position is the sagittal one. Stones almost always lie in the most dependent portion of the gallbladder which is the fundus in the erect position. This is the view that best shows

that region. In the transverse view the erect position is often of little value because the plane does not include the fundus (Fig. 6.19).

It is important to realize that stones can move slowly in the gallbladder. Therefore, we have found it useful to wait up to 30 min with the patient in either the decubitus or erect position before concluding that the intraluminal filling defect seen on the supine position failed to move. Failure to demonstrate movement of a small intraluminal gallbladder mass suggests that it may represent a polyp or stone adherent to the wall. The former is more likely if no acoustic shadow is cast (9).

A maneuver that can help identify small intraluminal stones when a loop of gas-filled bowel lies adjacent to the gallbladder and masks the acoustic shadows cast by the stones is to change the patient's position and immediately rescan the gallbladder. The sud-

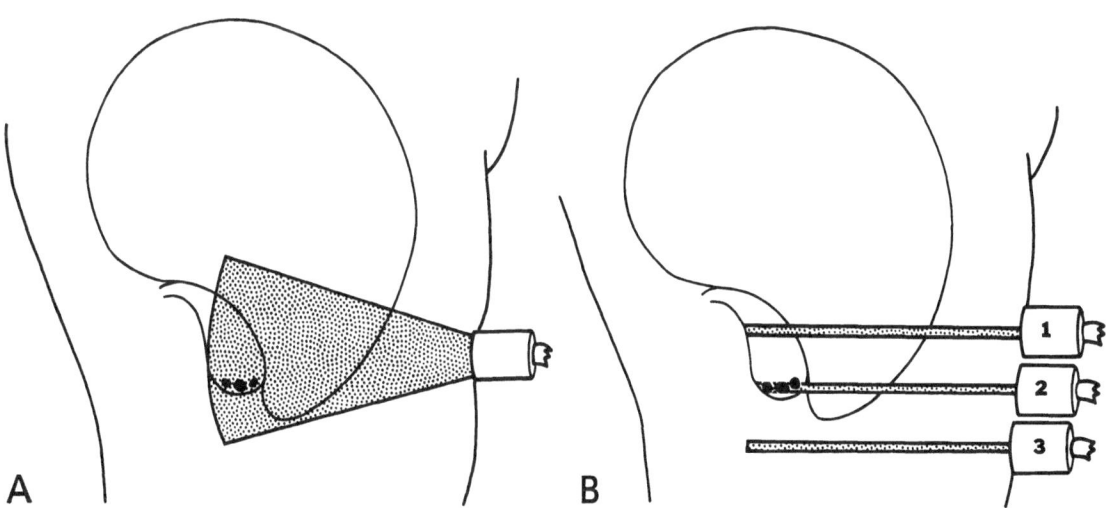

Fig. 6.19. Scanning in erect position. **A** Sagittal plane is the key view and most inferior portion of gallbladder must be included on image since stones usually settle to dependent surface. **B** Transverse planes are more difficult for detecting stones because the stones are seen on only one level, i.e., plane (2) just above the most dependent surface of the gallbladder. A slight tilt of the beam above (1) or below (3) this plane will miss the stones.

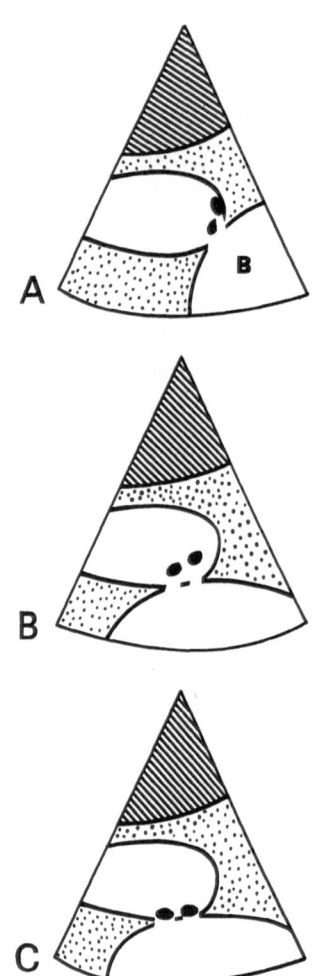

Fig. 6.20. Maneuver for differentiating small stones from gas-filled bowel loop adjacent to gallbladder. All views are sagittal. **A** Patient erect for several minutes. Stones fall to fundus but then acoustic shadows are difficult to distinguish from loop of gas-filled bowel (*B*). **B** Patient placed supine and gallbladder immediately rescanned. Stones fall away from inferior wall and are briefly surrounded by bile. **C** Several minutes later stones settle to posterior wall and again become difficult to identify because of underlying loop of gas-filled bowel.

den change in position causes the stones to fall away from the wall into the lumen. When the patient is rapidly rescanned in the new position, the stones can be seen surrounded by bile for a brief period before they resettle against the dependent wall. To perform this maneuver we first examine the patient erect in the sagittal plane and then rapidly rescan again in the same plane after the patient assumes the supine position (Fig. 6.20).

4. PATHOLOGIC CONDITIONS

A. Gallstones

With the advent of real-time ultrasound scanning equipment, the accuracy of detecting gallstones by ultrasound is very similar to that of oral cholecystography (10). As a result, we and other authors (11) are advocating that ultrasound replace oral cholecystography as the initial examination for demonstrating gallbladder calculi.

The ultrasonic diagnosis of gallstones is pathognomonic when mobile echo-producing structures within the lumen of the gallbladder that cast acoustic shadows are identified (12). Even stones as small as 3 mm cast acoustic shadows behind them if the stones are centered in the beam (Fig. 6.21A) and at the focal zone of the beam. When the stone is at the edge of the beam or out of the focal zone, echoes from tissues deep to the stone are produced that appear behind the stone (Fig. 6.21B) and obscure the acoustic shadowing (13). This effect is similar to the appearance of echos within a cyst when the ultrasound beam encompasses both the cyst and some adjacent solid tissue (Fig. 3.6).

When the gallbladder is contracted and almost entirely filled with stones, the fluid-filled gallbladder lumen may not be iden-

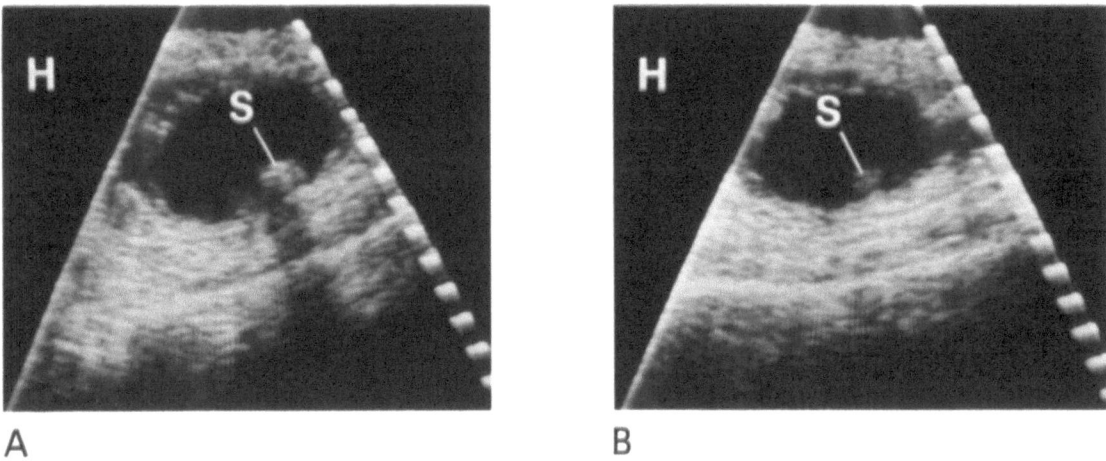

Fig. 6.21. Effect of beam position upon detection of acoustic shadow cast by gallstone (S). **A** Stone centered within beam; shadow cast. **B** Stone at edge of beam; no shadow cast.

tifiable. Instead, one may only see in the region of the inferior surface of the right lobe of the liver a localized area of acoustic echoes (representing stones in the gallbladder) with a sharp acoustic shadow behind them (Fig. 6.22). This abnormality will maintain a constant relationship to the liver as the patient shifts position. Although it is strongly suggestive of stones (12), it is by no means diagnostic since on occasion a gas-filled loop of bowel can produce a similar appearance. Gas in the biliary tree can

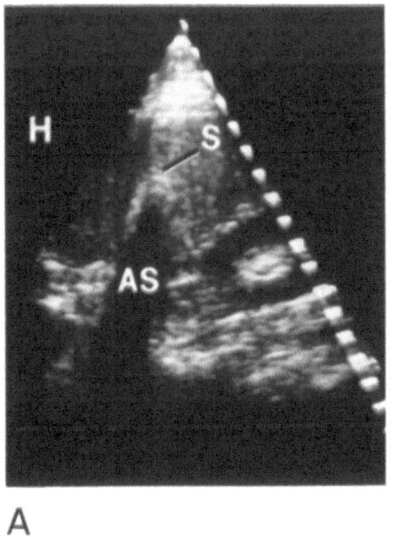
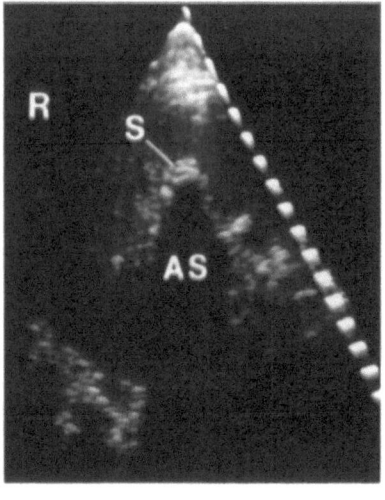

Fig. 6.22. Gallbladder completely filled with stones. Strong echoes reflected from upper surface of stones (S) and acoustic shadow (AS) is cast by stones. Sagittal (**A**) and transverse (**B**) planes.

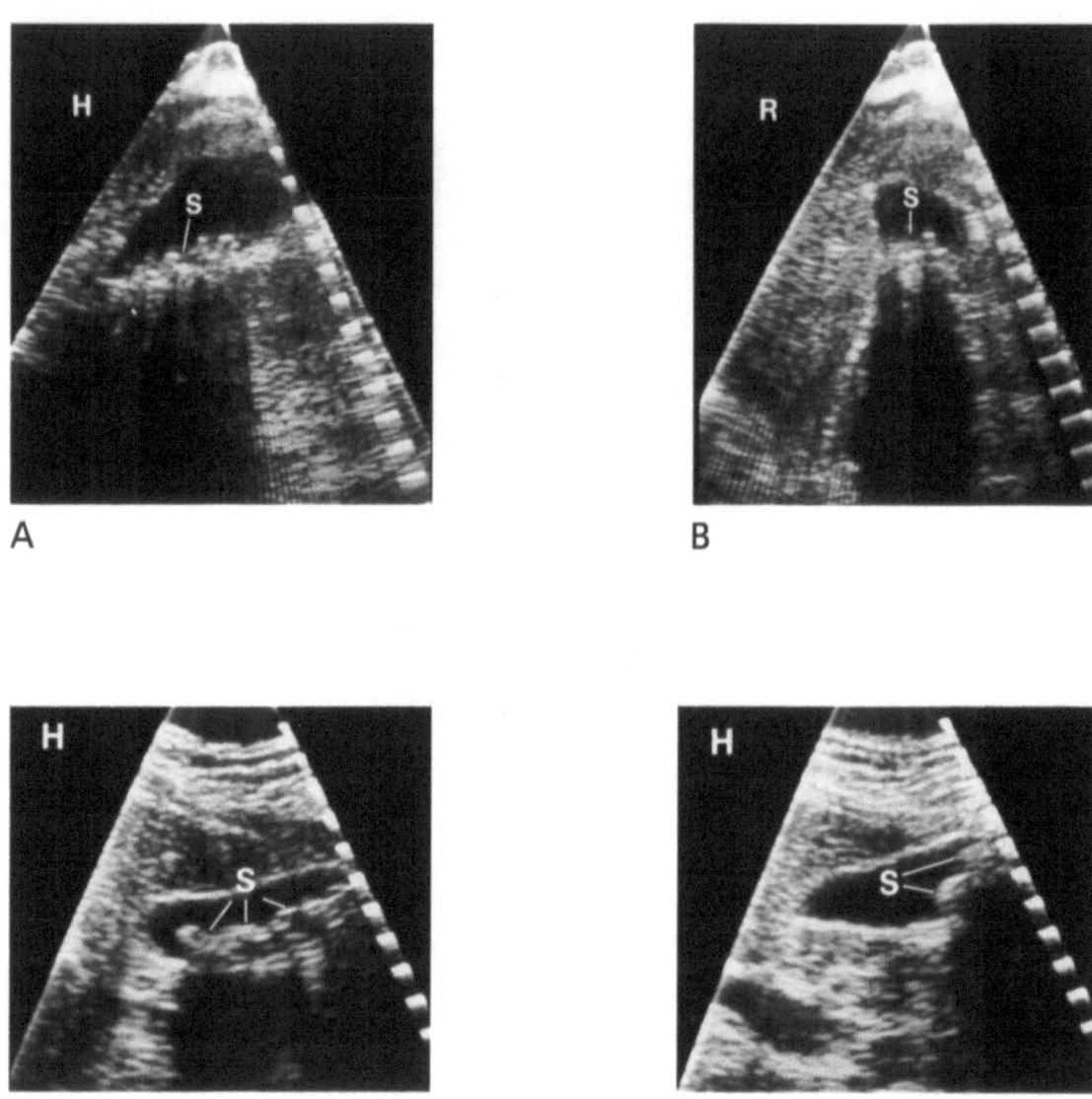

Fig. 6.23. Spectrum of gallstones. **A** and **B** Supine sagittal and transverse views. Cluster of small stones (*S*) layered on posterior wall. **C** and **D** Sagittal supine and erect views. Cluster of stones shifts from posterior wall with patient supine (*C*) to inferior wall with patient erect (*D*). **E** and **F** Sagittal supine and erect views. Impacted 1-cm stone in neck of gallbladder. No change from supine (*E*) to erect (*F*) position.

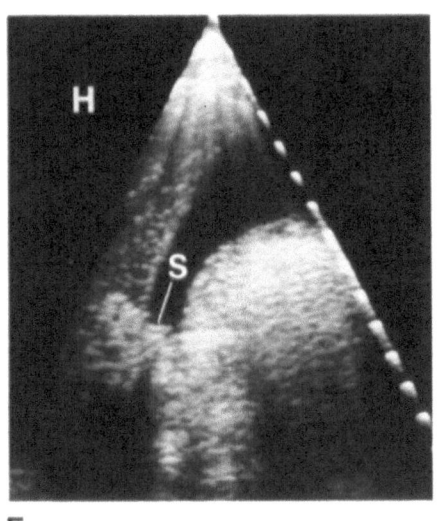

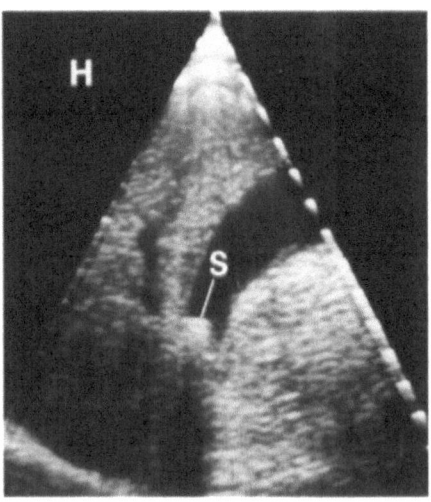

E

F

Fig. 6.23. E, F.

produce a similar appearance with the patient supine but should shift location when the patient is erect. However, the failure to visualize the gallbladder on oral cholecystography or intravenous cholangiography coupled with the above ultrasonic findings is strongly suggestive of stones in a contracted gallbladder. Furthermore, the acoustic shadow cast by a gas filled loop of bowel usually does not produce as sharp margins as that cast by a stone.

The ultrasonic appearance of gallstones depends upon their size and number (Fig. 6.23). Stones may be freely mobile (Fig. 6.23C and D) or impacted in the gallbladder neck (Fig. 6.23E and F). Since they are usually heavier than bile, stones rest upon the most dependent surface of the lumen. However, occasionally gallstones may be seen floating within the bile (Fig. 6.24), if their specific gravity is less than that of bile. Floating stones may also be seen if an ultrasound study is done when contrast material from oral cholecystographic agents is within the gallbladder. The oral contrast agents increase the specific gravity of the bile and can cause stones to float (14).

B. Biliary Ductal Dilatation

Dilated bile ducts are identified by noting the presence of tubular structures parallel to the intrahepatic branches of the portal system (15) (Fig. 6.25A and B), and/or by observing an increased number of usually tortuous tubular channels within the central portion of the liver (Fig. 6.25C), especially adjacent to the major branches of the portal veins (14). Dilatation of portal branches does not produce a similar appearance. In addition, areas of acoustic enhancement may be identified behind the dilated bile ducts (16) because bile often attenuates the ultrasound beam to a lesser degree than adjacent liver tissue and blood in vessels. Occasionally, when the acoustic properties of bile equal those of blood, no increased acoustic transmission is seen behind dilated bile ducts.

Dilatation of the biliary system may be uniform or focal within the liver depending upon the cause of the obstruction. For example, a focal mass may obstruct the main bile duct to only one lobe (6). Even when the site of obstruction is in the common duct and, therefore, affects the entire system,

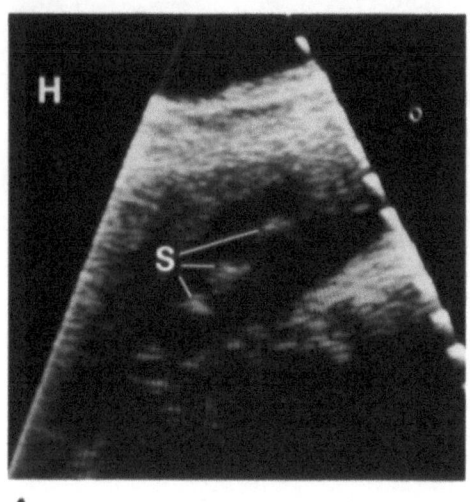
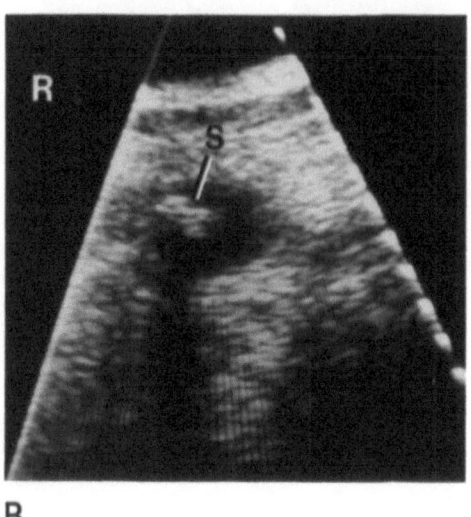

A   B

Fig. 6.24. Floating gallstones (*S*) in sagittal (**A**) and transverse (**B**) views with patient supine.

dilatation may be disproportionate. The common duct may show a proportionally greater increase in caliber than that of the intrahepatic radicals (1).

When dilated ducts are identified, it is important to try to trace the ducts to the point of obstruction in an attempt to define the cause such as a stone in the distal common duct (Fig. 6.26) or a tumor mass encasing the common duct (Fig. 6.27).

Ultrasound has been reported to be a more sensitive method for detecting biliary obstruction than elevation of the serum bilirubin level, since dilatation of the bile ducts can occur before the bilirubin rises (25). The levels of alkaline phosphatase is a more sensitive indicator of biliary dilatation and may be elevated when the bilirubin level is still normal (6).

C. Acute Cholecystitis

The normal gallbladder wall is under 2 mm in thickness (17). When the gallbladder wall

becomes thicker, especially when there is a hyporeflective layer within the wall (19), the diagnosis of acute cholecystitis should be strongly considered (Fig. 6.28). Intraluminal stones may or may not be present. This hyporeflective layer is believed to represent subserosal edema and necrosis (18).

D. Gallbladder Tumors

Cancer of the gallbladder is a much rarer condition than gallstones, but should be suspected when an irregular nonshifting intraluminal mass is detected within the gallbladder that partially or completely fills the lumen (19). This mass may be associated with acoustic shadows thereby suggesting a combination of tumor and gallstone (20). Occasionally, a similar picture may occur when a combination of stones and inflammatory debris is present within the gallbladder. Differentiation from gallbladder carcinoma is not possible in such circumstances.

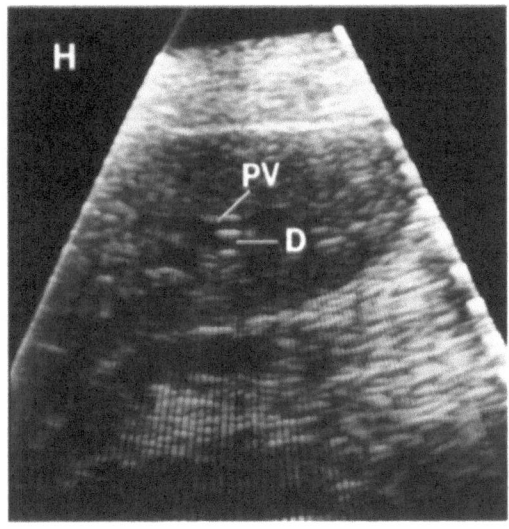

A

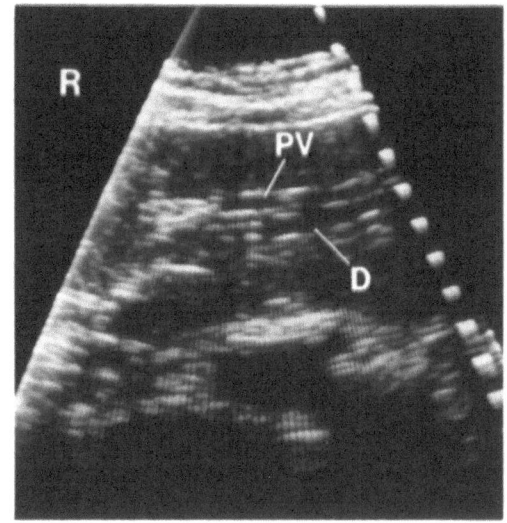

B

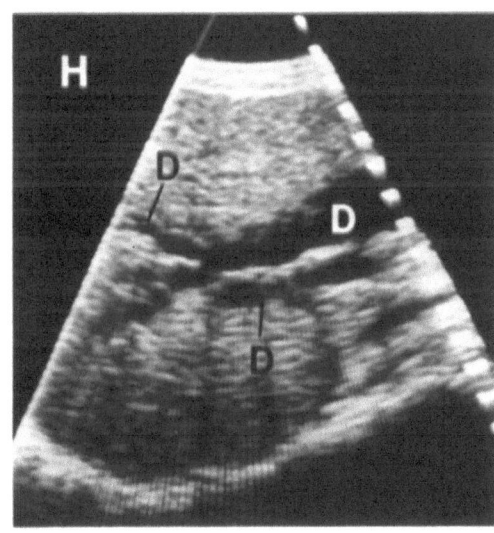

C

Fig. 6.25. Dilated intrahepatic bile ducts. **A** and **B** Dilated ducts (*D*) seen as tubular structures adjacent and parallel to portal veins (*PV*). **A** Transverse scan; left lobe. **B** Sagittal scan; right lobe. **C** Dilated ducts seen as cluster of dilated and tortuous channels in central part of liver in another patient.

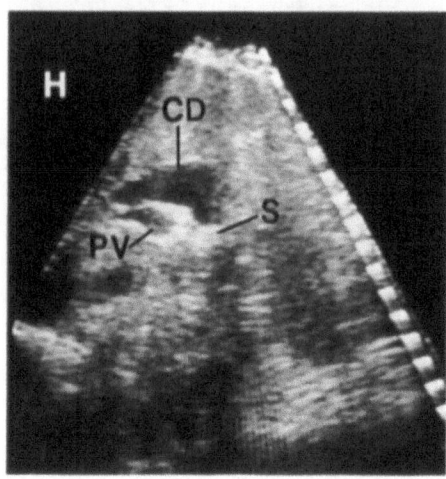

Fig. 6.26. Stones (*S*) in distal common duct (*CD*) producing ductal dilatation. *PV,* portal vein. Sagittal view.

E. Biliary Sludge

Occasionally, a layer of low amplitude echoes that cast no acousitc shadows may be seen in the dependent portion of the gall-

bladder. This reflective layer moves very slowly when the patient's position is changed suggesting that it is composed of a very viscous material. It can be seen in patients who have fasted for several days (usually acutely ill patients on intravenous fluids) or in gallbladders that are obstructed from tumor or stones (Fig. 6.29). Until recently the cause of these echoes was not clear. Some investigators (21, 22) thought they were produced by bile of abnormally high viscosity, whereas others postulated that crystalline material within the bile was the cause (23). In an excellent paper, Filly et al. (24) showed that the echoes were caused by a combination of bile pigment granules (mainly calcium bilirubinate) and cholesterol crystals. The presence of sludge according to these authors suggests a pathologic state but not necessarily biliary pathology since sludge is present in patients who are quite ill and fasting from other causes, such as pancreatitis and bowel obstruction.

F. Gallbladder Versus Localized Ascites

The visualization of a fluid-filled space between the right lobe of the liver and right kidney that is arcuate in configuration with sharply angled margins should not be confused with the gallbladder. This space represents the accumulation of a small amount of ascites. Likewise, ascites can be seen as an echo-free space inferior to the gallbladder. Ascites can be differentiated from the normal gallbladder because the margins of the ascitic collection have sharp angles where the fluid fills recesses between the liver and kidney, whereas the gallbladder has a round or oval configuration in cross section and a fusiform appearance sagittally (see Chapter 9).

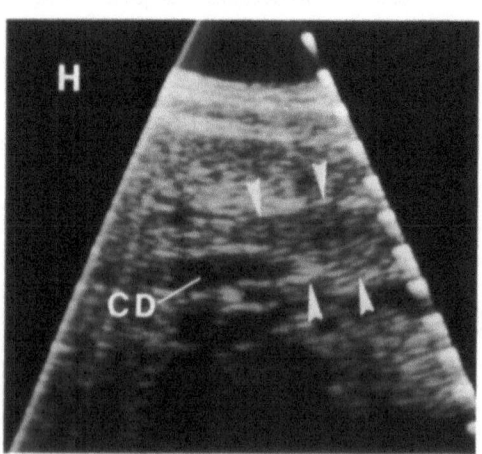

Fig. 6.27. Carcinoma (*arrowheads*) within pancreatic head obstructing and dilating common duct (*CD*).

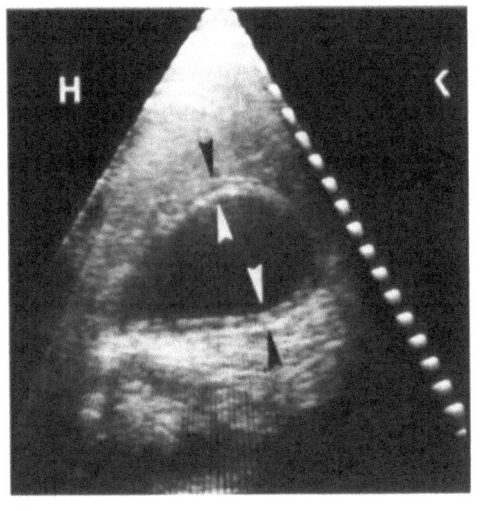

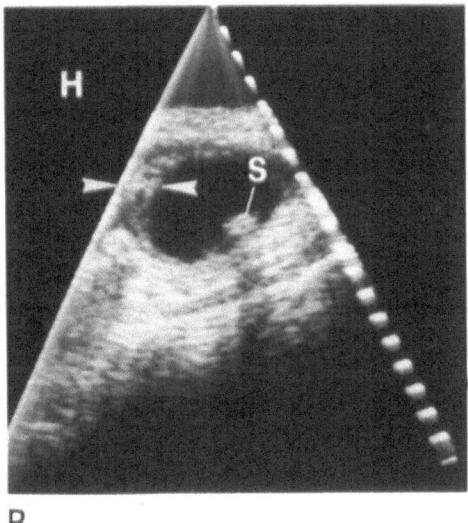

Fig. 6.28. Acute cholecystitis. Sagittal views. Gallbladder walls are thickened (*arrows*) and contain hypoechoic layer within the walls. **A** Acalculous cholecystitis; no stones identified. **B** Cholecystitis and cholelithiasis. Stones (*S*) present.

5. STATIC VERSUS REAL-TIME IMAGING OF BILIARY SYSTEM

We believe that real-time instrumentation is the preferred method for imaging the gallbladder and common bile duct and for detecting dilated intrahepatic bile ducts.

What real-time scanners lack in resolution (as compared to articulated arm contact scanners), they compensate for by their ability to continuously scan the entire volume of the organ, thereby increasing the chances of seeing small structures (gallstones and dilated ducts) that may be missed between sections of the contact scanner.

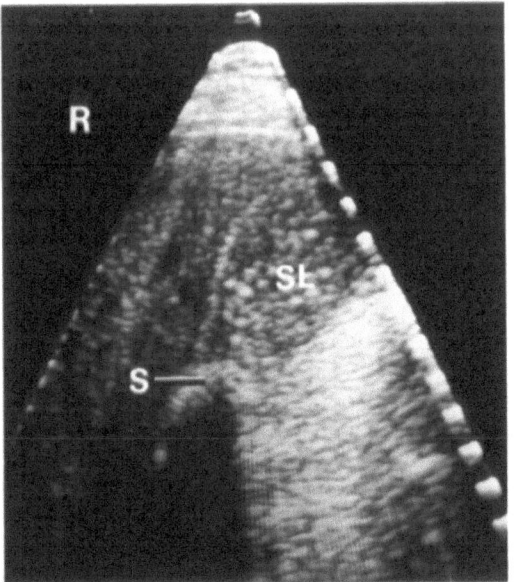

Fig. 6.29. Sludge (*SL*) in gallbladder that is obstructed by stone (*S*) impacted in neck. Sagittal view.

References

1. Cooperberg PL, Li D, Wong P, Cohen MM, Burhenne HJ (1980) Accuracy of common hepatic duct size in the evaluation of extrahepatic biliary obstruction. Radiology 135:141–144

2. Sample WF, Sarti DA, Goldstein LI, Weiner M, Kadell BM (1978) Gray-scale ultrasonography of the jaundiced patient. Radiology 128:719–725

3. Parulekar SG (1979) Ultrasound evaluation of common bile duct size. Radiology 133:703–707

4. Behan M, Kazam E (1978) Sonography of the common bile duct: value of the right anterior oblique view. Am J Roentgenol 130:701–709

5. Graham MF, Cooperberg PL, Cohen MM, Burhenne HJ (1980) The size of the normal common hepatic duct following cholecystectomy: an ultrasonographic study. Radiology 135:137–139

6. Zeman R, Tayler KJW, Burrell MI, Gold J (1980) Ultrasound demonstration of anicteric dilatation of the biliary tree. Radiology 134:689–692

7. Elyaderani MK, Skolnick ML, Weinstein BJ (1979) Ultrasonic detection and aspiration confirmation of intra-abdominal fluid collections. Surg Gynecol Obstet 149:529–430

8. McCune BR, Weeks LE, O'Brien TF, Martin JF (1977) "Pseudostone" of the gallbladder: ultrasound findings and case report. Gastroenterology 73:1149–1151

9. McIntosh DMS, Penney HF (1980) Gray-scale ultrasonography as a screening procedure in the detection of gallbladder disease. Radiology 136:725–727

10. Krook PM, Allen FH, Bush WH, Malmer G, MacLean MD (1980) Comparison of real-time cholecystosonography and oral cholecystography. Radiology 135:145–148.

11. Cooperberg PL, Pon MS, Wong P, Stoller JL, Burhenne HJ (1979) Real-time high resolution ultrasound in the detection of biliary calculi. Radiology 131:789–790

12. Crade M, Taylor KJW, Rosenfield AT, deGraaff CS, Minihan P (1978) Surgical and pathologic correlation of cholecystosonography and cholecystography. Am J Roentgenol 131:227–229

13. Filly RA, Moss AA, Way LW (1979) In vitro investigation of gallstone shadowing with ultrasound tomography. J Clin Ultrasound 7:225–262

14. Scheske GA, Cooperberg PL, Cohen MM, Burhenne HJ (1980) Floating gallstones: the role of contrast material. J Clin Ultrasound 8:227–231

15. Conrad MR, Landay MJ, Janes JO (1978) Sonographic "parallel channel" sign of biliary tree enlargement in mild to moderate obstructive jaundice. Am J Roentgenol 130:279–286

16. Laing FC, London LA, Filly RA (1978) Ultrasonographic identification of dilated intrahepatic bile ducts and their differentiation from portal venous structures. J Clin Ultrasound 6:90–94

17. Finberg HJ, Birnholz JC (1979) Ultrasound evaluation of the gallbladder wall. Radiology 133:693–698

18. Marchal GJF, Casaer M, Baert AL, Goddeeris PG, Kerremans R, Fevery J (1979) Gallbladder wall sonolucency in acute cholecystitis. Radiology 133:429–433

19. Yeh HC (1979) Ultrasonography and computed tomography of carcinoma of the gallbladder. Radiology 133:167–173

20. Yum HY, Fink AH (1980) Sonographic findings in primary carcinoma of the gallbladder. Radiology 134:693–696

21. Conrad MR, Janes JO, Dietchy J (1979) Significance of low level echoes within the gallbladder. Am J Roentgenol 132:967–972

22. Simeone JF, Mueller PR, Ferrucci JT, Harbin WP, Wittenberg (1980) Significance of nonshadowing focal opacities at cholecystosonography. Radiology 137:181–185

23. Glancy JJ, Goddard J, Pearson DE (1980) In vitro demonstration of cholesterol crystals' high echogenicity relative to protein particles. J Clin Ultrasound 8:27–29

24. Filly RA, Allen B, Minton MJ, Bernhoft R, Way LW (1980) In vitro investigation of the origin of echoes within biliary sludge. J Clin Ultrasound 8:193–200

25. Weinstein BJ, Weinstein DP (1980) Biliary tract dilatation in the nonjaundiced patient. Am J Roentgenol 134:899–906

7
Pancreas

The pancreas is one of the more difficult solid intraabdominal organs to completely delineate by ultrasound because portions of it are often obscured by overlying gas-filled stomach or colon. Thus, a variety of scanning windows and several different patient positions may be needed to completely visualize this organ.

1. ANATOMY

The pancreas, shaped like the letter "J" lying on its side, is located in the upper central retroperitoneal region, and is sandwiched between the anteriorly located intraperitoneal organs of the upper abdomen—the liver, stomach, spleen, and possibly colon—and the posteriorly located major retroperitoneal vessels and left kidney (1, 2) (Figs. 7.1–7.5). To the right of the pancreas lies the second portion of the duodenum. The extent to which the liver, stomach, or transverse colon lies anterior to the pancreas depends upon the patient's body habitus and phase of respiration at the time of scanning.

There is considerable variation in the total length of the pancreas, the exact plane of its long axis, and its thickness. It is composed of three major regions: the head, body, and tail. The head, which forms the short and vertical limb of the "J," lies to the right side of the vertebral column and contains a medial extension—the uncinate process—while the body and tail form the long and transversely oriented part of the "J." The body lies in front of the vertebral column and follows its arcuate configuration. After descending along the left side of the vertebrae, the body continues as the tail which crosses between the stomach and upper pole of the left kidney, and extends for a variable distance toward the spleen.

There are several criteria for defining a normal pancreas: (1) measurements of the thickness of the head, body, and tail; (2) the shape of the gland; and (3) the level of echoes reflected by the pancreatic parenchyma.

There is no precise agreement in the literature as to what constitutes the upper limits of normal pancreatic size. Rather, dimensions as measured in the transverse plane range from 2.5 to 3.5 cm for the head, 1.75 to 2.5 cm for the body, and 1.5 to 3.5 cm for the tail (2, 3, 4, 5, 6, 7). de Graaff et al. (5) believe that more accurate measurements of pancreatic dimensions can be obtained in

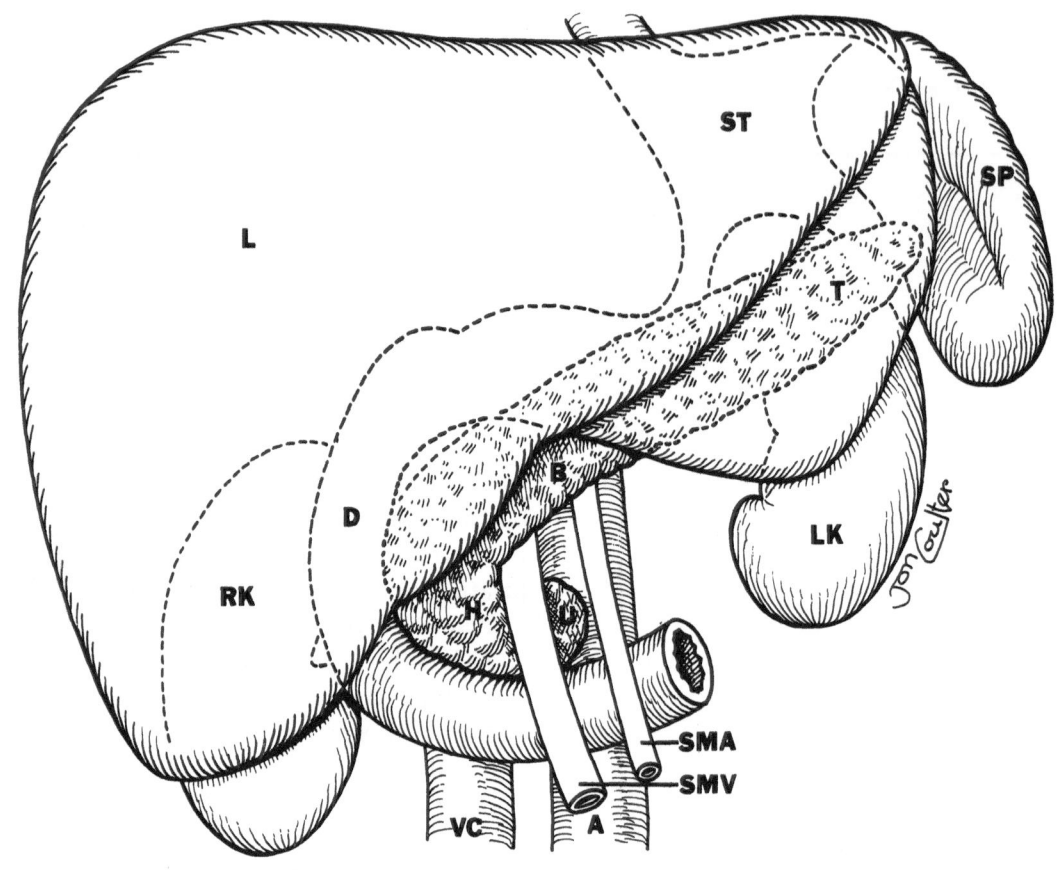

Fig. 7.1. Relationships of pancreas to adjacent upper abdominal structures. *L,* liver; *D,* duodenum; *RK,* right kidney; *LK,* left kidney; *H,* head, pancreas; *B,* body, pancreas; *T,* tail, pancreas; *U,* uncinate process, pancreas; *ST,* stomach; *SP,* spleen; *VC,* vena cava; *A,* aorta; *SMA,* superior mesenteric artery; *SMV,* superior mesenteric vein.

the sagittal views because one cannot be sure that the thickest part of each region of the pancreas was imaged in the transverse plane.

Instead, greater emphasis is being placed on overall shape of the gland as a criterion for normality rather than on absolute dimensions (2, 3). The normal contours should show a gradual tapering in the size or smooth transition from one region to the other, with the width of the head being the largest. Any localized widening or bulging should be suspected of being a pathologic mass even if its dimensions are within normal limits for that region of the pancreas, especially if it also contains echoes of lower intensity than the remainder of the pancreas.

The echo levels of the normal pancreas are equal to or greater than those of the normal liver (8), and the pattern is usually coarser than that of the liver as well (Fig. 7.4B).

It is important to emphasize that the head may extend vertically for several centimeters below the level of the body and tail so one should appreciate that the transverse plane which shows the body and tail well may really include little or no portion of the head. In order to fully image the head, additional scans may be required for several centimeters below the level that best shows the body and tail region (Fig. 7.4E).

When bowel overlies pancreas, the ability

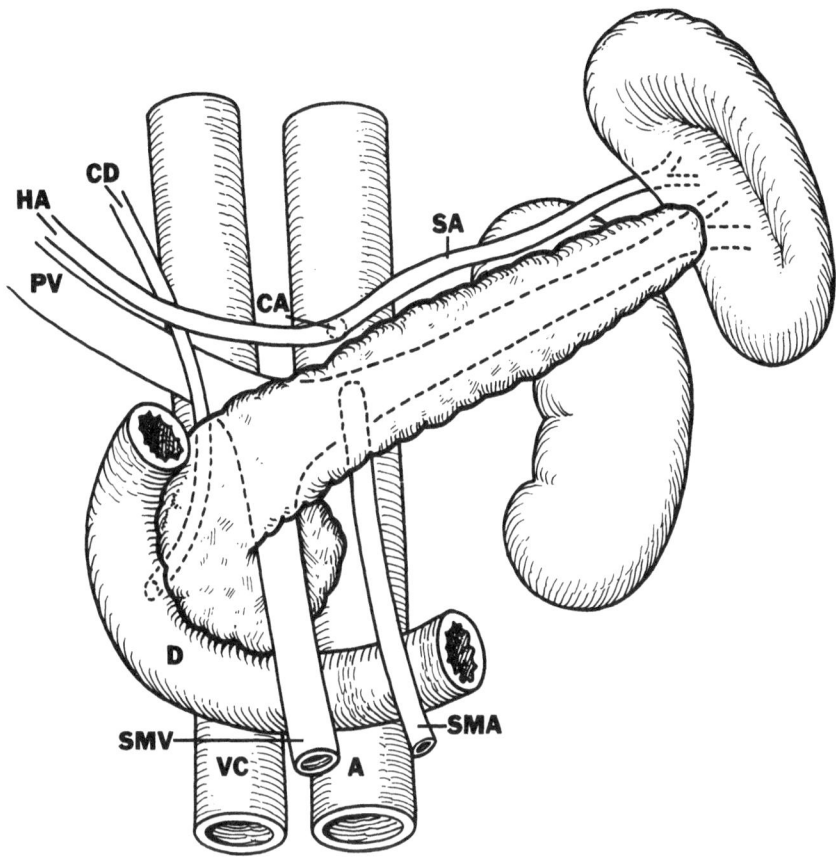

Fig. 7.2. Relationships of pancreas to adjacent vessels. *D*, duodenum; *CD*, common duct; *PV*, portal vein; *HA*, hepatic artery; *A*, aorta; *CA*, celiac axis; *SA*, splenic artery; *SMA*, superior mesenteric artery *SMV*, superior mesenteric vein; *VC*, vena cava.

of ultrasound to visualize the pancreas in the supine position depends upon whether the bowel contains intraluminal gas. Those regions of the pancreas posterior to gas-filled stomach or colon or immediately adjacent to gas-filled duodenum (Fig. 7.6) cannot be adequately seen. The tail is the region most frequently obscured because of gas in the gastric fundus and body.

There are several vascular landmarks adjacent to the pancreas that help identify the gland (Figs. 7.2–7.5). The most consistent of these and the most prominent is the splenic vein which courses along the posterior surface of the body and tail of the pancreas (Figs. 7.2, 7.3B, and 7.4B). At the junction of the head and body (the neck region), the splenic vein joins with the su-

perior mesenteric vein (SMV) to form the portal vein which then continues into the liver (Fig. 7.4A). Posterior to the head of the pancreas lies the inferior vena cava (IVC) (Fig. 7.2). The superior mesenteric artery (SMA) and SMV, which run perpendicular to the long axis of the pancreas, lie inferior to the splenic vein and just anterior to the aorta and vena cava. The SMA is either directly anterior to the aorta or slightly to the left, while the SMV is to the right of the SMA. Thus, at the level of the pancreas, the SMA and SMV lie posterior to the gland. However, the uncinate process of the pancreas, a medial extension of the pancreatic head, lies adjacent to or even extends posterior to the SMA and SMV (Figs. 7.2 and 7.4B and E). Inferior to the pancreas the

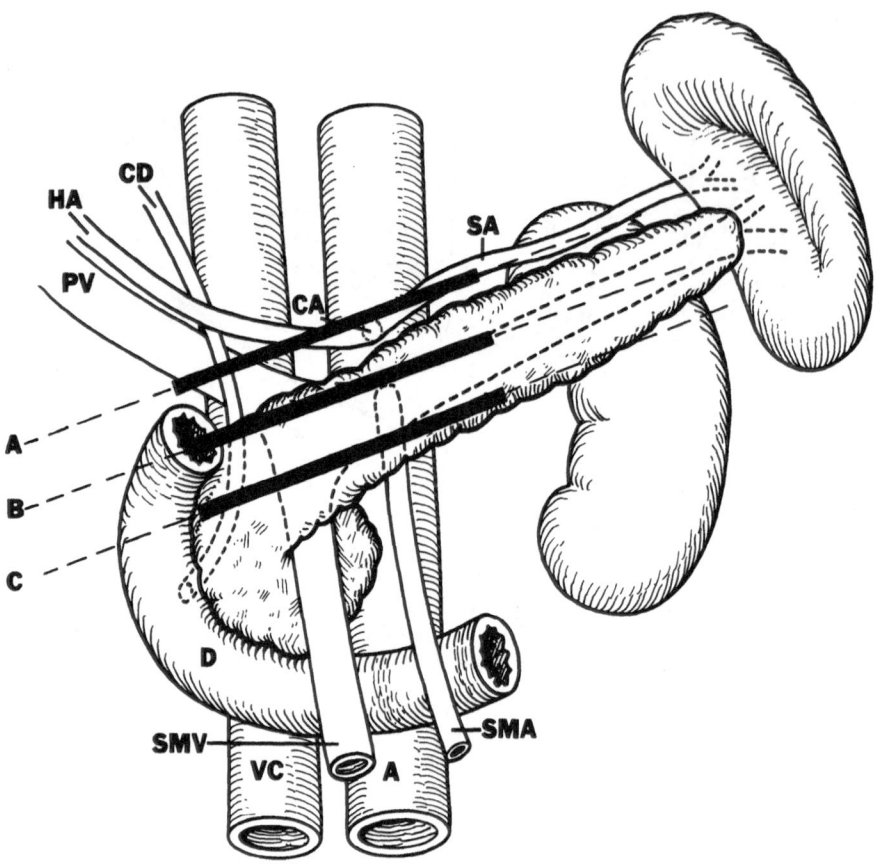

Fig. 7.3. Normal peripancreatic vasculature as displayed serially in diagonally oriented scans and related to anatomic sketch in Fig. 7.2. Plane of each scan identified by dashed line. Solid central portion of dashed line defines extent of ultrasound image. **A** Through celiac axis (*C*). Hepatic (*HA*) and splenic (*SA*) arteries. **B** Through upper edge of pancreatic body (*B*). Splenic vein (*SV*) and origin of superior mesenteric artery (*SMA*). **C** Through head (*H*) and body (*B*) of pancreas. Superior mesenteric artery (*SMA*), superior mesenteric vein (*SMV*), left renal vein (*LRV*). *A*, aorta; *VC*, vena cava; *L*, liver.

SMA and SMV course anteriorly to lie above the transverse portion of the duodenum (Fig. 7.2). In transverse section the SMA and SMV appear as two circles with the thicker-walled artery lying to the left of the vein (Fig. 7.4E).

The celiac axis, another constant vascular landmark, takes origin from the aorta within a centimeter above the SMA. The main trunk of the celiac axis runs anteriorly and is just superior to the pancreas. The axis then splits into splenic and hepatic branches which run along or adjacent to the superior surface of the pancreas. They are best seen

in the region of the body and proximal tail (Figs. 7.2, 7.3A, and 7.5A).

The common bile duct maintains an intimate relationship with the pancreatic head. It crosses anterior to the portal vein and then runs through the posterior portion of the pancreatic head and into the second part of the duodenum that lies just lateral to the pancreatic head (Fig. 7.2). On transverse views of the pancreas, the common duct can be seen in cross section as a circular structure lying in the posterior portion of the head (Fig. 7.4D). In the right parasagittal view, the duct is seen in its long axis anterior to

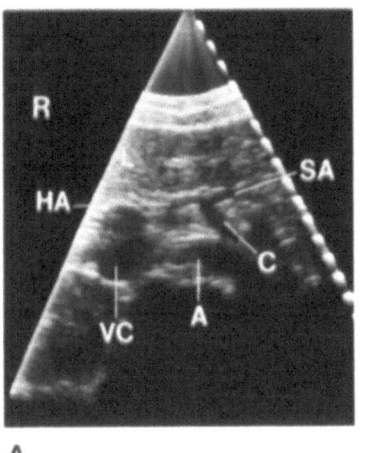 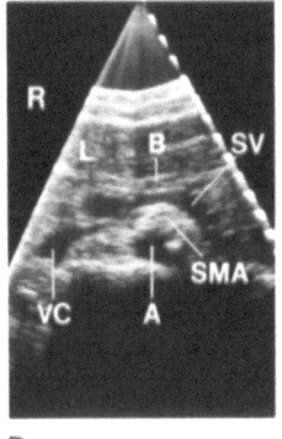 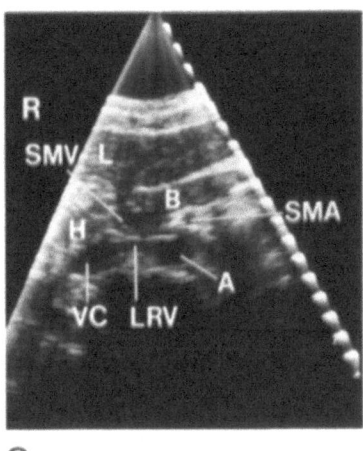

A   B   C

Fig. 7.3. (cont.)

the portal vein (Fig. 7.5D). (See Chapter 6 for further discussion of the common duct.)

Another normal ductal structure that can sometimes be seen is the pancreatic duct. It is best visualized in transverse scans where the pancreatic body crosses the vertebral column. In order to definitely identify this duct, one must demonstrate the splenic vein as well in the same section so as to differentiate the duct from the vein. The normal duct is seen either as a single highly reflective line running through the central portion of the body of the pancreas (9, 10) or as two parallel lines with an echo-free space in between having an intraluminal diameter less than 2 mm (Fig. 7.7) (10, 11). Diameters greater than 2 mm are considered dilated, although specific types of pathology cannot be related to a specific size of the duct (9, 12).

2. IMAGING TECHNIQUES

The major limitation to pancreatic imaging is the presence of overlying gas-filled bowel. This limitation can be overcome by finding ultrasonic windows free of intervening bowel, by applying pressure to collapse or displace bowel, by changing patient position or phase of respiration to displace bowel away from the pancreas, or by instilling fluids within the bowel to change a gas-filled structure to a fluid-filled ultrasonic window.

A. Supine Position

Our approach to pancreatic imaging begins with the patient supine. Since the long axis of the pancreas has a "J" or arcuate shape, the entire gland may not lie in one plane. Several changes in the transducer position may be necessary to view the entire gland. The head may represent one segment, the body and proximal tail a second, and the distal tail a third. Even if the entire long axis of the pancreas were in one plane, the small fields of view of some real-time scanners may preclude imaging the entire pancreas on one scan.

After the pancreas is identified in the transverse plane, a series of sagittal views is obtained starting with a midsagittal plane. The transducer is then moved to the right of the midline to examine the head (Fig. 7.5A–C) and an attempt is made to identify the common bile duct as it traverses through the head (Fig. 7.5D). Next, the transducer is moved to the left of the midline to obtain a series of cross sections through the body and tail. The splenic vein should be seen in cross

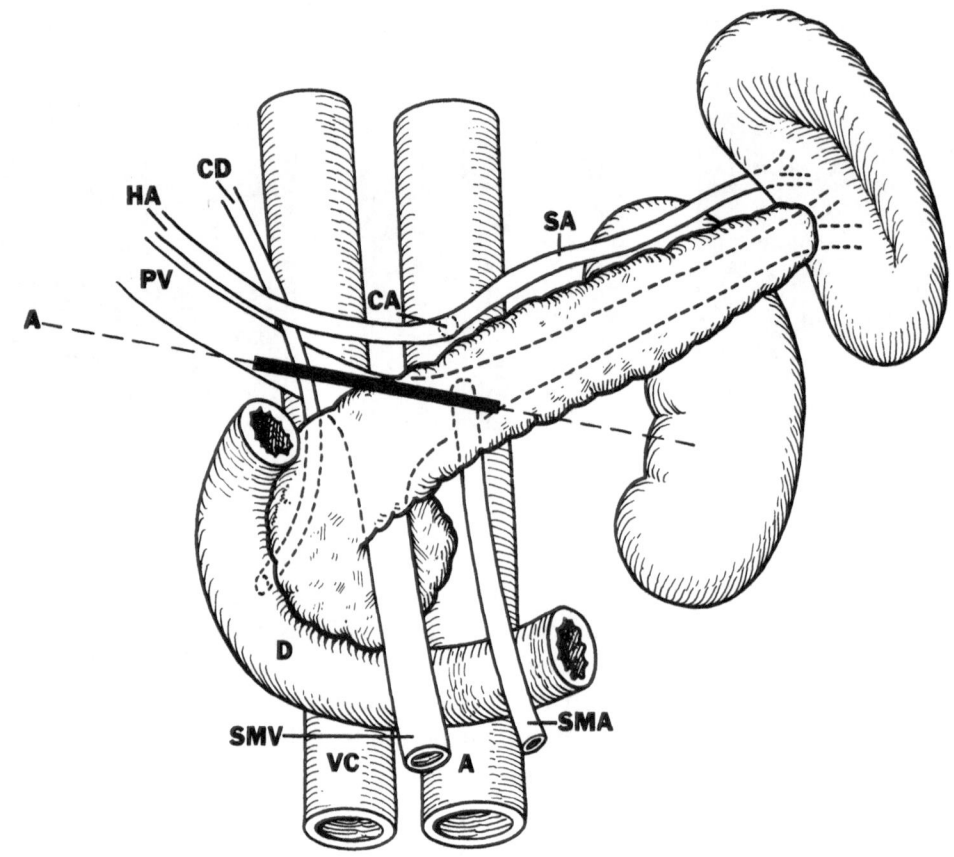

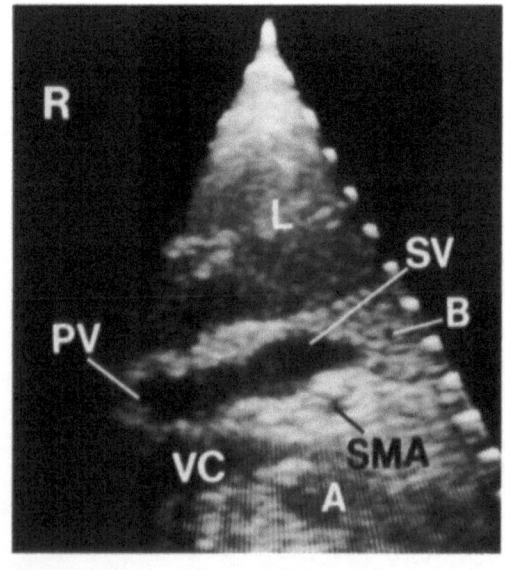

A

Fig. 7.4. A.

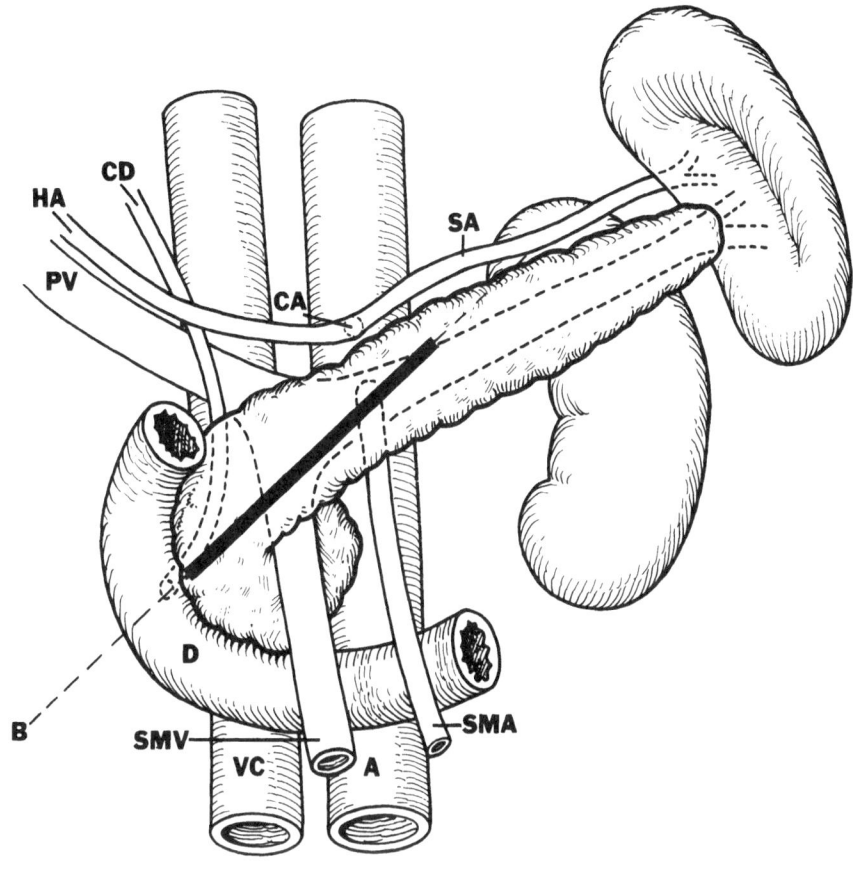

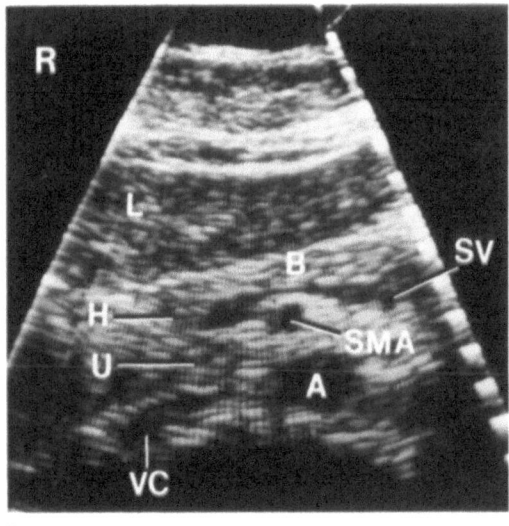

B

Fig. 7.4. B.

Fig. 7.4. Transducer rotated around transverse plane into different diagonal planes so as to optimally display specific portions of pancreas and peripancreatic structures. Scan planes are related to anatomic sketch in the same manner as in Fig. 7.3. Key is the same as for Figs. 7.1–7.3. **A** Portal vein and its junction with splendic vein. **B** Head and body of pancreas. **C** Body and tail of pancreas. **D** Common duct within pancreatic head. **E** Uncinate process wrapped around superior mesenteric vein. (Figure continued on pages 146, 147, 148.)

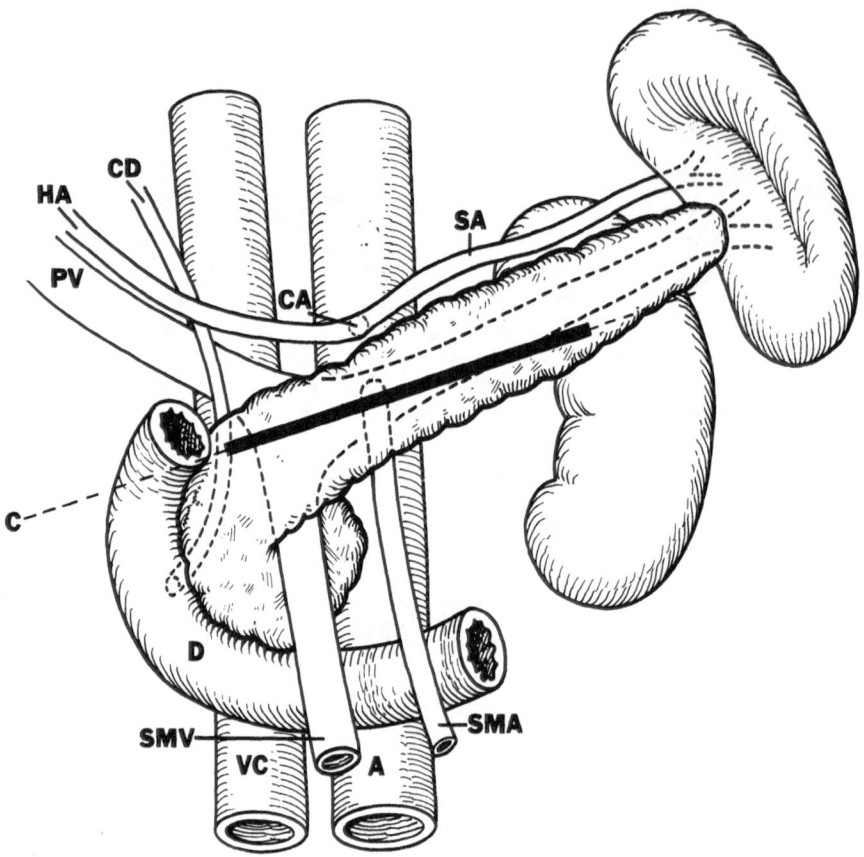

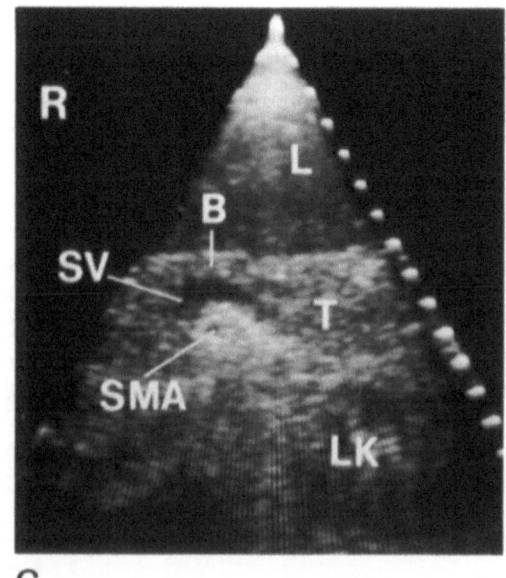

Fig. 7.4. C.

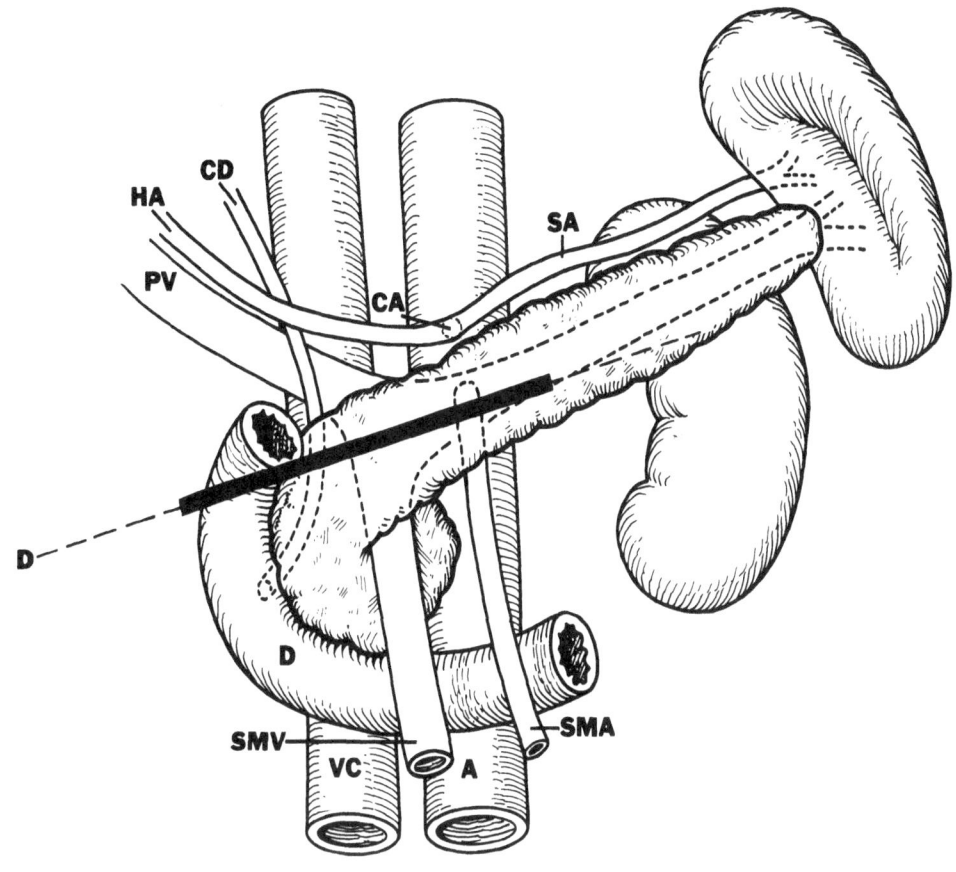

Fig. 7.4. (See legend on page 145. 7.4. E on page 148.)

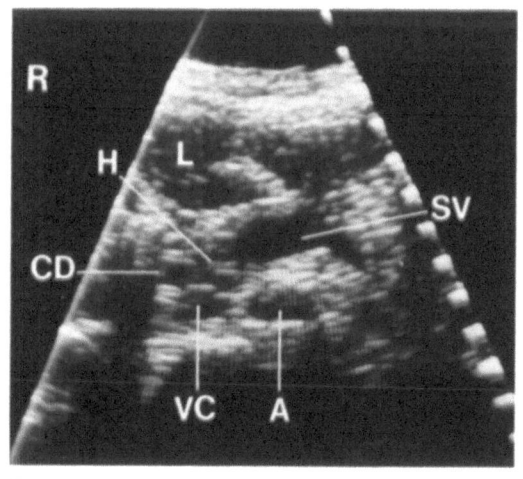

Fig. 7.4. D.

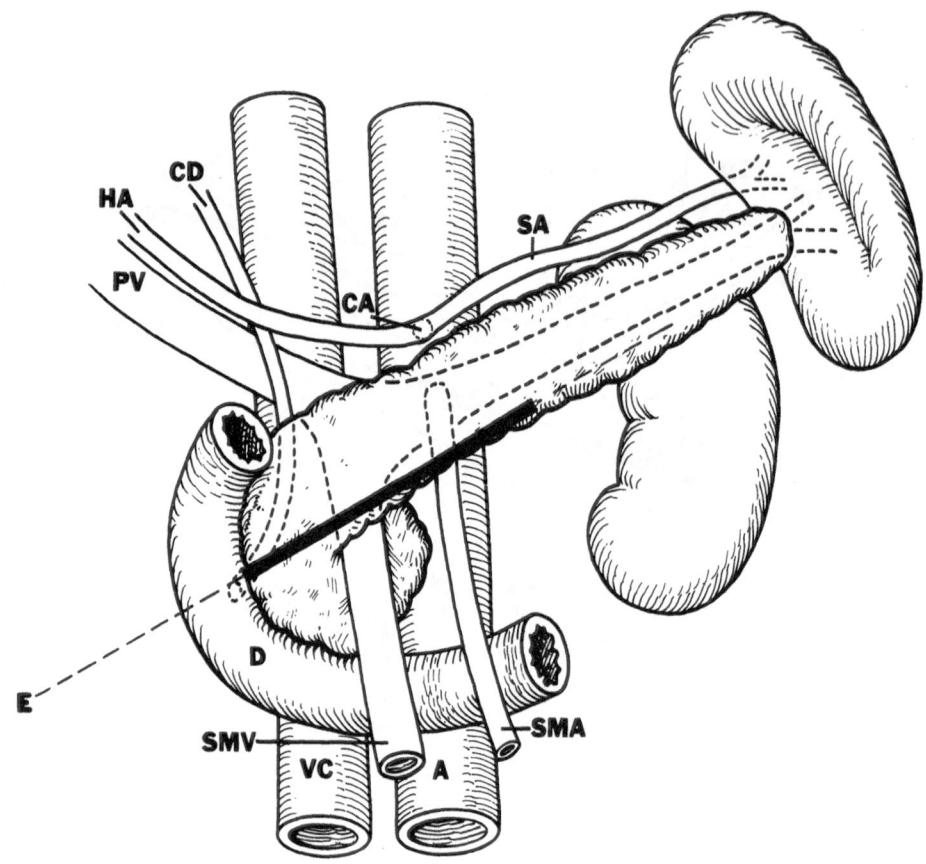

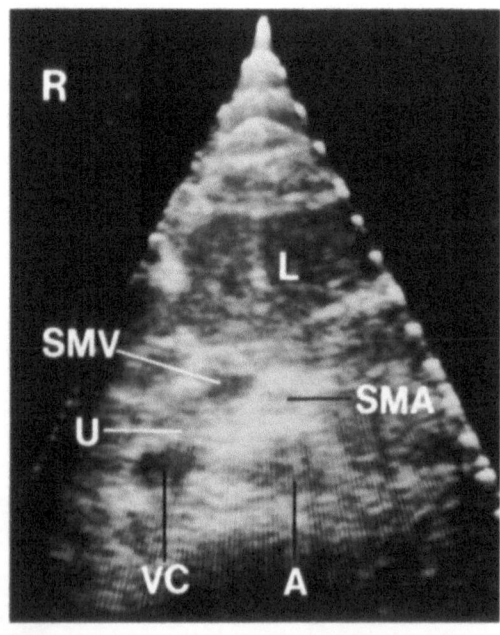

E

Fig. 7.4. E. (See legend on page 145.)

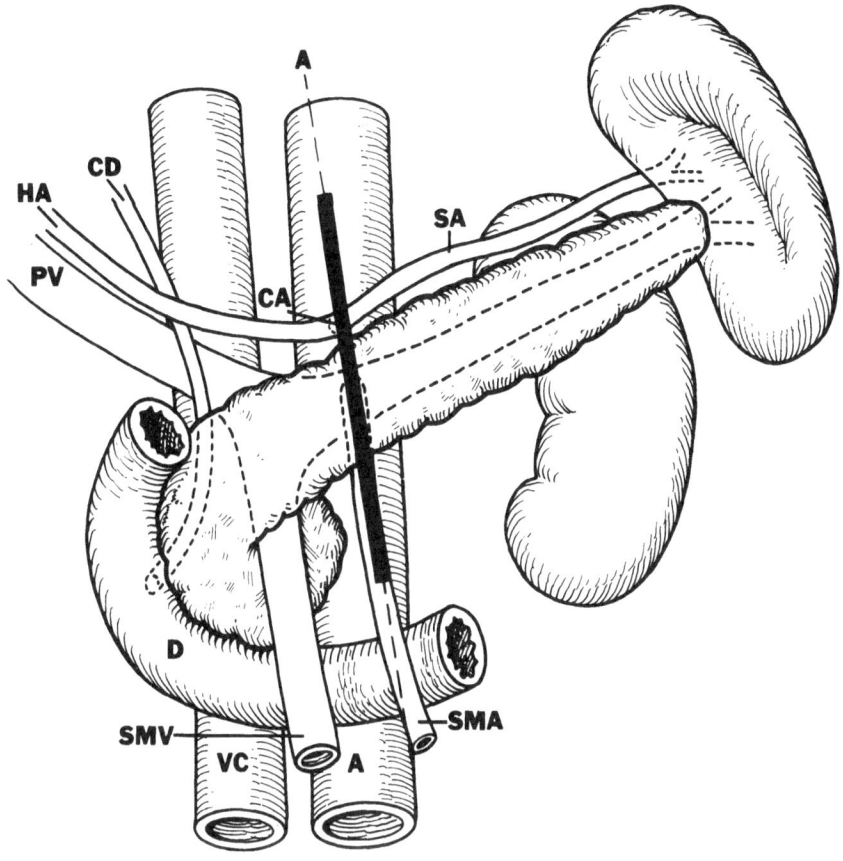

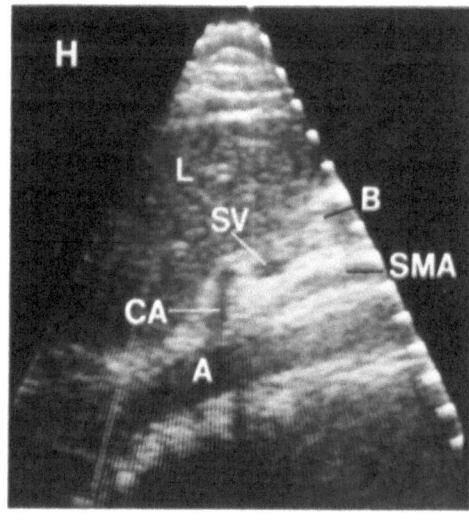

A

Fig. 7.5. A.

Fig. 7.5. Serial parasagittal scans relating pancreas and peripancreatic structures to anatomic sketch. Method of relating scans to sketch is the same as for Figs. 7.3 and 7.4. Key is the same as for Figs. 7.1–7.3. **A** Midsagittal plane through aorta and celiac axis, superior mesenteric artery, and pancreatic body. **B** Right parasagittal plane through uncinate process of pancreas and third portion of duodenum. **C** Plane through pancreatic head. **D** Plane through common duct traversing into pancreatic head. **E** Left parasagittal scan through tail of pancreas. (Figure continued on pages 151, 152, 153.)

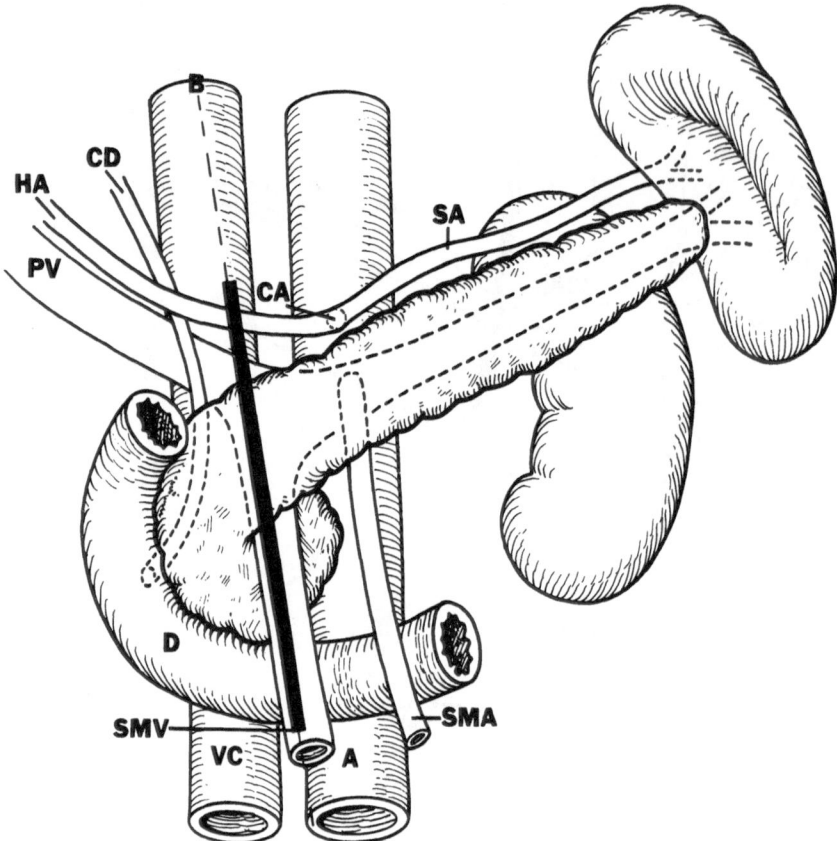

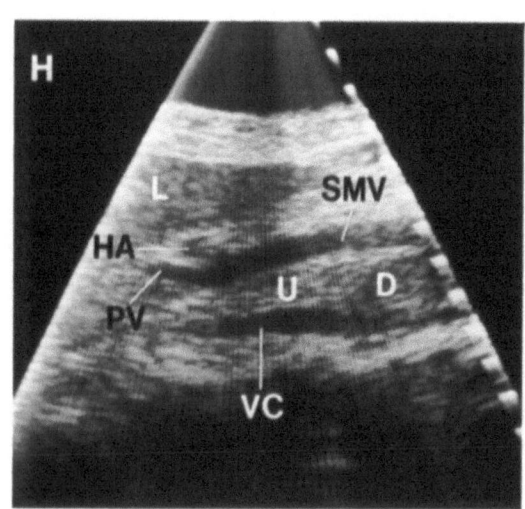

B

Fig. 7.5. B.

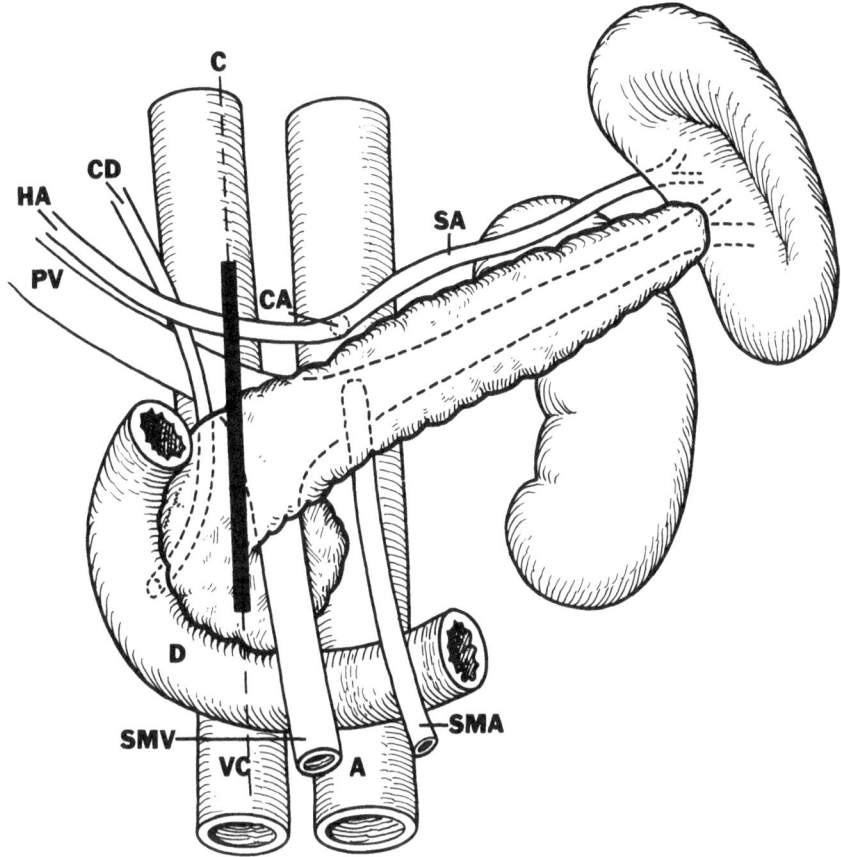

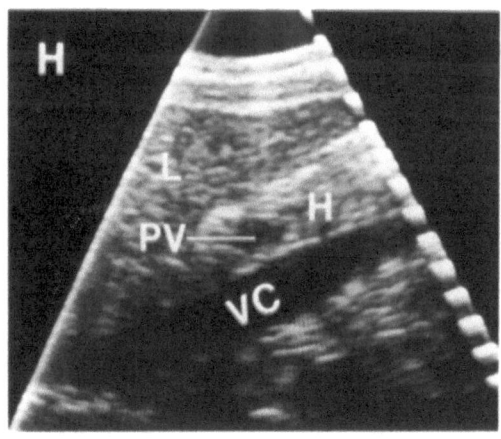

C

Fig. 7.5. C.

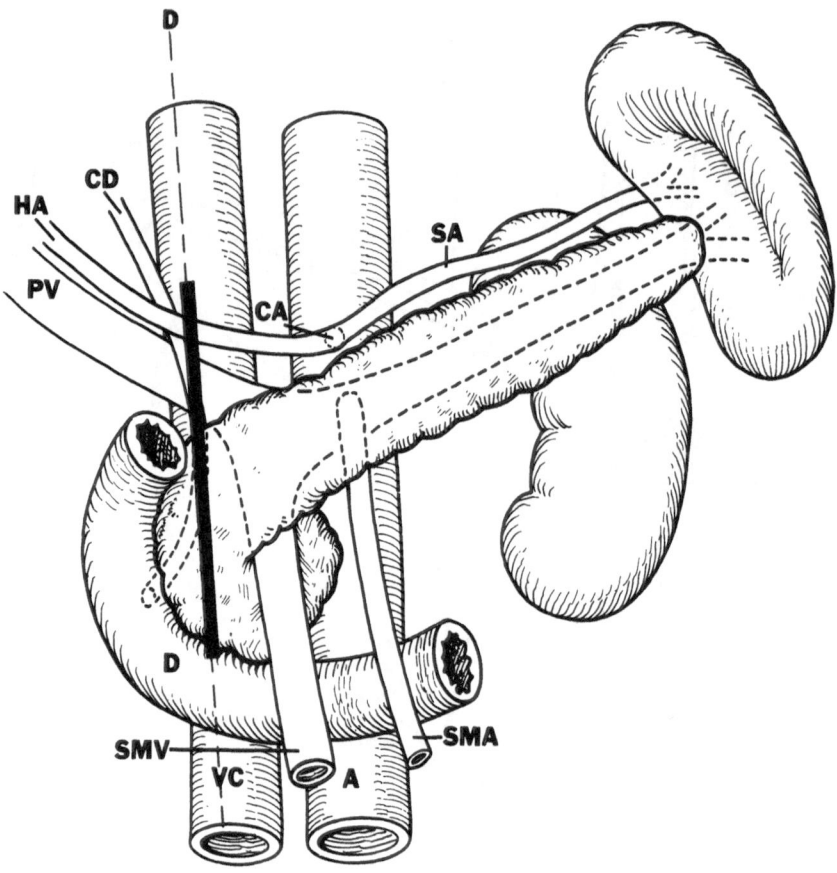

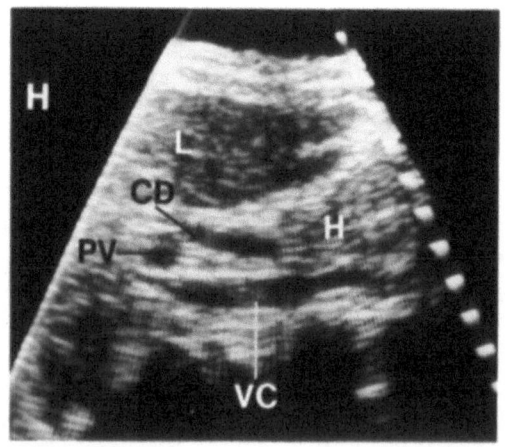

D

Fig. 7.5. D.

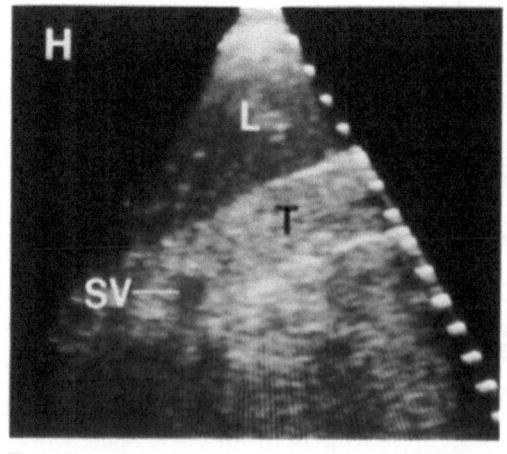

E

Fig. 7.5. E.

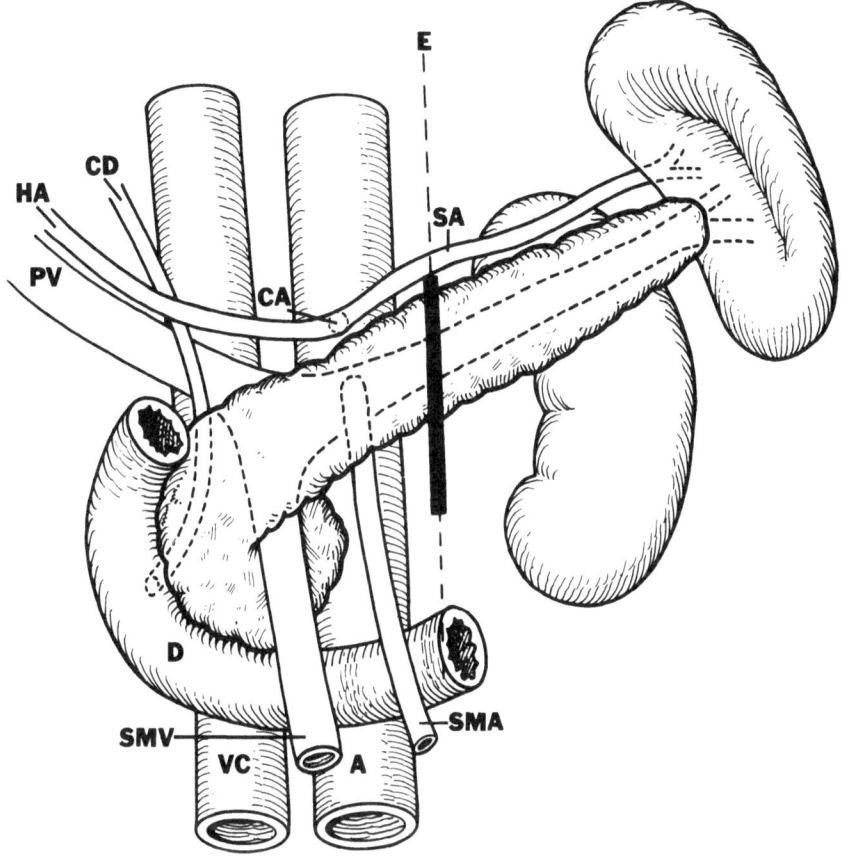

Fig. 7.5. (See legend on page 150.)

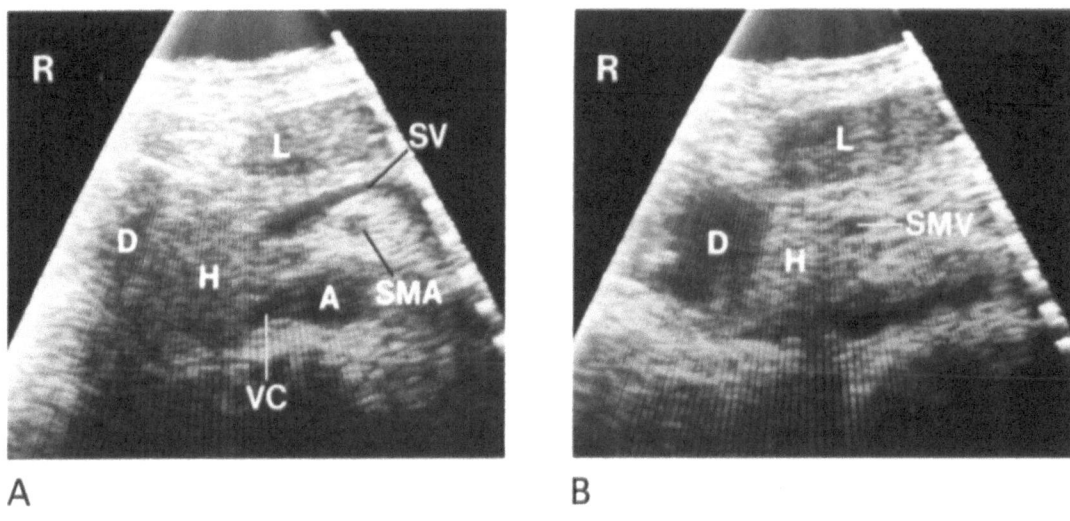

Fig. 7.6. Effect of duodenal contents upon the quality of the image of the pancreatic head in transverse plane. Key is the same as in Figs. 7.1–7.3. **A** Gas in duodenum (*D*) obscures the lateral margin of the pancreatic head (*H*) and accurate size of head cannot be determined. **B** Fluid in duodenum. Lateral margin of pancreatic head is visible. Head appears of normal size.

section behind the pancreas to accurately identify this part of the gland (Fig. 7.5E).

B. Respiratory Maneuvers

In order to improve visualization of the pancreas in the supine position (if portions of it are obscured by overlying gas-filled bowel) repeat scanning should be attempted in deep inspiration in the hope that the liver will descend over the pancreas. Sometimes deep inspiration may make pancreatic imaging more difficult than quiet breathing because the patient may actually move the liver superiorly with deep inspiration (because of expansion of the rib cage) (Fig. 5.3A). If this occurs, the patient should then be instructed to push out his upper abdomen by contracting the diaphragm to force the liver inferiorly ("belly out" maneuver; Fig. 5.3B). If neither of these maneuvers proves completely successful, the patient can be examined in the erect position. Now gravity may help to cause the liver to descend over the pancreas and the stomach contents to shift.

Gas which was previously lying in the antrum and obscuring the pancreas with the patient supine will rise to the cardia with the patient erect and be replaced by fluid that previously was in the cardia.

C. Prone Position

These respiratory and positional maneuvers are best for examining the head, body, and proximal tail region. When the stomach is filled with a considerable amount of gas, the distal tail region can usually not be seen from the anterior abdominal approach whether the patient is erect or supine. Then one may have to resort to using the left kidney as a window for viewing the tail of the pancreas. The patient can be prone (13) or erect. The tail of the pancreas is seen deep to the left kidney. Transverse scans show the long axis of the pancreas and parasagittal scans image the tail in cross section (Fig. 7.8). Sometimes the tail of the pancreas can be seen if the patient is scanned transversely in the decubitus position, left side up, be-

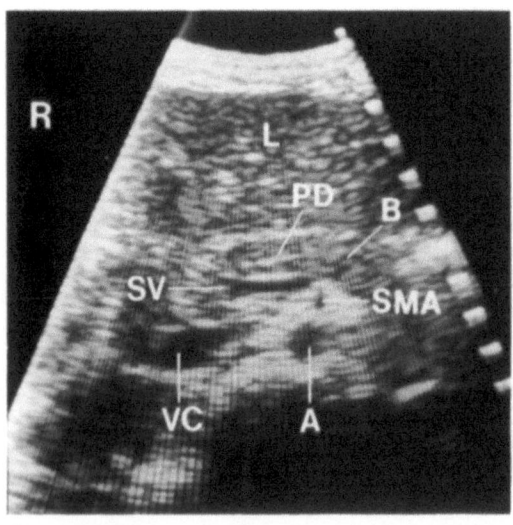

A

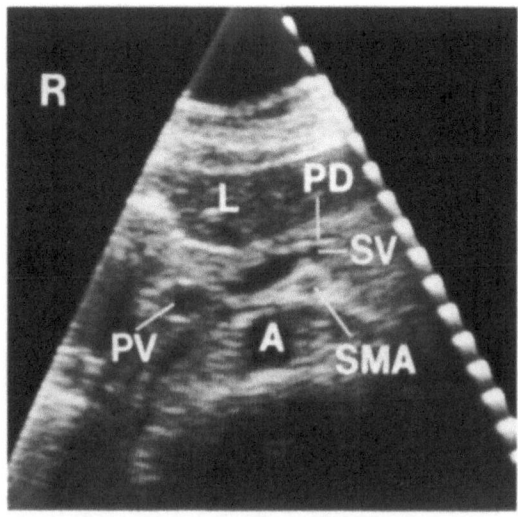

B

Fig. 7.7. Normal pancreatic ducts (*PD*); transverse planes. Key is the same as in Figs. 7.1–7.3. **A** Single line; presumably collapsed duct. **B** Double line; duct less than 2 mm in diameter.

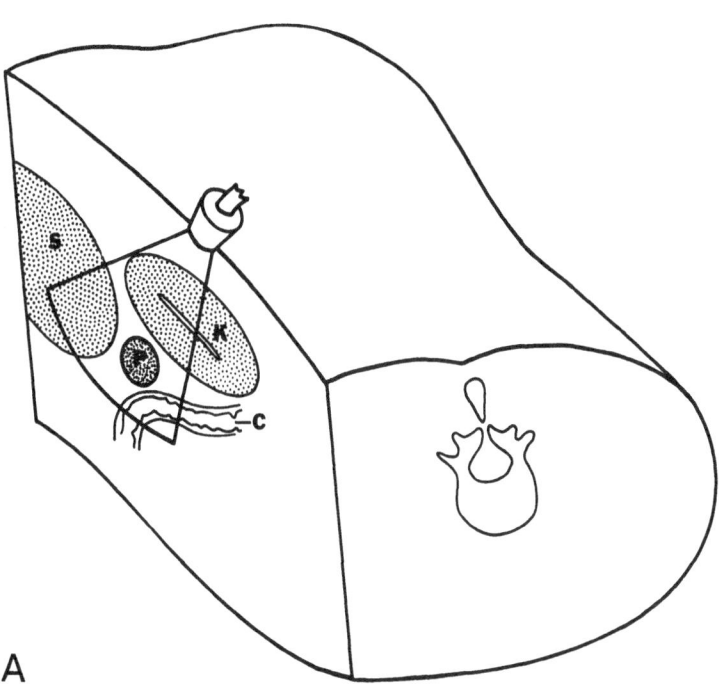

A

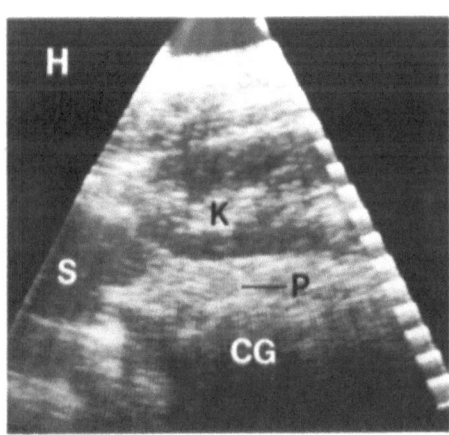

B

Fig. 7.8. Imaging of pancreatic tail using left kidney as window. Patient is prone or erect and plane is parasagittal. Pancreatic tail is anterior to upper pole of kidney. Fluid when present in adjacent colon may be confused with a pancreatic pseudocyst unless patient is examined in both prone and erect positions. Appearance of pseudocyst remains constant in both positions, but colonic fluid is replaced with gas in erect position. **A** Sketch; prone position. **B** Trapezoid scan; prone position. *K,* kidney; *P,* pancreas; *S,* spleen; *C,* colon; *CG,* gas-filled colon.

cause the spleen moves medially and displaces overlying gas-filled bowel.

D. Eliminating Gas in Overlying Bowel

Gas in bowel overlying the pancreas, especially overlying the head and body, may be minimized or eliminated by increasing pressure on the anterior abdomen in order to compress the bowel and thereby express the gas. This pressure can be effectively applied by pressing more firmly with the transducer against the skin. However, do not press to the point of producing patient discomfort. Pain can produce anxiety and increase the amount of air that the patient may swallow, thereby defeating the purpose of the above maneuver.

If the pancreas is still obscured despite the various maneuvers to displace gas-filled bowel overlying it, one can then resort to maneuvers that will replace the intraluminal gas with intraluminal fluid. A simple ma-

neuver is to fill the stomach with a large amount of fluid so as to both eliminate the gas and enlarge the size of the fluid-filled acoustic window overlying the pancreas. Although water may be the easiest fluid to obtain, it is not preferred because the acoustic absorption of water is much less than that of the adjacent liver and spleen. Therefore, a region of the pancreas over which the fluid-filled stomach lies will have a greater intensity of ultrasound reaching it than regions overlaid with liver. Thus, the intensity of echoes reflected by the portions of the pancreas deep to the liver will be weaker than that reflected by the gland lying deep to the stomach and one may have to frequently change time-gain compensation settings to correct for the difference in sound attenuation by liver and water-filled stomach. Therefore, a more appropriate fluid would be one that attenuates sound to a greater degree than water. Kossoff and his associates (14) recommend a mixture consisting of a 1% solution of methylcellulose with a flavor-

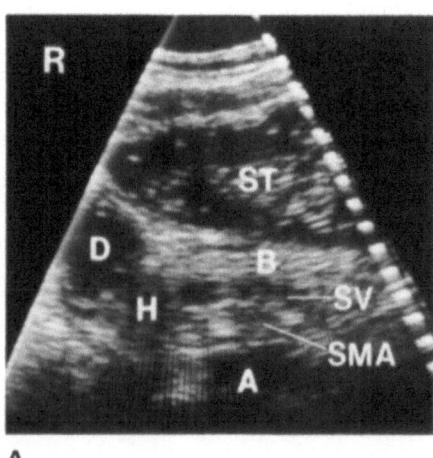

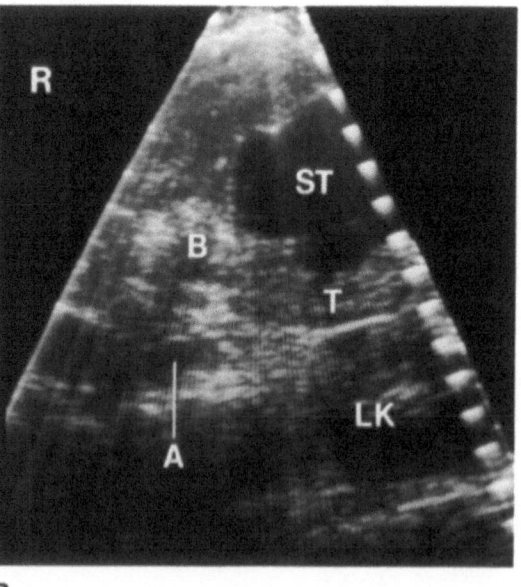

Fig. 7.9. Use of fluid-filled stomach to improve pancreatic visualization. Patient is erect. **A** Transverse scan through head and body. **B** Transverse scan through body and tail. *ST*, stomach; *D*, duodenum; *H*, pancreatic head; *B*, pancreatic body; *T*, pancreatic tail; *SV*, splenic vein; *LK*, left kidney; *A*, aorta.

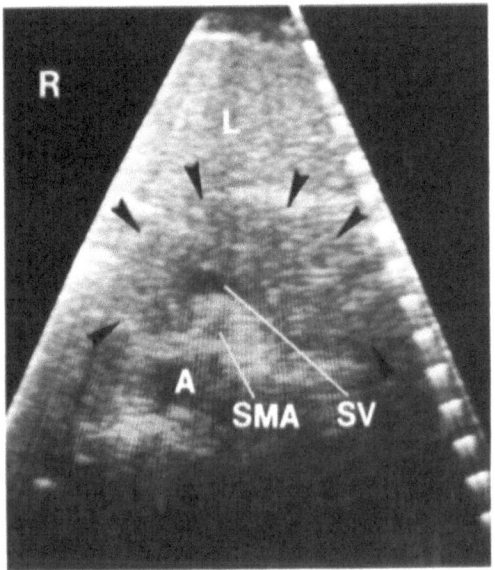

Fig. 7.10. Acute pancreatitis. Pancreas (*arrowheads*) is diffusely enlarged and contains lower level echoes than liver (*L*). Transverse scan. *SV,* splenic vein; *A,* aorta; *SMA,* superior mesenteric artery.

ing agent such as orange or strawberry syrup to mask the taste of methylcellulose. The

patient is encouraged to drink about four to six cups of this fluid which should be given cold to be most palatable. Other recommendations are tomato juice, orange juice, and milk in similar quantities. The disadvantage of milk is that it produces contraction of the gallbladder, and one may want to examine the gallbladder when the pancreas is being studied. Our experience has been mainly limited to tomato and orange juices since they are easy to obtain, have good patient acceptance, and require no preparation.

The patient can be examined in a supine or in a right or left posterior oblique position (15) but preferably should be in the erect position (16, 17) when the fluid-filled stomach is used, since it is almost impossible to completely fill the stomach with fluid and eliminate all the air. In the horizontal (supine or oblique) position a bubble might persist despite the large quantity of fluid below the bubble and defeat the attempt to visualize the tail (Fig. 3.14A). We have found that this maneuver is quite useful especially when the gas-filled stomach obscures the tail (Fig. 7.9) or when the gas-filled duo-

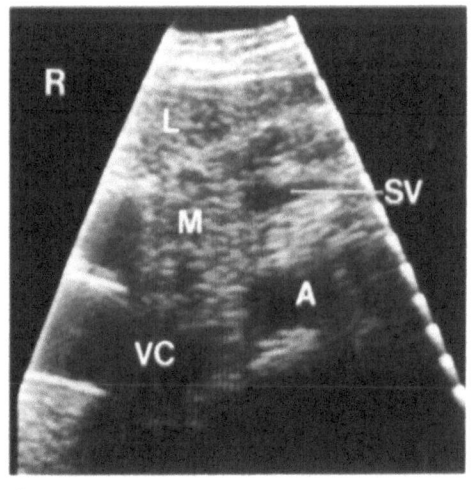

A

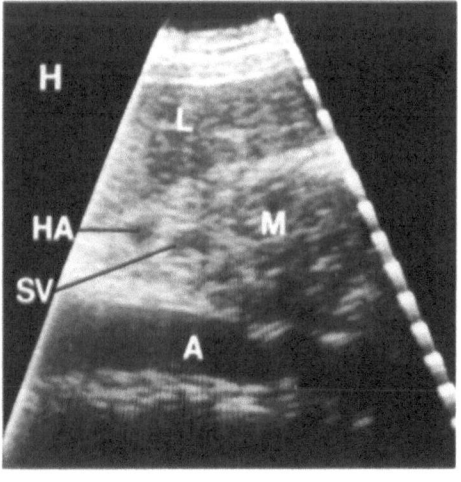

B

Fig. 7.11. Chronic pancreatitis. Focal inflammatory mass in head of pancreas indistinguishable from carcinoma on ultarsound scans. **A** Tranverse scan. **B** Right parasagittal scan. *M,* mass; *L,* liver; *SV,* splenic vein; *A,* aorta; *VC,* vena cava; *HA,* hepatic artery.

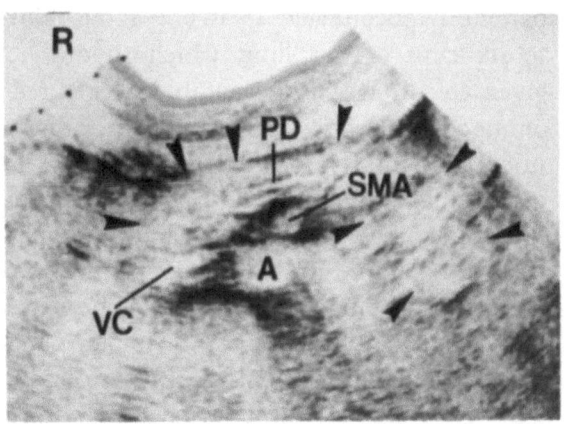
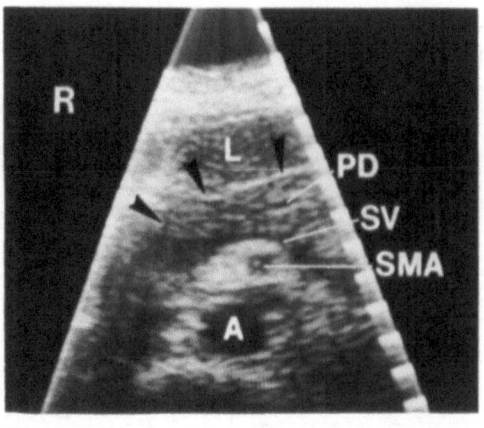

Fig. 7.12. Slightly dilated pancreatic duct (*PD*) in patient with pancreatitis. Comparison between contact scanner (**A**) and trapezoid scanner (**B**) images in the transverse plane. Pancreas is not enlarged and echo levels are not reduced below that of liver. *L,* liver; *SV,* splenic vein; *SMA,* superior mesenteric artery; *arrows,* pancreas; *A,* aorta; *VC,* vena cava.

denum obscures the lateral margin of the pancreatic head (Fig. 7.6).

3. PANCREATIC DISEASE

Pancreatic disease falls basically into two categories: diffuse disease and focal disease. The former is produced by inflammatory processes and the latter by cystic or solid masses.

A. Pancreatitis

Ultrasonically detectable diffuse pancreatic disease occurs in acute pancreatitis when the pancreas becomes edematous. When the gland swells, the normal slightly cobble-stoned surface is stretched out and becomes smoother. Thus, the capsule of the gland becomes more distinct and easier to identify. The intrapancreatic echoes become reduced

because of the greater accumulation of fluid within, and the gland uniformly increases in size (Fig. 7.10) (2). There may also be dilatation of the pancreatic duct (9). Ultrasonic signs of pancreatitis may persist for days or weeks (18), while the serum amylase may remain elevated for only one or two days (19). Thus, if there is a several-day lag between the onset of symptoms and the ultrasound study, the ultrasound may be effective in making the diagnosis in spite of a normal level of amylase.

Chronic pancreatitis is a more difficult diagnosis to make by ultrasound than acute pancreatitis. The gland may be of normal size, or smaller or larger than normal. The intensity of the pancreatic echoes within the entire gland may be greater than that of the normal pancreas, especially in an atrophic gland (2). However, it is often difficult to determine when pancreatic echoes are more reflective than normal.

Chronic pancreatitis may also present as a focal mass of reduced reflectivity (Fig. 7.11) that cannot be differentiated from pancreatic

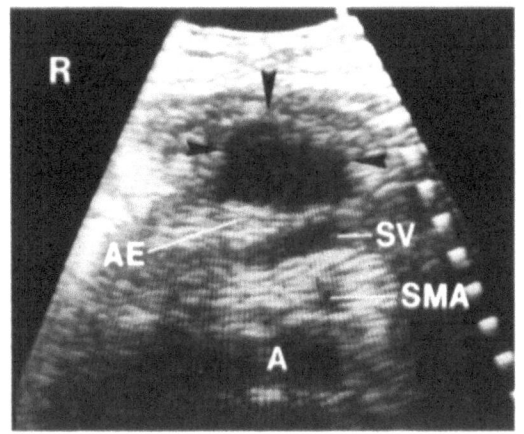

A

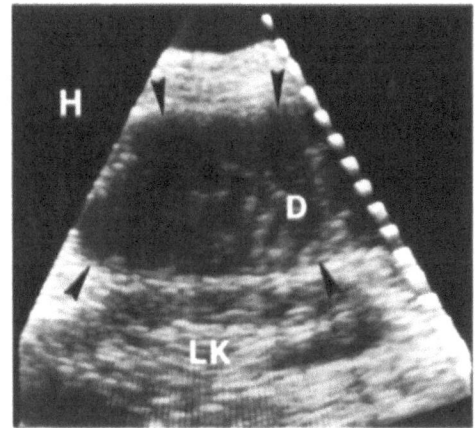

B

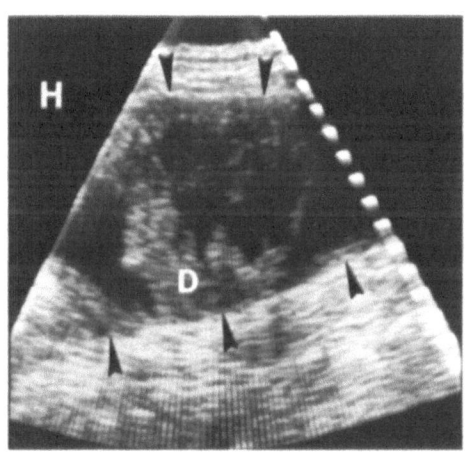

C

Fig. 7.13. Pancreatic pseudocysts (*arrowheads*). **A** Transverse scan of pseudocyst located in body of pancreas. Pseudocyst fluid contains weak internal echoes. A moderate amount of acoustic enhancement (*AE*) is present deep to pseudocyst. **B** and **C** Left parasagittal scans in plane of and lateral to kidney demonstrating large pseudocyst that contains regions of strong internal echoes produced by tissue debris (*D*) within pseudocyst. *SV*, splenic vein; *SMA*, superior mesenteric artery; *LK*, left kidney; *A*, aorta.

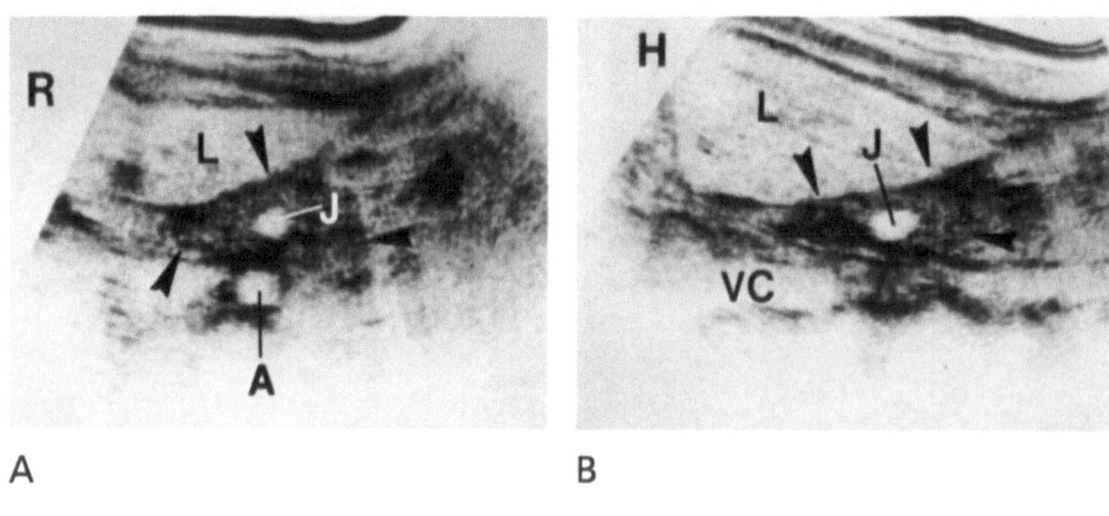

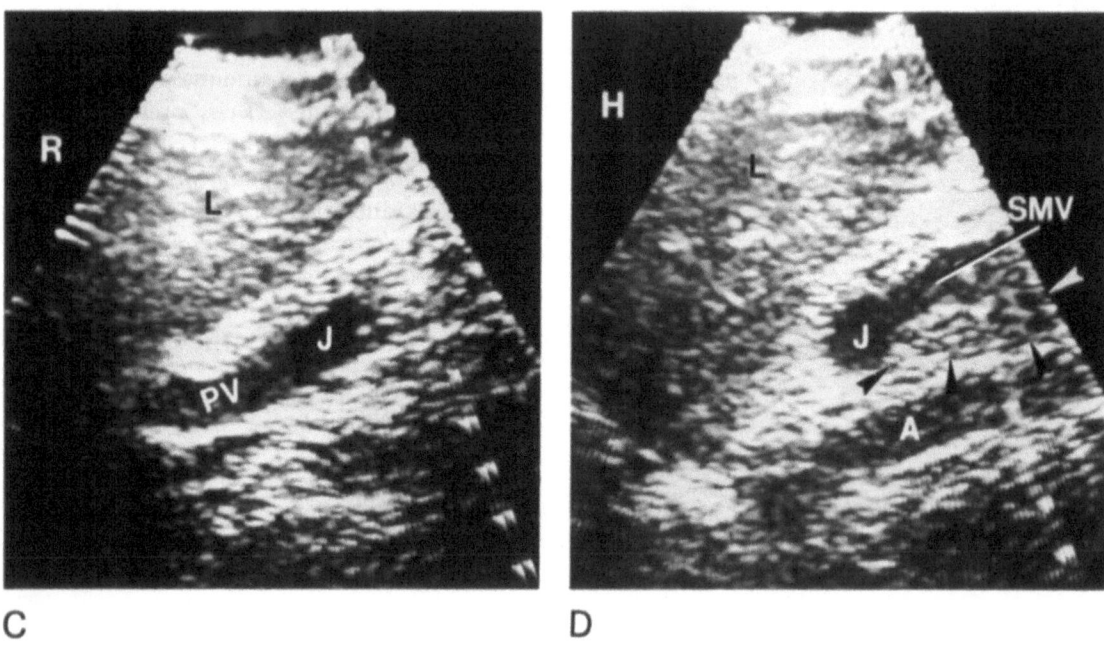

Fig. 7.14. Prominent junctional region (*J*) formed at confluence of splenic and superior mesenteric veins (*SMV*) to form portal vein (*PV*). Contact scan images in transverse (**A**) and sagittal (**B**) planes interpreted as small pseudocyst in pancreatic head (*arrowheads*) because portal and superior mesenteric veins could not be demonstrated in continuity with junctional region. Real-time scans in transverse (**C**) and sagittal (**D**) planes demonstrate this venous continuity. *L*, liver; *A*, aorta; *VC*, vena cava.

carcinoma solely on the basis of imaging techniques (20). The incidence of concomitant carcinoma in patients with calcific pancreatitis has been reported to be as high as 25% (21). Therefore, when a focal mass is detected, percutaneous aspiration under ultrasonic guidance may be advisable so as to obtain a cytologic diagnosis (see Chapter 10).

There are two signs that are helpful in the identification of chronic pancreatitis: (1) the visualization of a dilated pancreatic duct (7, 9, 12) (Fig. 7.12); and (2) the detection of intrapancreatic calcifications as evidenced by scattered discrete areas of high level reflectivity with acoustic shadows behind (20). The presence of concomitant biliary dilatation suggests the existence of an ampullary mass or stone impacted in the ampulla even if the obstructing lesion is not seen by ultrasound.

B. Pseudocysts

Pancreatic pseudocysts are identified as fluid-filled mass lesions either in or adjacent to the pancreas. Their internal architecture is quite variable. Their walls may appear smooth or irregular. The cavities may be echo free or contain echoes reflected from debris produced by digested tissue (Fig. 7.13). The intensity of the zone of acoustic enhancement can also vary depending upon the amount of protein and tissue debris within the cavity. If there is a considerable amount of tissue debris, or perhaps debris mixed with blood, much more sound will be absorbed and scattered by this material and the zone of acoustic attenuation may be reduced or absent.

After a single pancreatic pseudocyst is detected, others should be searched for both in the region of the pancreas and elsewhere

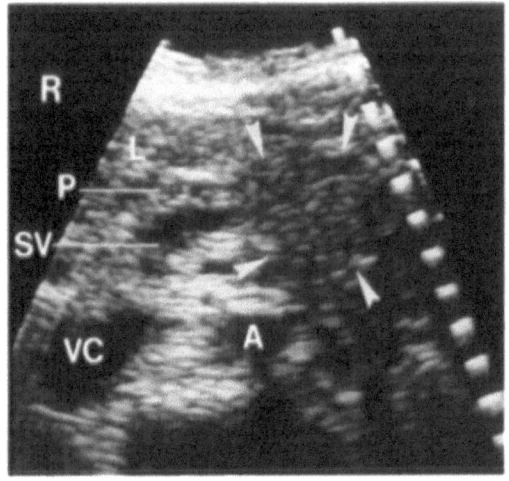
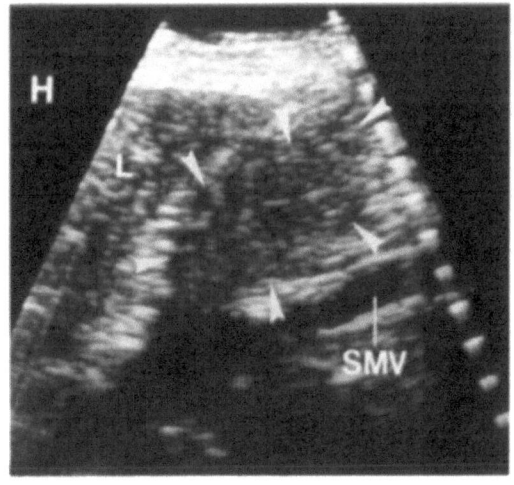

Fig. 7.15. Pancreatic carcinoma. Focal mass (*arrowheads*) extends beyond confines of the normal pancreas and contains reduced internal echoes as compared to normal gland. Mass located in pancreatic body. Transverse (**A**) and sagittal (**B**) scans. *L*, liver; *P*, normal pancreas; *SV*, splenic vein; *VC*, vena cava; *A*, aorta; *SMV*, superior mesenteric vein.

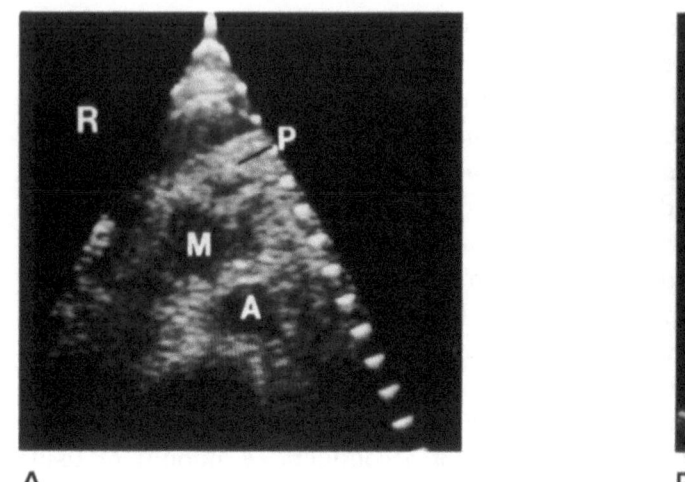
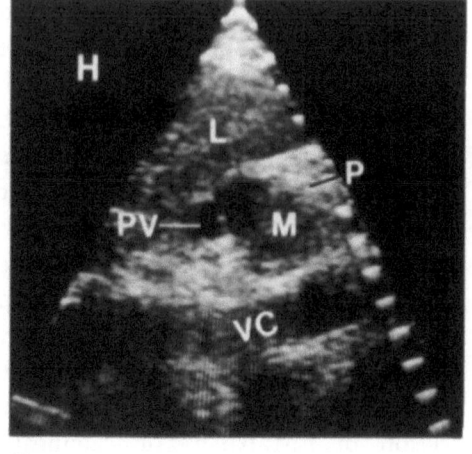

A   B

Fig. 7.16. Pancreatic carcinoma. Focal mass (*M*) within confines of normal pancreatic head. Mass identified only because it contains lower intensity echoes than surrounding normal pancreas (*P*). Transverse (**A**) and sagittal (**B**) scans. *A*, aorta; *PV*, portal vein; *VC*, vena cava, *L*, liver.

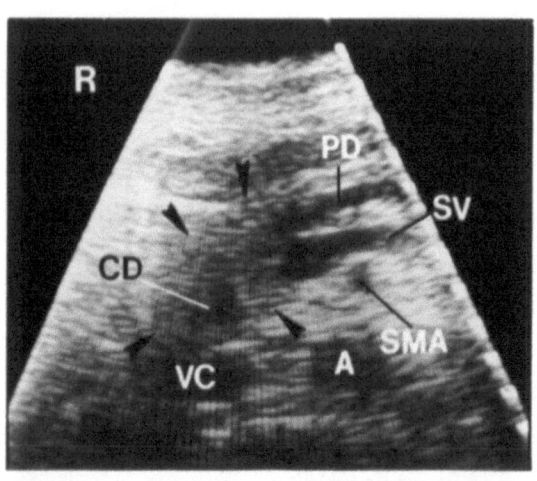
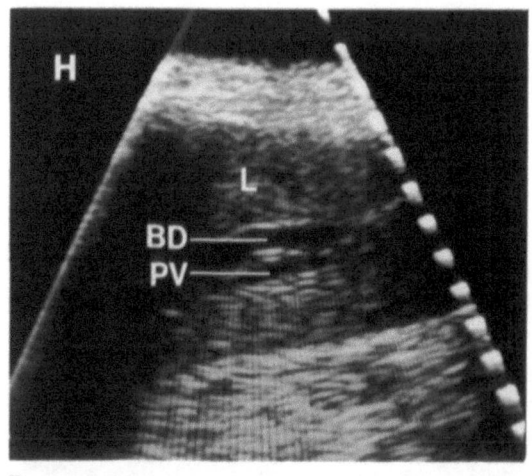

A   B

Fig. 7.17. Carcinoma in the head of the pancreas producing obstruction of both the pancreatic duct and biliary system. **A** Transverse scan through pancreatic head and body. Tumor (*arrowheads*) encases common duct (*CD*) and obstructs pancreatic duct (*PD*). **B** Sagittal scan through liver demonstrating dilated bile ducts (*BD*). Extrapancreatic portion of common duct could not be visualized because of overlying gas-filled bowel. *L*, liver; *PV*, portal vein; *VC*, vena cava; *A*, aorta; *SV*, splenic vein; *SMA*, superior mesenteric vein.

in the upper and lower abdomen. Pancreatic enzymes can dissect along retroperitoneal tissue planes for some distance beyond the pancreas and thus form pseudocysts distant to the pancreas.

On occasion the junctional region in which the SMV and splenic vein meet to form the portal vein may be prominent. If on scans produced with an articulated arm contact scanner no continuity with the splenic vein or SMV has been seen, then the confluence may be mistakenly diagnosed as a small pancreatic pseudocyst (Fig. 7.14A and B). However, when a real-time scanner is used and the transducer is rotated around the confluence, its connection with the splenic vein and SMV becomes obvious and the diagnosis of pseudocyst is not substantiated (Fig. 7.14C and D).

C. Pancreatic Carcinoma

The typical appearance of pancreatic carcinoma is that of a focal mass within the pancreas which contains lower internal echoes than the adjacent normal pancreas (2). The mass usually projects beyond the confines of the normal pancreas to form either a discrete lesion or an ill-defined enlargement of one region of the gland (Fig. 7.15). However, a pancreatic carcinoma may be detected before it enlarges beyond the margins of the gland if a focal area of decreased echoes within normal parenchyma can be seen (Fig. 7.16). If the mass is located in the head, dilatation of the pancreatic duct, bile duct or both may be ancillary signs (Fig. 7.17). To confirm that the mass is a carcinoma, ultrasonically guided percutaneous aspiration biopsy can be used (see Chapter 10).

When a focal solid mass is identified within the pancreas, evidence of metastatic disease should be searched for. The liver should be examined for focal masses and the paraaortic and porta hepatis regions searched for enlarged nodes.

References

1. Skolnick ML, Royal DR (1976) Normal upper abdominal vasculature: a study correlating contact B scanning with arteriography and gross anatomy. J Clin Ultrasound 6:399–402
2. Johnson ML, Mack LA (1978) Ultrasonic evaluation of the pancreas. Gastrointest Radiol 3:257–266
3. Lawson TL (1978) Sensitivity of pancreatic ultrasonography in the detection of pancreatic disease. Radiology 128:733–736
4. Arger PH, Mulhern CG, Bonavita JA, Stauffer DM, Hale J (1979) An analysis of pancreatic sonography in suspected pancreatic disease. J Clin Ultrasound 7:91–97
5. de Graaff CS, Taylor KJW, Simonds BD, Rosenfield AJ (1978) Gray-scale echography of the pancreas. Radiology 129:157–161
6. Weill FS (1978) Ultrasonography of digestive diseases. CV Mosby, St. Louis
7. Cotton PB, Lees WR, Vallon AG, Cottone M, Croker JR, Chapman M (1980) Gray-scale ultrasonography and endoscopic pancreatography in pancreatic diagnosis. Radiology 134:453–459
8. Filly RA, London SS (1979) The normal pancreas: acoustic characteristics and frequency of imaging. J Clin Ultrasound 7:121–124
9. Weinstein DP, Weinstein BJ (1979) Ultrasonic demonstration of the pancreatic duct: an analysis of 41 cases. Radiology 130:729–734
10. Bryan PJ (1980) Appearance of normal pancreatic duct: a study using real-time ultrasonography. Presented at the American Institute of Ultrasound in Medicine Annual Meeting, New Orleans, Louisiana, September
11. Parulekar SG (1980) Ultrasonic evaluation of the pancreatic duct. J Clin Ultrasound 8:457–463
12. Ohto M, Saotome N, Saisho H, Tsuchiya Y, Ono T, Okuda K, Karasawa E (1980) Real-time sonography of the pancreatic duct: application to percutaneous pancreatic ductography. Am J Roentgenol 134:647–652
13. Goldstein HM, Katragadda CS (1978) Prone view ultrasonography for pancreatic tail

neoplasms. Am J Roentgenol 131:231–234

14. Warren PS, Garrett WJ, Phil D, Kossoff G (1978) The liquid-filled stomach—an ultrasonic window to the upper abdomen. J Clin Ultrasound 6:315–320

15. Crade M, Taylor KJW, Rosenfield AT (1978) Water distention of the gut in the evaluation of the pancreas by ultrasound. Am J Roentgenol 131:348–349

16. Jacobson P, Crade M, Taylor KJW (1978) The upright position while giving water for the evaluation of the pancreas. J Clin Ultrasound 6:353–354

17. MacMahon H, Bowie JD, Beezhold C (1979) Erect scanning of pancreas using a gastric window. Am J Roentgenol 132:587–591

18. Carey LC (1975) Acute and chronic pancreatitis. Surg Clin North Am 55:325–338

19. Doust BD, Pierce GD (1976) Gray-scale ultrasonic properties of the normal and inflamed pancreas. Radiology 120:653–657

20. Weinstein BJ, Weinstein DP, Brodmerkel GJ (1980) Ultrasonography of pancreatic lithiasis. Radiology 134:185–189

21. Skolnick ML, Dekker A, Weinstein BJ (1978) Ultrasound guided fine needle aspiration biopsy of abdominal masses. Gastrointest Radiol 3:295–302

22. Paulino-Netto A, Dreiling DA, Baronofsky ID (1960) The relationship between pancreatic calcification and cancer of the pancreas. Ann Surg 151:530–537

8
Retroperitoneum

The retroperitoneum as defined in this chapter covers the central retroperitoneal area from the diaphragm to the region of the aortic bifurcation. It includes the major vessels and perivascular soft tissues exclusive of the pancreas which was covered in the preceding chapter. (The more lateral retroperitoneal regions comprising mainly the kidneys and perirenal masses have been discussed in Chapter 4.) Below the level of the aortic bifurcation, retroperitoneal structures often cannot be seen by ultrasound because the overlying bowel may contain gas which prevents further ultrasound penetration. The only retroperitoneal structures in the lower abdomen that can be consistently im-

aged are those seen through the acoustic window of a full bladder.

As far as this chapter is concerned, the major emphasis will be placed on the study of the retroperitoneal vascular structures and adjacent lymph nodes. The vessels readily lend themselves to examination with real-time instrumentation because such instrumentation possesses two important characteristics for evaluating vascular structures: (1) the ability to differentiate larger arteries and veins by their intrinsic movements; and (2) the ability to identify a specific vessel through careful tracking of its course to determine its origin or termination.

1. ANATOMY

The most posterior vascular structures in the central retroperitoneum are the aorta and vena cava. The aorta lies either centrally over the vertebral column or slightly to the left, while the vena cava lies to the right of the aorta either over the right side of or just lateral to the vertebral column. The space between the posterior surface of the aorta and the anterior surface of the vertebral column in the normal subject is just several millimeters thick and usually is not appreciated by ultrasound. Rather, the aorta appears to lie on top of the vertebral column. When retroperitoneal pathology is present (e.g., enlarged nodes, hematomas), this space widens.

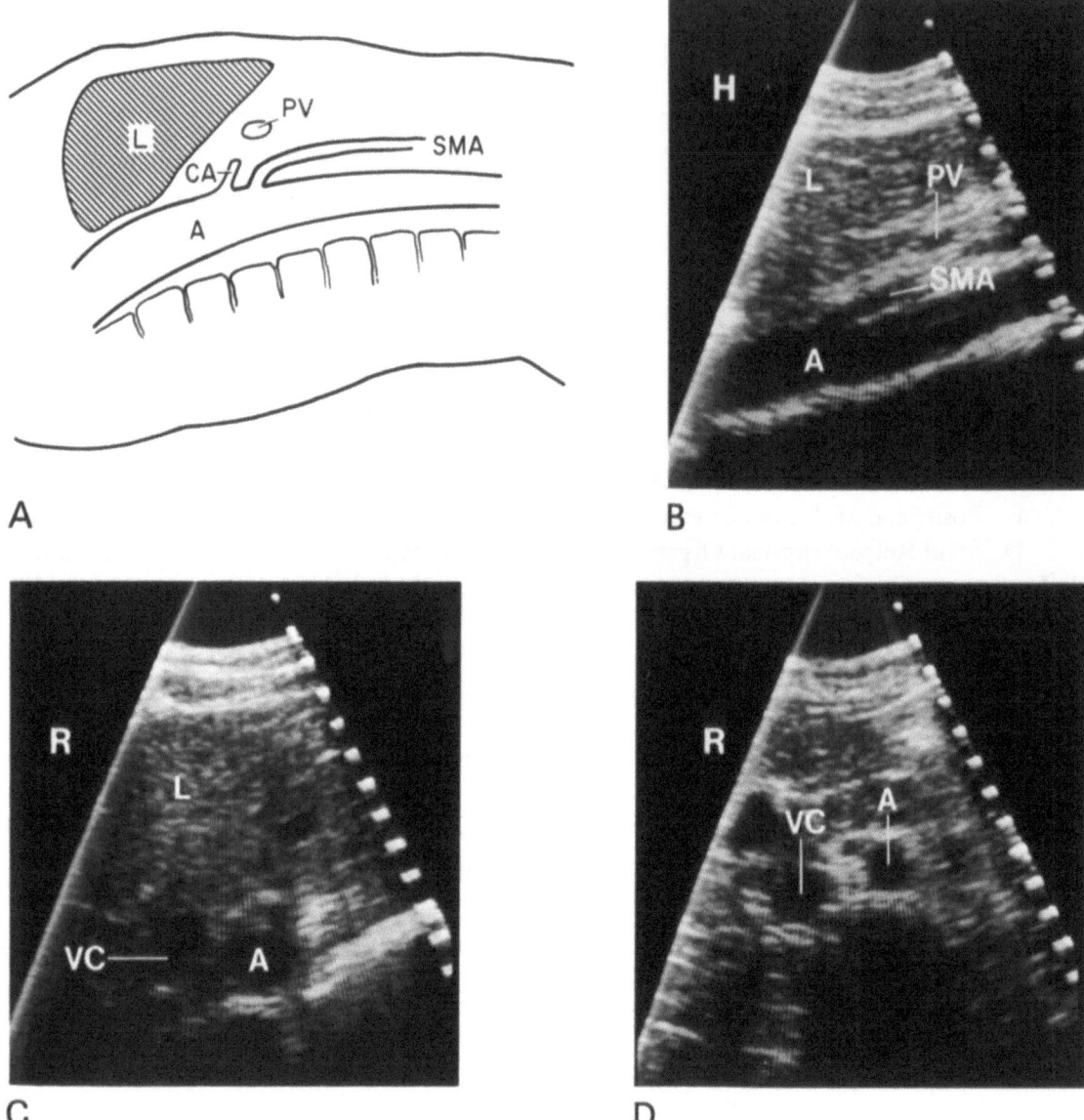

Fig. 8.1. A Normal aorta (*A*) has a gentle single convex anterior curve that parallels the lumbar curvature. Lumen gradually tapers as aorta extends from diaphragm to bifurcation. Superior mesenteric (*SMA*) and celiac (*CA*) arteries take origin from anterior wall. *PV*, portal vein; *L*, liver. **B** Midsagittal image of normal aorta. **C** Transverse scan of upper aorta. *VC*, vena cava. **D** Transverse scan of lower aorta. Note decrease in luminal diameter as compared to **C.**

The aorta parallels the contour of the lumbar vertebral column. On sagittal scans, the curvature of the aorta is a single arcuate line with the superior end most posterior (Fig. 8.1A and B). The diameter of the aorta is greatest at the superior end. It slowly and continuously tapers to the region of the bifurcation. On transverse scans the cross-sectional images of the aorta are basically circular with the diameters of the circles decreasing from a superior to inferior direction (Fig. 8.1C and D).

The spinal canal is usually not seen since ultrasound does not penetrate through vertebral bodies. However, sound does penetrate the cartilaginous intervertebral disks and when the beam is positioned over a disk space, a ringlike sonoreflective structure is seen posterior to the disk on a transverse view (Fig. 8.2A). The anatomic basis for this ringlike echo is not presently clear. It

may represent reflections from the margins of the cord itself or from the surrounding membranes. It is important to correctly differentiate this structure from the aorta because if it were interpreted to represent the aorta in cross section, then the space anterior to it might be interpreted as a mantle of enlarged nodes rather than an intervertebral disk. A transverse view at a slightly lower or higher level through the vertebral body (Fig. 8.2B) is helpful in differentiating aorta from spinal canal.

The configuration of the vena cava on sagittal scan is different from the aorta. It is composed of two curves: a major convex anterior curve paralleling that of the aorta and a minor convex posterior curve in the most superior region (Fig. 8.3). Thus, on sagittal scans the proximal end of the cava points superiorly whereas the proximal end of the aorta points inferiorly. The superior

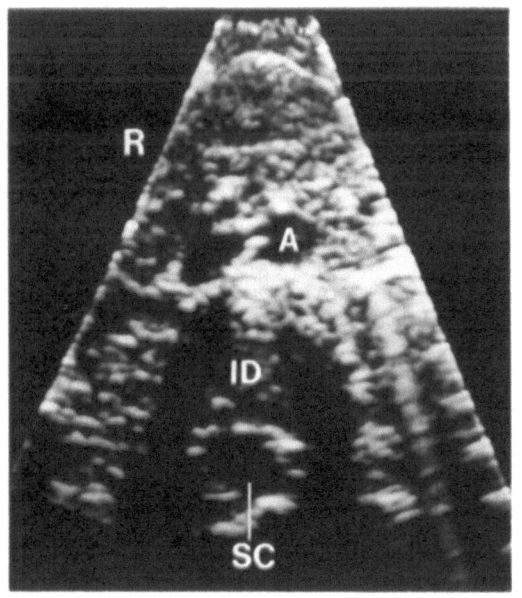

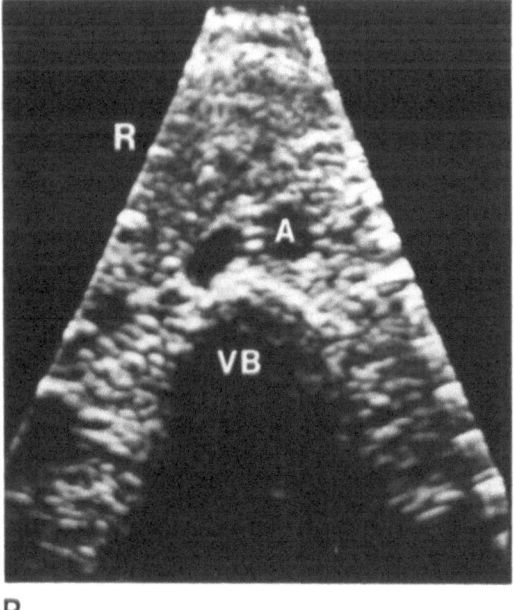

A   B

Fig. 8.2. Relationship of aorta to spinal canal. **A** Transverse section through intervertebral disk (*ID*). Spinal canal (*SC*) visualized posterior to disk because ultrasound is propagated through cartilaginous disk space. Spinal canal should not be confused with aorta. **B** Transverse scan several millimeters inferior to **A** at level of vertebral body (*VB*). Bone prevents sound transmission so spinal canal is not seen. Normal aorta (*A*) lies anterior to vertebral body.

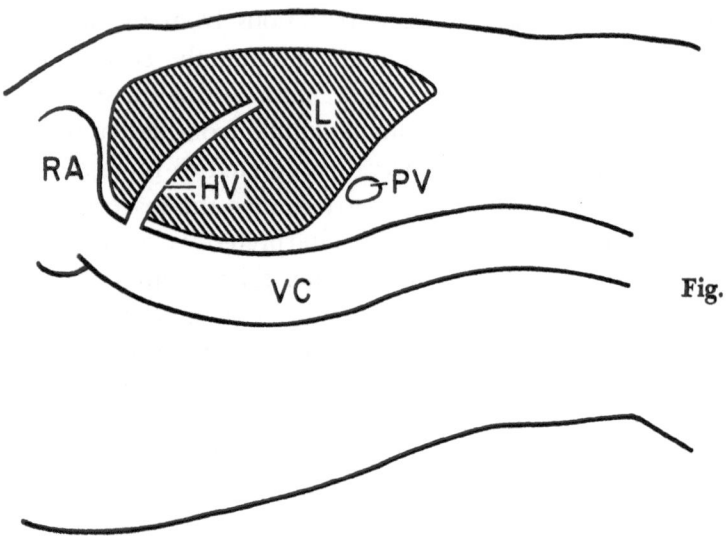

Fig. 8.3. The normal vena cava (*VC*) contains two curves: a major convex anterior one and a minor convex posterior one in the most superior region. *HV*, hepatic vein; *PV*, portal vein; *L*, liver; *RA*, right atrium.

end of the cava continues through the diaphragm into the right atrium. Although the vena cava also shows a decrease in transverse diameter in its more distal portion as compared to its cephalad region, there is not the continuous tapering that is seen in the aorta. The diameter of the cava is more variable because its thin wall readily conforms to changes in intraluminal or external pressures produced by different phases of respiration (Fig. 8.4). On transverse scans, when the intravascular pressure is high, the cava can assume a round configuration, whereas during quiet breathing when the cava is partially collapsed, it can assume an oval or even flat configuration.

A. Intrinsic Vascular Movements

The aorta demonstrates pulsatile movements synchronous with the heartbeat. The anterior wall shows greater anterior and posterior pulsatile movement than the posterior wall because the latter is limited in its movement by the vertebral column. The pulsatile movements seen in the aorta are difficult to observe in smaller arteries.

The movements of the vena cava are more complex. During the inspiratory phase of breathing, as the intrathoracic pressure be-

comes more negative, there is an increase in blood flowing through the cava. At the end of inspiration the cava reaches its maximum diameter (Fig. 8.4A). During expiration, as the intrathoracic pressure increases, there is a decrease in blood flowing through the cava and a decrease in its luminal diameter (Fig. 8.4B). In intermediate phases of breathing focal regions of greater and lesser diameter may be seen (Fig. 8.5). The cava can also be distended during a forced Valsalva maneuver. If the abdominal aorta touches the vena cava as sometimes occurs when there is an aneurysm or tortuosity of the aorta, then aortic pulsations can be transmitted to the cava and be superimposed upon the phasic caval changes in caliber associated with respiration.

B. Arteries Branching Off the Aorta

The major tributaries of the abdominal aorta that can be readily visualized as one progresses inferiorly from the diaphragm are the celiac axis, superior mesenteric artery (SMA), renal arteries, and common iliac arteries (Fig. 8.6). The main axis of the celiac artery originates from the anterior surface of the aorta and runs anteriorly (Fig. 8.7A). It bifurcates into the splenic artery (to the

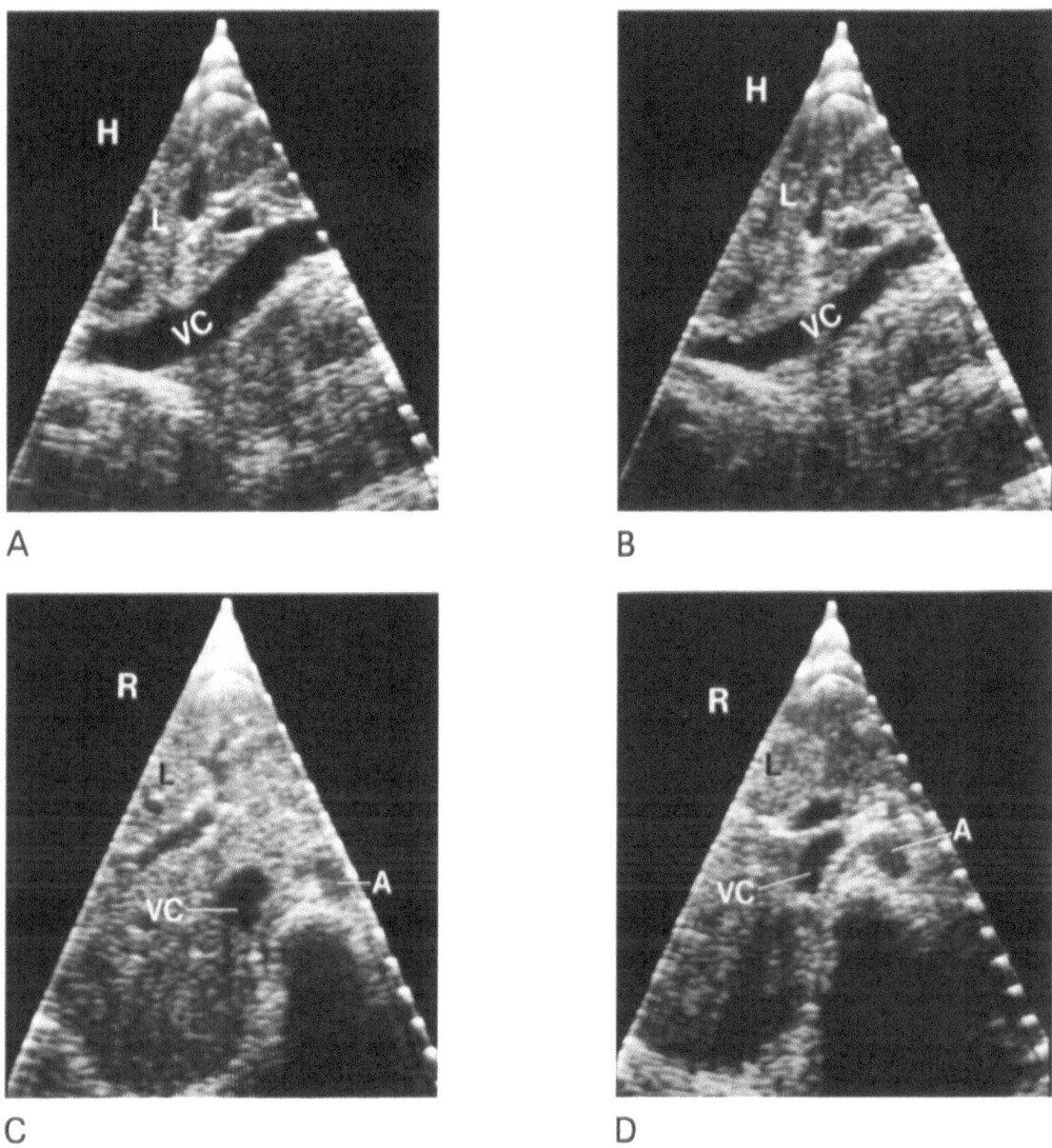

Fig. 8.4. Changes of vena caval (*VC*) diameter in different phases of respiration. Sagittal views in end inspiration (**A**) and during expiration (**B**). Transverse views in end inspiration (**C**) and during expiration (**D**). *L*, liver; *A*, aorta.

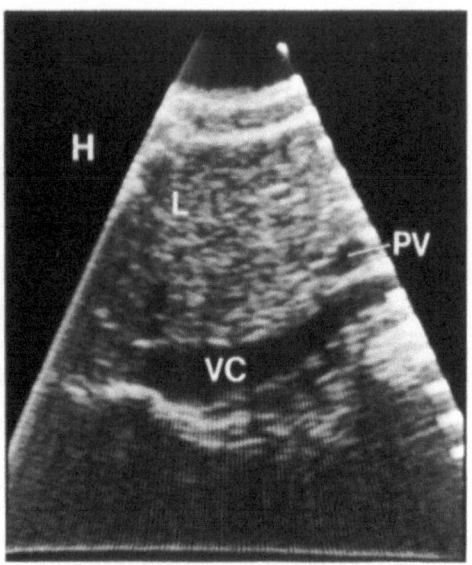

Fig. 8.5. Sagittal view of vena cava (*VC*) during intermediate phase of respiration. Superior portion of vessel is more dilated than inferior portion. Thin wall of cava allows rapid change in diameter in response to changing intraluminal and intraabdominal pressures which at any instant may not be uniform along its entire length. *L,* liver; *PV,* portal vein.

left) and the hepatic artery (to the right) (Fig. 8.7B). About 1 cm inferior to the origin of the celiac axis the SMA originates. Its course is first slightly anterior and then inferior paralleling the position of the aorta (Fig. 8.7A). Rarely, a vessel is seen branching to the right from the SMA just below its origin from the aorta. This vessel is the replaced right hepatic artery that originates from the SMA (Fig. 8.8) (1, 2). The renal arteries originate from the lateral or anterior lateral aspects of the aorta approximately 1 to 2 cm below the origin of the SMA. The right renal artery travels between the inferior vena cava (IVC) and vertebral column to the right kidney. The left renal artery parallels the curvature of the vertebral body and then continues to the left kidney (Fig. 8.8). We have not been able to visualize the inferior mesenteric artery. The iliac arteries, which originate at the aortic bifurcation,

course inferolaterally and lie anterior to the iliac veins. A coronal scanning plane with the patient positioned either supine or decubitus, left side down, may be used to show a long axis view of the aorta bifurcating into the iliac arteries (3). Transverse views of these vessels can be obtained by either placing the transducer on the anterior surface of the abdomen (Fig. 8.9), provided the overlying bowel is not gas filled, or on the right flank.

The tributaries of the vena cava that can be appreciated by ultrasound are the hepatic veins at the superior end, the renal veins in the midregion, and sometimes the iliac veins that join to form the cava at the inferior end. The hepatic veins drain into the cava from the right and left lobes in a radial pattern (Fig. 8.10). Their diameter can vary considerably as does the diameter of the cava

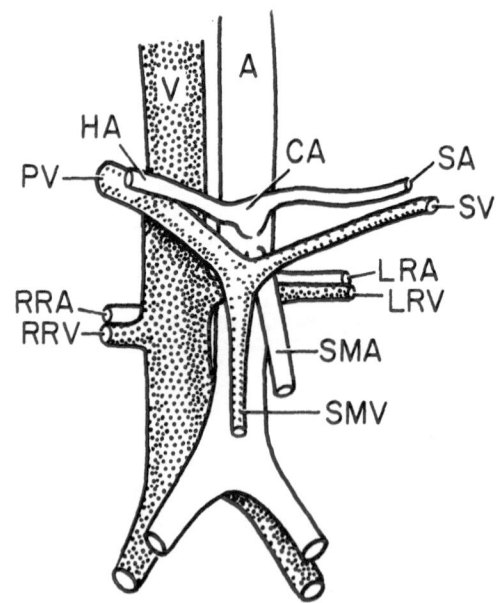

Fig. 8.6. Anatomic relationships of major retroperitoneal vessels. *A,* aorta; *VC,* vena cava; *RRA,* right renal artery; *RRV,* right renal vein; *LRA,* left renal artery; *LLV,* left renal vein; *CA,* celiac artery; *HA,* hepatic artery; *SA,* splenic artery; *PV,* portal vein; *SV,* splenic vein; *SMV,* superior mesenteric vein; *SMA,* superior mesenteric artery.

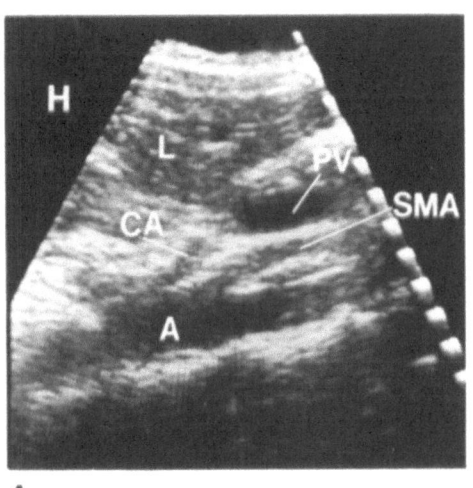
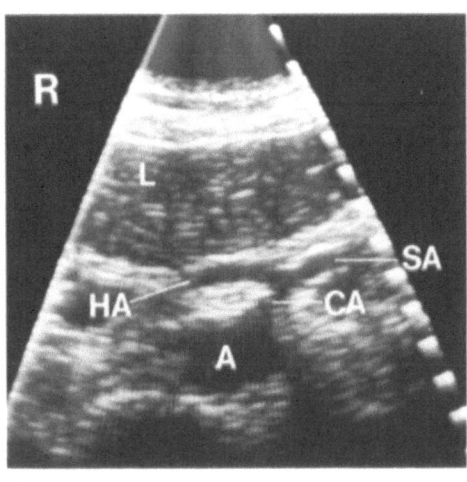

A   B

Fig. 8.7. **A** Sagittal view of aorta (*A*) with origin of celiac (*CA*) and superior mesenteric (*SMA*) arteries. Anterior to SMA is portal vein (*PV*). *L*, liver. **B** Transverse scan showing origin of celiac artery (*CA*) from aorta (*A*) and its branching into hepatic (*HA*) and splenic (*SA*) arteries. *L*, liver.

depending upon the phase of respiration or intravascular pressure. The right renal vein courses from the renal hilum into the vena cava entering along its right lateral aspect (Fig. 8.11). The left renal vein exits from the left renal hilum, parallels the left renal artery to its junction with the aorta, then crosses between the aorta and SMA to continue into the left lateral side of the vena cava (Fig. 8.12).

C. Positional Mobility of Vena Cava

Besides exhibiting intrinsic changes in shape related to blood flow, the vena cava can change anatomic position in normal subjects as a result of a change in patient position. With the patient in supine position, the cava lies to the right of the aorta. When the patient is shifted to decubitus position, left side down, the cava can assume a position anterior to the aorta (Fig. 8.13).

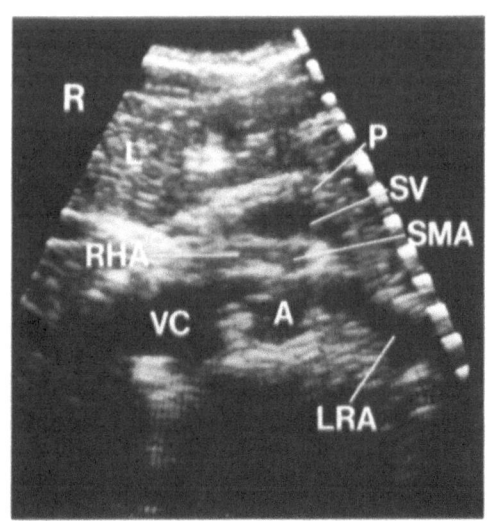

Fig. 8.8. Origin of replaced right hepatic artery (*RHA*) originating from superior mesenteric artery (*SMA*). Also a good example of left renal artery (*LRA*) originating from left side of aorta (*A*). *SV*, splenic vein; *VC*, vena cava; *L*, liver; *P*, pancreas.

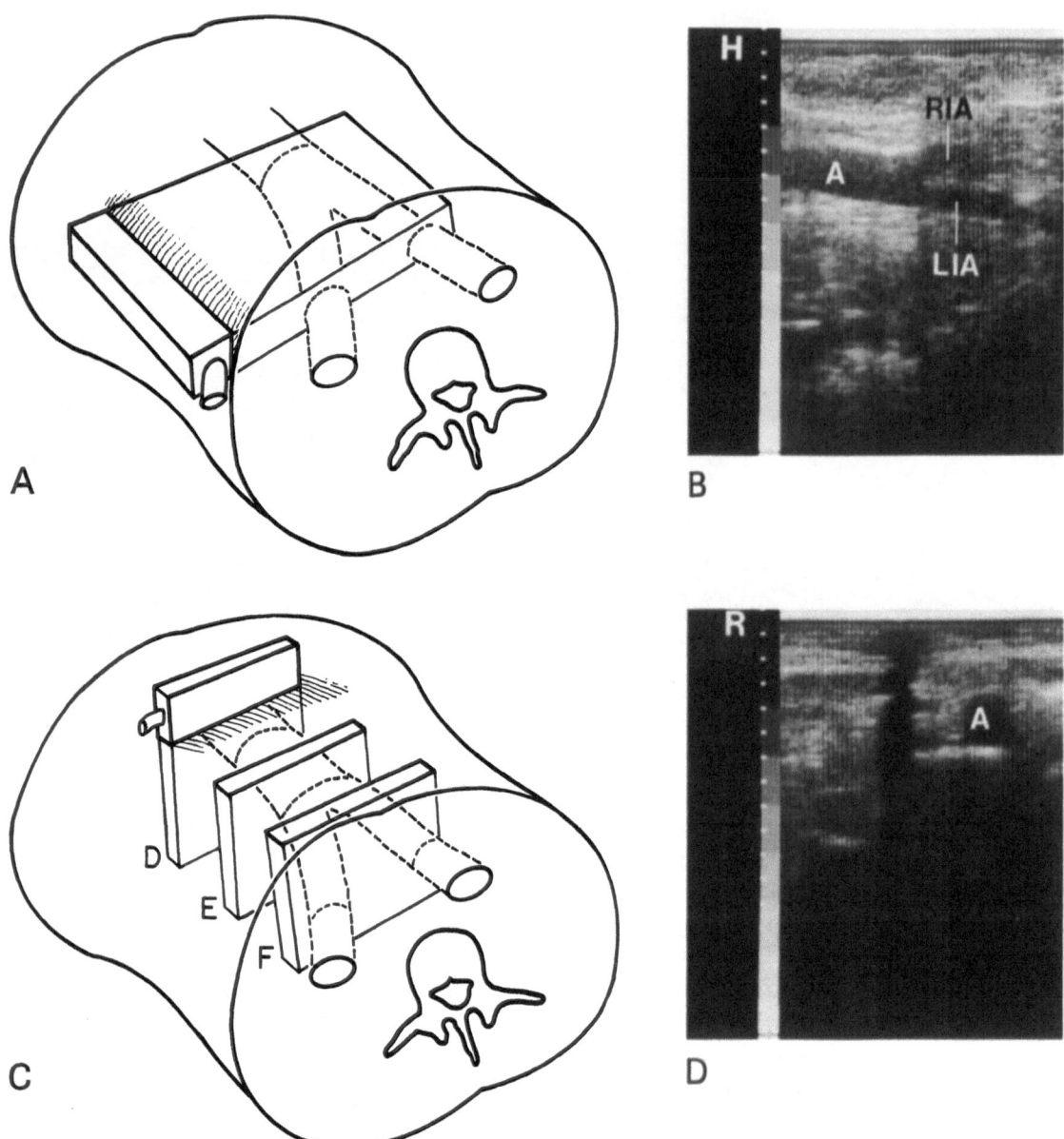

Fig. 8.9. Imaging of distal aorta and its continuity with the iliac arteries. **A** Long axis view obtained in coronal plane. Transducer is placed on right flank. **B** Coronal image at level of bifurcation. *A*, aorta; *RIA*, right iliac artery; *LIA*, left iliac artery. **C** Transverse sections. Transducer placed on anterior abdominal wall. **D** Level of distal aorta just above bifurcation. **E** At bifurcation (*arrow*). **F** Below bifurcation. Right (*RIA*) and left (*LIA*) iliac arteries.

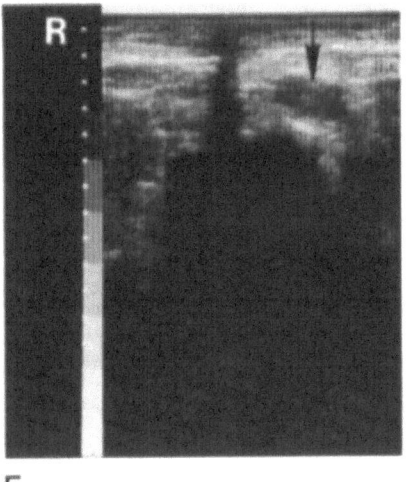

E

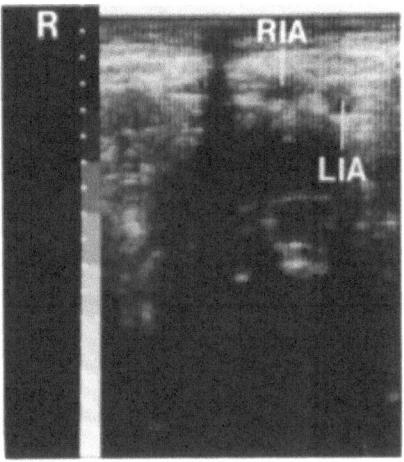

F

D. Solid Retroperitoneal Organs

Aside from the major vessels, the other central retroperitoneal structures of major clinical significance for the ultrasonographer are the perivascular lymph nodes which surround the aorta and vena cava. However, when these nodes are of normal size they are usually not seen by ultrasound.

Of much less clinical significance are the psoas muscles which are on either side of the vertebral column and can often be appreciated by ultrasound. In well-developed and muscular subjects, especially males, these muscles can be quite prominent. Occasionally one side may appear thicker in cross section than the other because the patient has developed that side of his body to a greater extent, or because he is lying in a twisted or curved manner on the examining table and thus has contracted one psoas muscle more than the other.

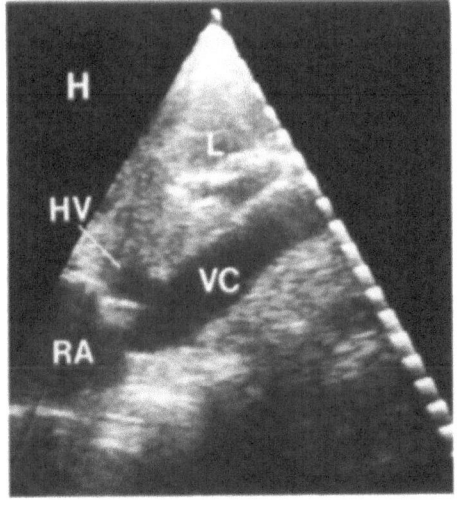

A

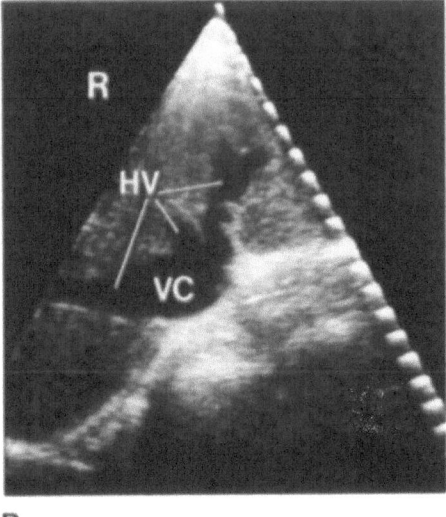

B

Fig. 8.10. Hepatic veins (*HV*) draining into vena cava (*VC*). Sagittal (**A**) and transverse (**B**) planes. *L*, liver; *RA*, right atrium.

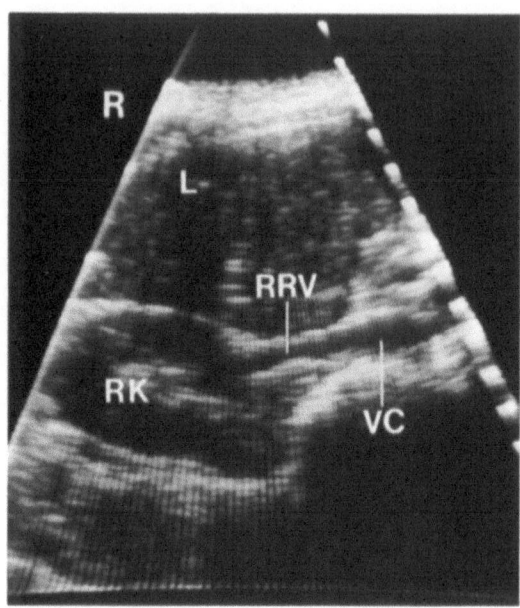

Fig. 8.11. Right renal vein (*RRV*) draining into vena cava (*VC*). Transverse plane. *L,* liver; *RK,* right kidney.

2. EQUIPMENT CHOICE

The choice of transducer head (size, shape, and beam pattern) can have a bearing on the success of the examination. Rectangular transducer assemblies (either consisting of linear arrays or several mechanically driven sector transducers which produce long trapezoid images) are very good for obtaining sagittal views of the aorta and cava (Fig. 8.14), especially when the patient is thin and these vessels are superficial, and for transverse views when the abdominal surface is flat or slightly convex anteriorly. However, they are more difficult to use when tracking vessels, and especially when obtaining transverse views of these vessels in patients with a concave abdominal configuration (Fig. 2.16A). On the other hand, the sector and small trapezoid transducer designs, while being very effective in tracking vessels and in obtaining transverse views, do not produce as satisfactory an examination of the long axis of the aorta and cava because only a short segment of the aorta or cava can be seen on any one sagittal view (Fig. 8.14B). To overcome the deficiencies of the rectangular transducer head for transverse scanning, the concave configuration of the abdomen can be changed to a flat or convex configuration by having the patient volun-

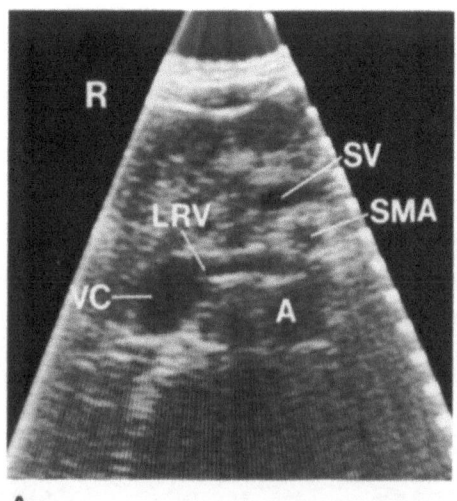

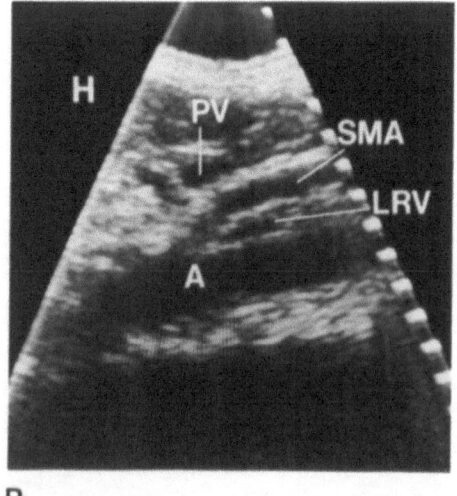

Fig. 8.12. Left renal vein (*LRV*) interposed between superior mesenteric artery (*SMA*) and aorta (*A*) in transverse (**A**) and sagittal (**B**) planes. *PV,* portal vein; *VC,* vena cava; *SV,* splenic vein.

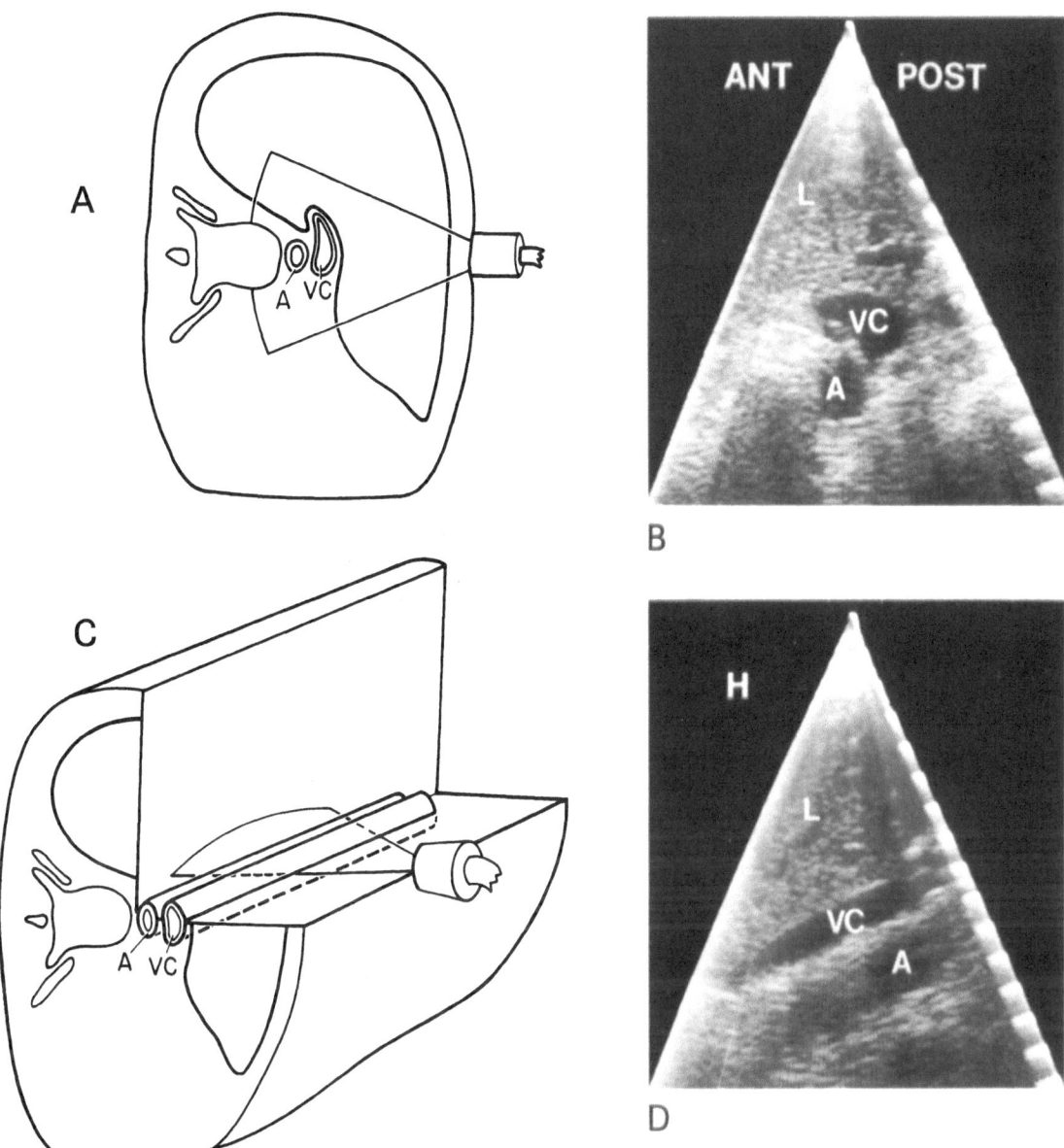

Fig. 8.13. Vena cava lying anterior to aorta in patient positioned decubitus, left side down. **A** Transducer positioned for transverse scan. **B** Corresponding image. **C** Transducer positioned for sagittal scan. **D** Corresponding image. *A,* aorta; *VC,* vena cava; *L,* liver. *ANT,* anterior; *POST,* posterior.

tarily distend the abdomen using the "belly out" maneuver (Fig. 5.3). The sagittal view limitations of the sector scanner and to a lesser extent that of the linear array can be overcome by obtaining partially overlapping sagittal views to delineate the full extent of the aorta and cava. If desired, these views can be cut and pasted adjacent to each other to produce one continuous image (Figs. 8.15 and 8.20).[1]

3. SCANNING TECHNIQUE

We prefer to begin the examination in the sagittal plane. The initial scan is midsagittal in order to define the long axis of the aorta and the origins of the SMA and celiac axis (Figs. 8.1B and 8.7A). The transducer is then slowly swept to the right revealing first the superior mesenteric vein (SMV) inserting into the portal vein and next the vena cava with hepatic veins terminating into the superior end (Fig. 8.10A; see also Fig. 7.5). When examining vascular structures, the transducer should be kept over the vessel through several cardiac and respiratory cycles so as to appreciate the intrinsic movements of that vessel as an aid to differentiating arteries from veins (Fig. 3.9). The previously described rocking maneuvers (Fig. 3.5) should be used to optimally orient the transducer perpendicular to the front and back walls of the vessel under observation.

Following the parasagittal scans, transverse scans are performed beginning at the diaphragm and working inferiorly. In the transverse plane both the aorta and vena cava are usually viewed simultaneously. Sometimes, however, one vessel is more clearly seen than the other. In the most

---

[1] With some newer design linear array systems, two images can be frozen on the monitor and displayed adjacent to each other to produce one image of double length so as to eliminate the need for pasting two figures adjacent to each other.

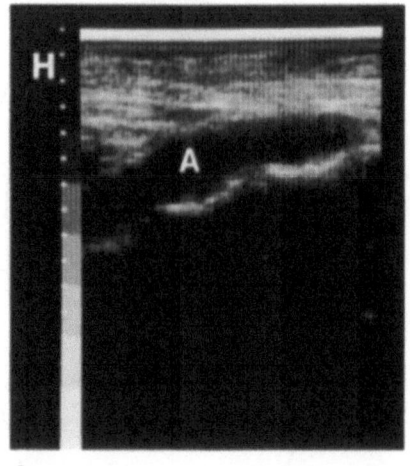

A

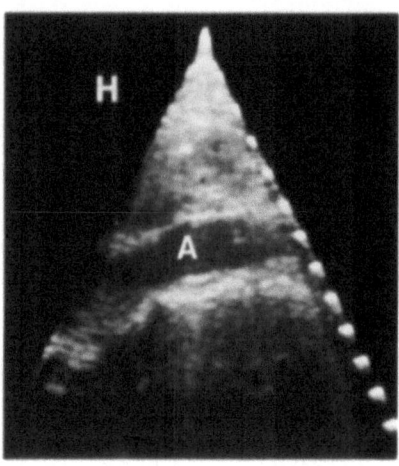

B

Fig. 8.14. Comparison between length of aorta (*A*) seen with linear array (**A**) and sector scanner (**B**). (Linear array made by Advanced Diagnostic Research Corp)

superior cuts the IVC is better visualized because the plane of the cava is more perpendicular to the ultrasound beam than is the plane of the aorta (Fig. 8.16). In a plane through the superior portion of the liver the terminations of the multiple hepatic veins into the cava are seen (Fig. 8.10B). If the transducer is angled slightly more cephalad, the chambers of the heart are appreciated (Fig. 5.2A). The transducer is then slowly and continuously moved inferiorly while attempting to maintain the beam

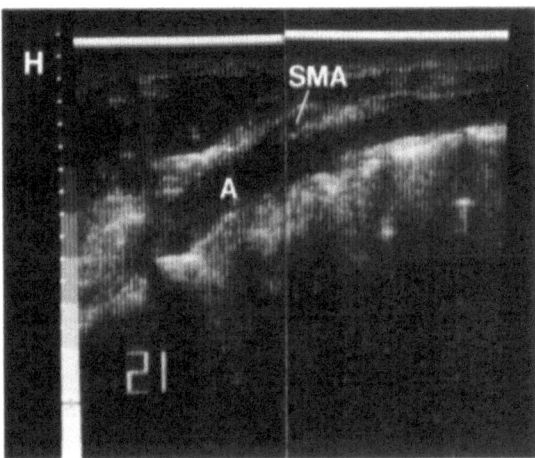

Fig. 8.15. Long composite image of a normal aorta (*A*) produced by overlapping photographs of two adjacent fields. *SMA,* superior mesenteric artery. (Linear array–ADR corp).

roughly perpendicular to the front and back walls of the aorta and cava. The various branches of the aorta and cava and portions of the portal system are appreciated during this sweeping maneuver. At times when specific branches are tortuous, especially those of the celiac axis and the splenoportal system, the operator may have to perform a series of tracking maneuvers by rotating and angling the transducer as it is moved above a particular vessel so as to identify the vessel by determining that it is a branch of a known larger vessel (Fig. 3.7). If a real-time scanner has a choice of frame rates, the highest frame rate should be used during this procedure in an attempt to determine whether the vessel is an artery or vein by its wall motions.

4. PATHOLOGY

A. Aorta

Ultrasound plays a major role in differentiating a normal from an aneurysmally di-lated aorta. In thin patients with lax abdominal musculature and with a prominent lumbar lordosis, a normal abdominal aorta can be within 2 cm of the anterior abdominal wall. Both the aorta and the underlying vertebral column can be easily palpated, and at times the clinician can confuse the mass effect created by the combination of the aorta and vertebral column with an aortic aneurysm. Prior to the advent of ultrasound imaging, arteriography was the diagnostic method of choice.

Besides differentiating a normal from an aneurysmally dilated aorta, ultrasound is very valuable for the follow-up studies of patients with known aneurysms to determine if interval changes have occurred. In both of these applications, real-time equipment, especially linear arrays or similar large field imaging instrumentation, can perform examinations more rapidly than can contact scanners.

Measuring Aneurysms

For this purpose it is important to develop a standardized procedure for measuring the aortic diameter so as to accurately quantify change in diameter. The antero-posterior diameter of the aneurysm should be measured only in the sagittal view; the width can only be measured in the transverse view. The anteroposterior diameter is the shortest distance between the luminal surfaces of the anterior and posterior walls at their maximum separation. Since the aorta is seen in profile on the sagittal scan, this distance is easy to determine (Fig. 8.17A). On the transverse scan, the anteroposterior distance depends on the tilt of the scan plane through the aorta. It is more difficult to accurately control the tilt with real-time than with contact scanners because in the latter instrument the plane in which the scan is performed is set by the position of the scanner arm assembly which can only be changed by releasing locks on the arm assembly. As the tilt of the transverse plane is increased, the anteroposterior diameter is

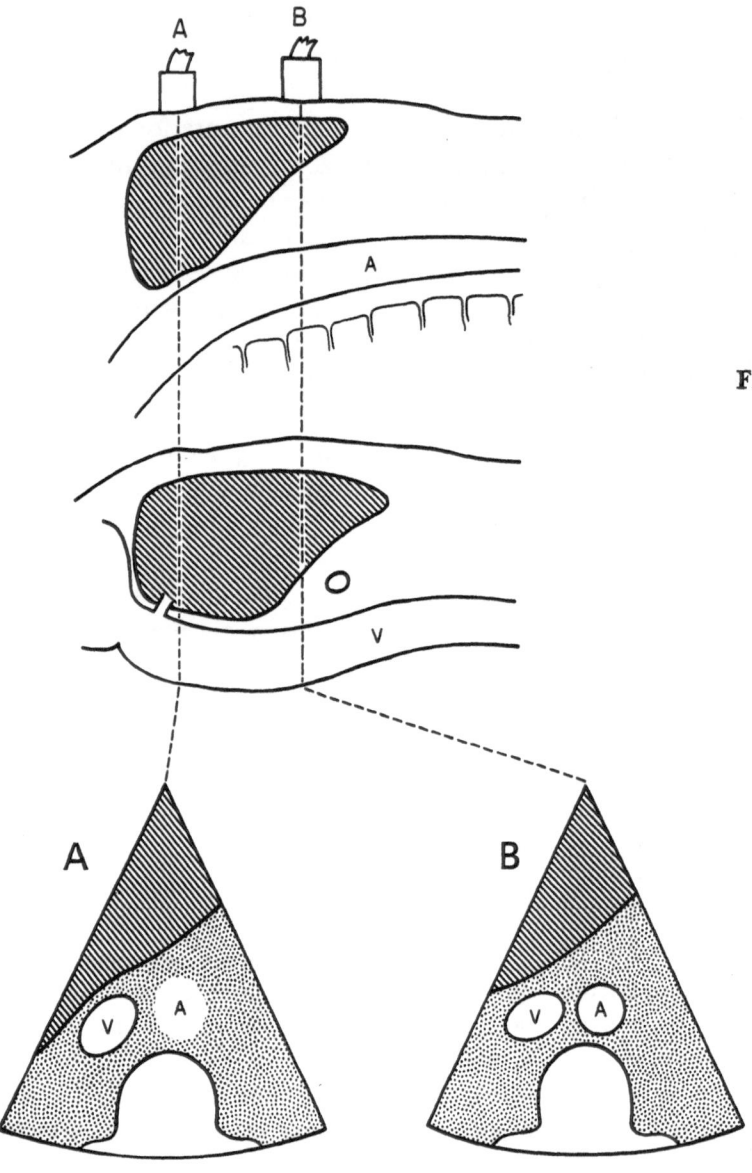

Fig. 8.16. Visualization of vessel walls is determined by orientation of ultrasound beam to these walls. Planes *A* and *B* are two transverse planes through the aorta (*A*) and vena cava (*V*). In plane (**A**) the caval wall is clearly delineated because the ultrasound beam is perpendicular to it while the aortic wall is not clearly seen because the beam is nonperpendicular. In plane (**B**) both the aortic and caval walls are well seen because the ultrasound beam is perpendicular or almost perpendicular to them.

increased and the aortic cross-sectional appearance becomes more oval.

By contrast, the width of the aorta stays constant in the transverse plane regardless of the tilt of the plane so that aneurysmal width can be accurately measured in transverse plane (Fig. 8.17B).

Imaging Aneurysms

To accurately delineate the shape and diameter of the aorta, especially when tortuous, it is imperative that the examiner move his transducer in a tracking manner to follow the various twists and curves of the aorta so as to truly appreciate its configuration and diameter. Therefore, instead of performing a series of parasagittal scans in planes parallel to each other, one might obtain a series of scans in which the planes actually intersect each other as the transducer follows the curves of the aorta (Fig. 8.18A). If the operator has difficulty in following the course of a tortuous aorta in the sagittal plane, a series of transverse aortic images produced by sweeping the transducer in a superior to inferior direction along the

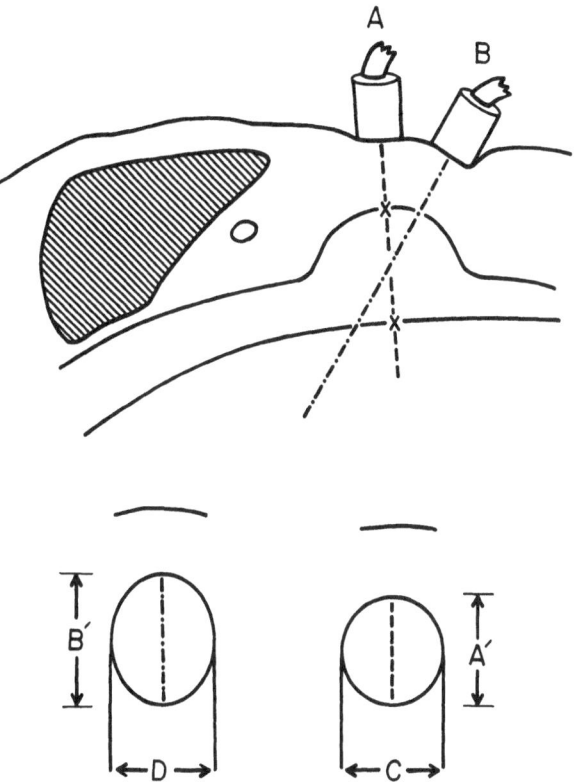

Fig. 8.17. Measuring diameters of aortic aneurysm. Anteroposterior diameter is shortest distance (**A**) between the anterior and posterior walls at their widest point. Transverse views cannot be used to measure anteroposterior diameter because the transducer may not be oriented along the shortest anteroposterior diameter (**B**) and the resultant image will give an incorrectly great A–P diameter (compare **B'** to **A'**). Transverse diameters of the aneurysm can be measured from the transverse images regarding of their inclination to the long axis of the aorta since this diameter is independent of beam inclination (compare D to C).

midsagittal plane may clarify the anatomy. By keeping the transducer centered on the midsagittal plane while observing the position of the aorta to this plane at various levels, one can determine the course of the aorta (Fig. 8.18B).

The major pathologic changes involving the abdominal aorta are ectasia, tortuosity, and aneurysmal dilatation (Fig. 8.19).

As the body ages, there may be loss of the normal tapering of the aortic diameter as the aorta progresses inferiorly from the diaphragm to the iliac bifurcation. The aorta instead may generally widen or become ectatic and appear as a tube of approximate constant diameter from its proximal to distal regions (Fig. 8.19B).

As the degenerative process progresses, the aorta may also increase in length. Since the aorta is anchored at several points by branching vessels, the increase in aortic length produces a tortuous appearance with regions of the aorta lifted away from the vertebral column (Fig. 8.19C). This increased space between the aorta and vertebral column should not be confused with elevation produced by enlargement of retroaortic nodes. Regions of aortic elevation as a result of tortuosity are quite discrete and much more localized than those produced by enlarged nodes. Furthermore, no other signs of nodal enlargement as discussed below are present.

Aortic aneurysm (Figs. 8.19D and 8.20), another effect of degenerative changes within the aorta, refers to a localized region of luminal dilatation that is greater than that of the aorta more proximal to it. There is a continuum of pathologic changes from ectasia to aneurysmal dilatation. By strictest definition, any area of loss of normal tapering is in fact dilatation in reference to the more proximal region. In our clinical practice, dilatation of the aorta under 3 cm in the adult is usually not considered significant (assuming a normal aortic diameter of 2 to 2.5 cm). In aneurysmal dilatation, tortuosity may also exist. Aneurysmal dilatation may involve a long segment and show a gradual

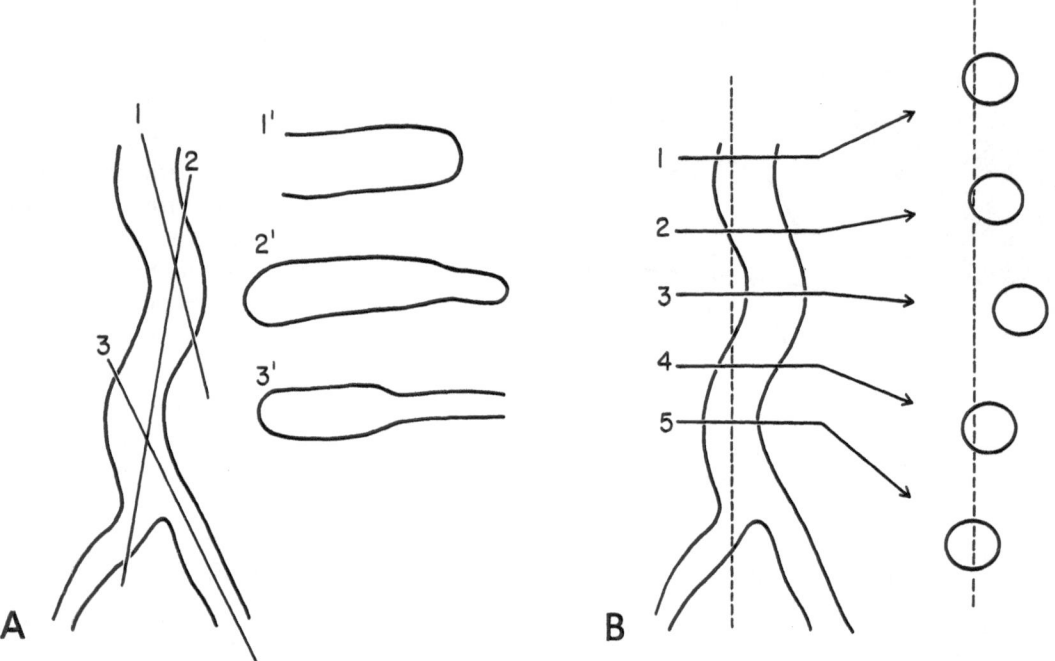

Fig. 8.18. Determining the course of a tortuous aorta. **A** Sagittal planes. Position and rotation of the transducer are varied to follow aortic curves. *1*, *2*, and *3* indicate the different positions in which the transducer must be placed to image the upper, middle, and lower portions of the aorta, respectively. The partial images of the aorta produced in each of these positions are illustrated in sketches *1'*, *2'*, and *3'*. **B** Transverse planes. Transducer swept along midsagittal plane (*dotted lines*) to produce a series of transverse images (*1–5*). Tortuosity of aorta determined by relating its transverse position to the midsagittal plane.

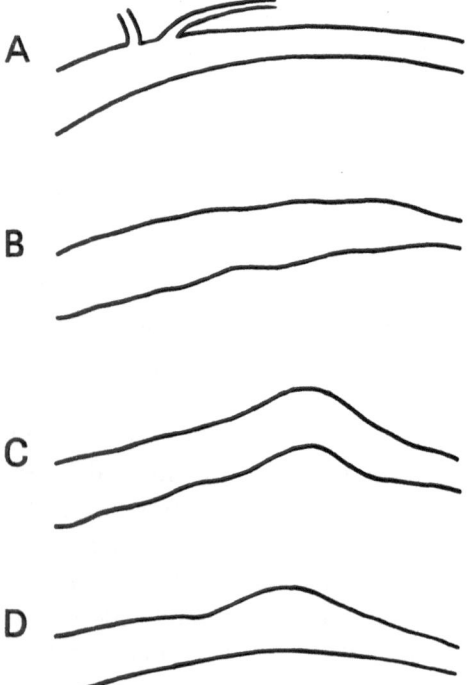

Fig. 8.19. A Normal abdominal aorta. Lumen gradually tapers from superior to inferior end. **B** Ectatic aorta. **C** Tortuous aorta. **D** Aortic aneurysm.

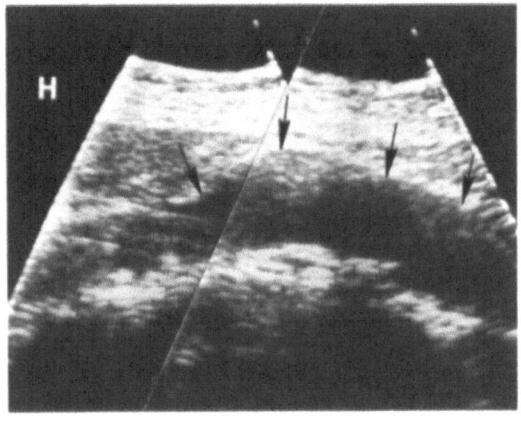
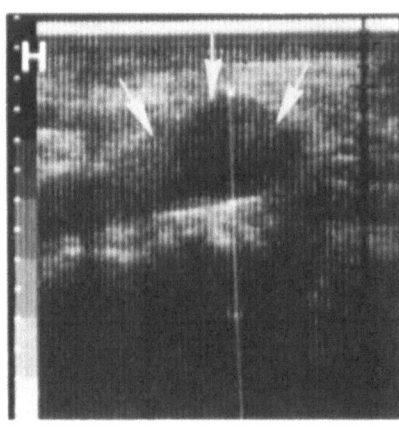

A

B

Fig. 8.20. Aortic aneurysm. **A** Fusiform aneurysm (*arrows*). Two adjacent fields of view partially overlapped to demonstrate a greater longitudinal view of the aneurysm. (Prototype Matzuk Trapezoid Scanner) **B** Saccular aneurysm (*arrows*). (Linear array manufactured by Advanced Diagnostic Research Corporation.)

change in contour from the normal to dilated region (fusiform aneurysm) (Fig. 8.20A) or affect a localized region of a wall to produce a discrete expansion (saccular aneurysm) (Fig. 8.20B).

At times a saccular aneurysm may be difficult to appreciate on sagittal scanning if the sac projects only sideward from the right or left lateral wall. The sagittal scans may show a normal appearance to the aorta. The aneurysmal region may be imaged as a cystic mass in a parasagittal plane adjacent to the aorta but the connection between the aneurysm and the aortic lumen may not be appreciated. In such a situation the transverse scan is crucial, since only in this plane can the connection between the aortic lumen and the aneurysm be seen on one plane (Fig. 8.21).

If no luminal continuity can be detected between the aorta and an adjacent cystic mass in a patient who presents with sudden abdominal pain and who has degenerative aortic changes, the diagnosis of a localized hematoma from a self-limited aortic leak should be considered. If the patient has had a prior aortic aneurysm resection and insertion of an aortic graft, then these ultrasound findings should suggest the possibility of a self-limited leak at the suture line between the graft and aorta.

Clot in Aneurysms

Intraaortic clot is more readily appreciated with real-time than with contact scanning equipment (Fig. 8.22). The beam of the real-time transducer can be more precisely adjusted to be perpendicular to the interface between the clot and column of moving blood than can that of the contact scanner so as to detect this low level reflective interface (as compared to reflectivity of aortic wall). Very slight changes in beam angulation in both the sagittal and transverse planes can result in the visualization or nonvisualization of this interface (Fig. 8.23). Low level echoes are seen within the clot while the moving column of blood is echo free. In our experience, clot is mainly seen along the anterior and lateral walls of the aorta. The clot usually fills the aneurysm so

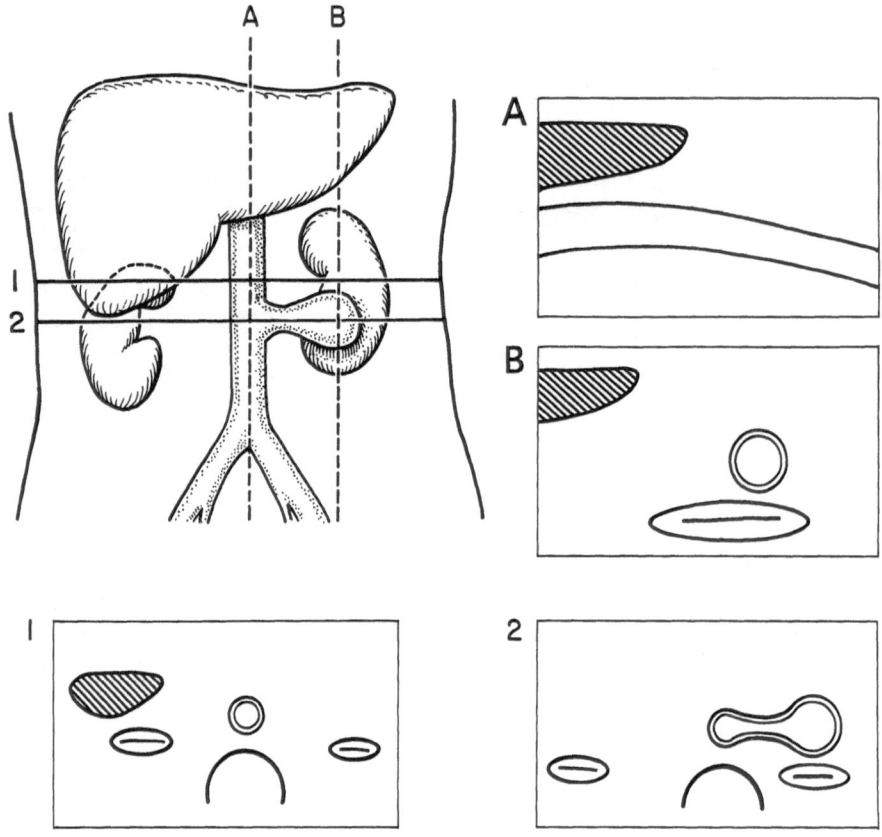

Fig. 8.21. Localized saccular aneurysm projecting from one side of aorta. **A** Sagittal plane through aorta shows normal aortic lumen. **B** Parasagittal plane through aneurysm shows sac. No connection seen with aortic lumen. *1,* transverse plane above level of aneurysm shows a normal aorta. *2,* transverse plane through neck of aneurysm shows continuity of aneurysm with aortic lumen.

as to form an inner surface that is in continuity with the nondilated aortic walls superior and inferior to the level of the aneurysm (Fig. 8.24). In noncalcified aortic aneurysms containing clot, ultrasound has an advantage over arteriography since arteriography may not detect the aneurysm because the radiopaque contrast material visualizes only the channel containing the moving column of blood. Since clot fills the aneurysm to the position of the moving column of blood, the aneurysmal dilatation may not be appreciated on arteriography.

Occasionally a flap of tissue moving within the aortic lumen synchronous with the heartbeat is detected (Fig. 8.25) which is indicative of an intimal dissection.

We have not been successful in delineating the relationship of the renal arteries to the aneurysm and, therefore, do not use ultrasound to determine whether the renal arteries are involved in the aneurysm. Occasionally the relationship of the SMA to the aneurysm can be seen, and if the aneurysm is large, the SMA may be displaced anteriorly.

B. Vena Cava

Caval pathology is much less common than aortic disease. Because the cava is a more pliable vascular structure than the aorta, adjacent focal mass lesions such as enlarged

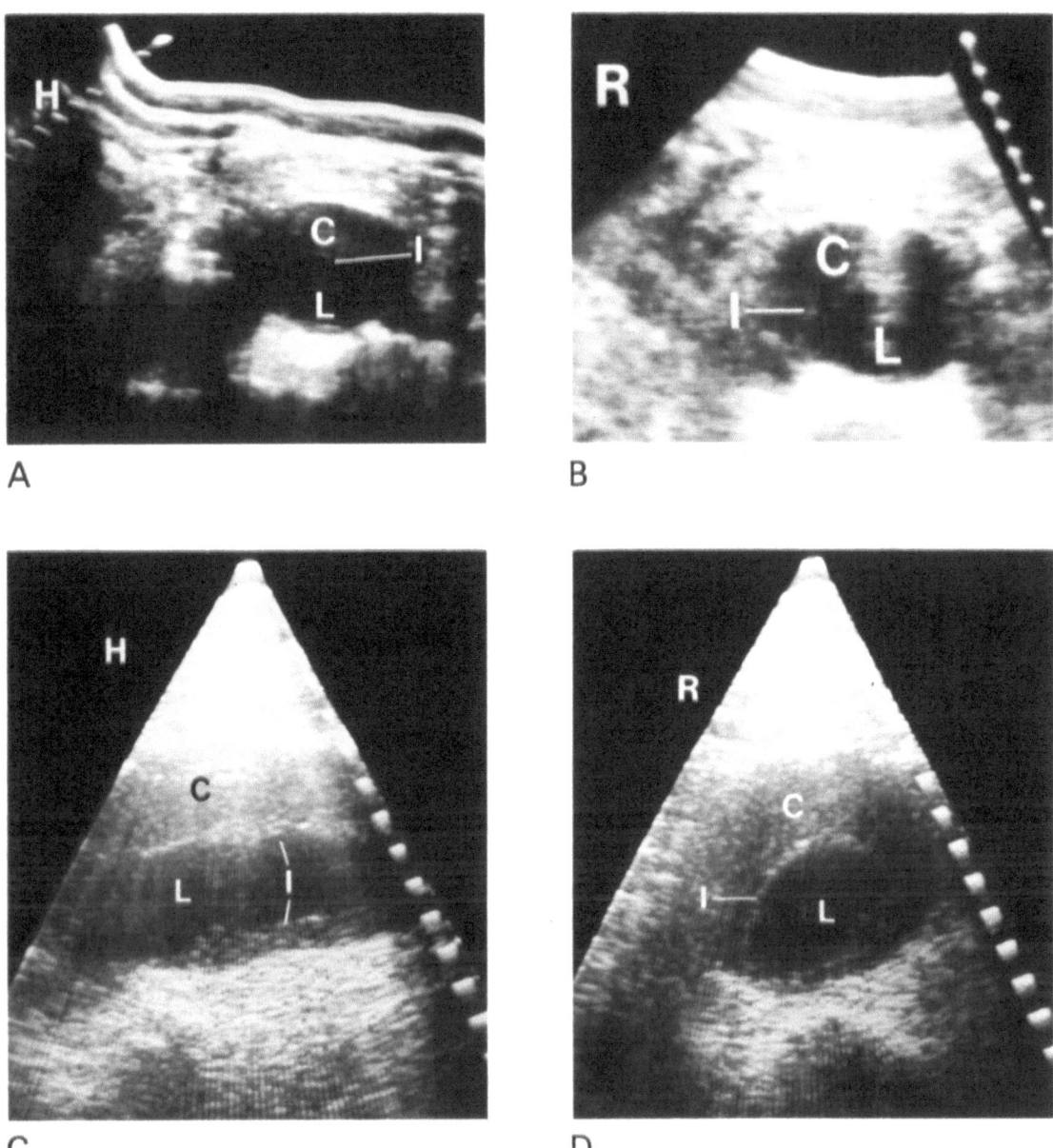

Fig. 8.22. Clot within aortic aneurysm. Echoes within clot (*C*) and interface (*I*) between clot and aortic lumen (*L*) are more clearly shown in real-time than in contact scans because a real-time transducer can be more readily positioned perpendicular to the blood-clot interface than can a contact scanner transducer. Contact scans in sagittal (**A**) and transverse (**B**) planes. Real-time scans in sagittal (**C**) and transverse (**D**) planes.

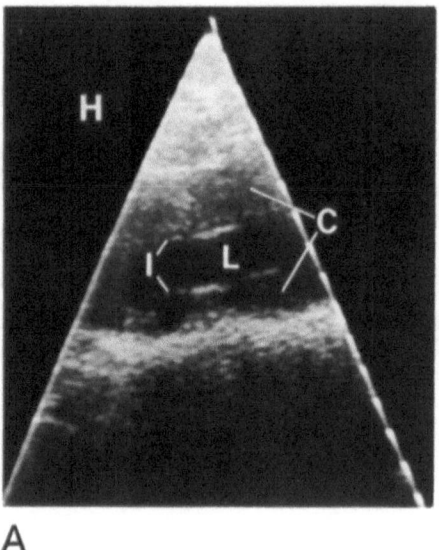

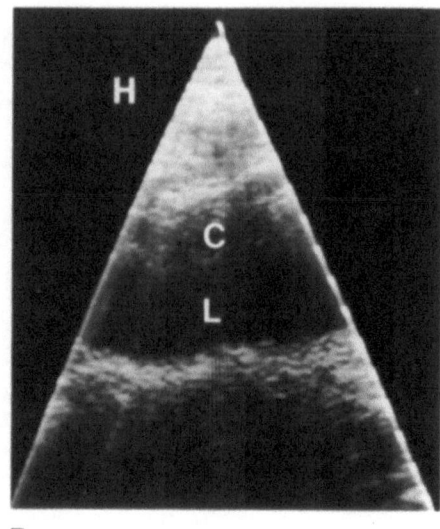

Fig. 8.23. As a result of minimal changes in the orientation of the ultrasound beam to the aorta, the interface between the clot and the lumen may be visualized (**A**) or not visualized (**B**). Same key as in Fig. 8.22.

nodes or an enlarged right adrenal gland (4) which lies just posterior to the cava can indent the wall and produce marginal distortions. Intraluminal mass lesions representing bland clot or metastatic tumor extensions from renal carcinoma can also be detected. In fact, whenever a solid mass lesion is detected within a kidney, especially within the right one, the cava should be carefully examined for intraluminal tumor extension (Fig. 4.24).

Pathologic changes in caval movement can also be appreciated which may suggest cardiac disease. A distended vena cava that shows no change with respiration in a patient who is not straining or suspending respiration suggests an abnormality such as right heart failure that impedes the return of blood to the right atrium (Fig. 5.16). On the other hand, gross insufficiency of the tricuspid valve may produce pulsatile movements of the caval wall that are synchronous with heart-beat rather than with respiratory movements.

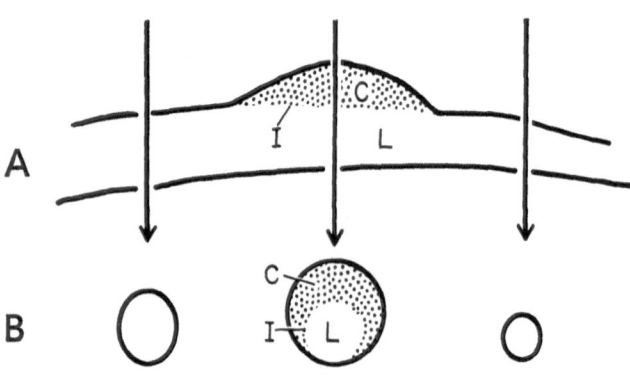

Fig. 8.24. Interface between clot and lumen usually appears in the position at which the aortic wall would have been if there had been no aneurysm. **A** Sagittal view. **B** Transverse views above, through, and below level of aneurysm. Same key as in Fig. 8.22.

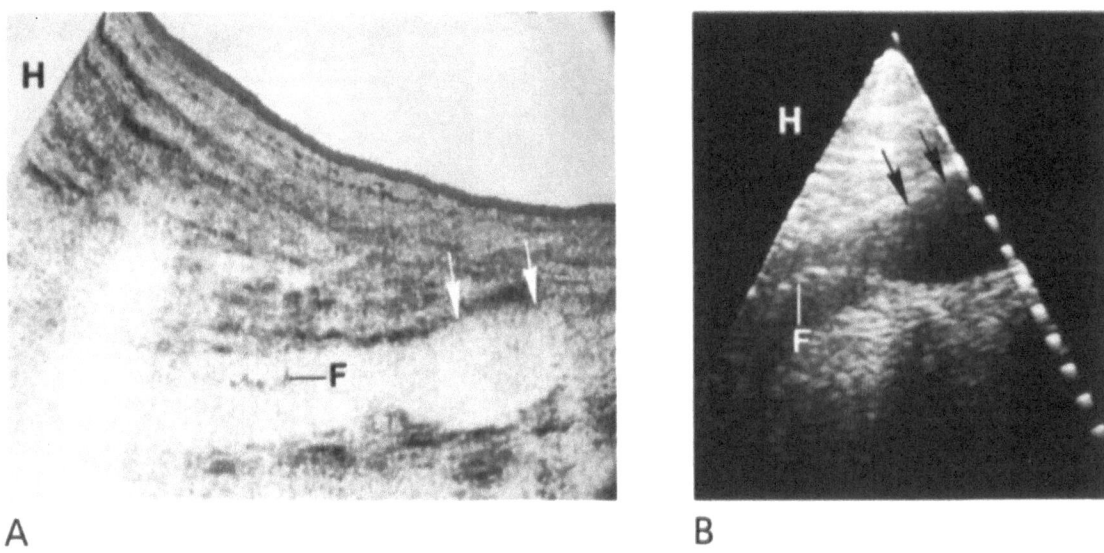

Fig. 8.25. Aortic dissection proximal to sacular aneurysm *(arrows)*. Sagittal view. **A** Contact scan. Intimal flap *(F)* oscillating within lumen. **B** Real-time scan.

C. Enlarged Paravascular Lymph Nodes

Since lymph nodes normally lie circumferentially around the aorta and the cava, when there is generalized enlargement of these nodal groups a circumvascular ring of solid tissue may be seen surrounding the aorta and cava (Fig. 8.26A and C). In sagittal view (Fig. 8.26A) the echo-free aorta is seen as two parallel lines surrounded by a zone of low reflective tissue comprising the enlarged nodes. On transverse scan (Fig. 8.26C) the aortic lumen appears like the hole within a doughnut, with the doughnut representing the enlarged nodes. Slight changes of ultrasound beam orientation can have a crucial effect in visualizing or not visualizing the interface between the nodes and aorta in a manner similar to that of detecting the interface between the aortic lumen and clot (Fig. 8.26B and D). Since the caval walls are soft, the enlarged paracaval nodes may collapse the cava so that its lumen may not be as well identified within the surrounding mantle of nodes as is the aortic lumen. In many cases there is not uniform enlargement

of all perivascular nodes but only focal nodal enlargement so the complete doughnut appearance is not seen (Figs. 8.27 and 8.28). The SMA may be anteriorly displaced from its normal position just anterior and parallel to the aorta by intervening enlarged nodes (Fig. 8.29). In our experience, the nodes anterior to the vessels are more frequently enlarged than those posterior and, in addition, anterior nodes are usually of greater size.

Prominent hypertrophic arthritic spurs that project anteriorly from vertebral bodies can anteriorly displace the aorta to produce a localized widening only of the retroaortic space which can be mistaken for enlarged retroaortic nodes. These spurs may lift the aorta several millimeters to a centimeter away from the vertebral column. Therefore, when the only suggested sign of enlarged paravertebral nodes is a widening of the retroaortic space, lateral lumbar vertebral films should be examined to see if hypertrophic spurs are present (5).

Enlarged paraaortic nodes are not the only cause of a soft tissue mass surrounding

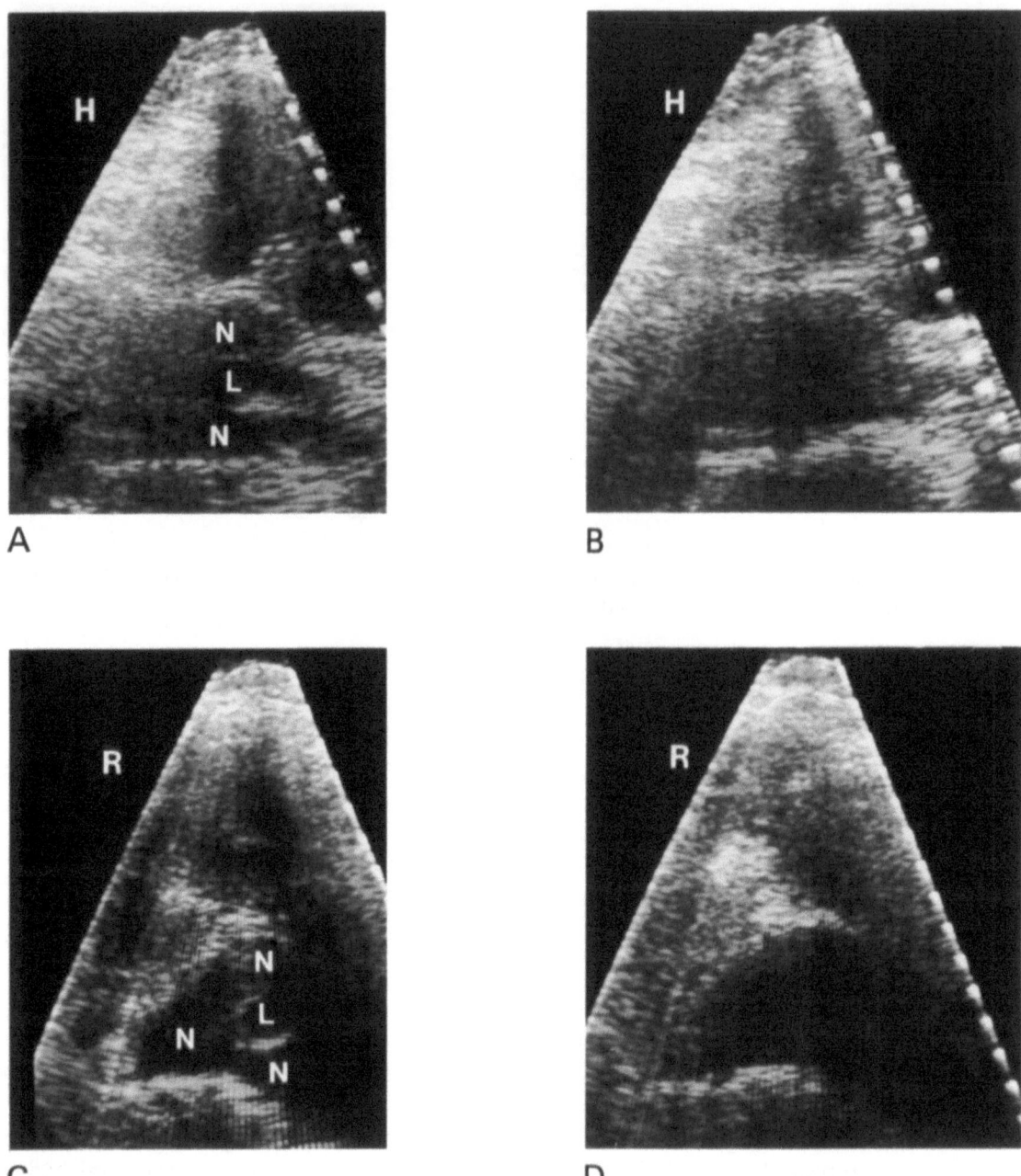

Fig. 8.26. Enlarged lymph nodes circumferentially encasing aorta. **A** and **B** Sagittal planes. **C** and **D** Transverse planes. Slight changes in orientation of the ultrasound beam result in visualization (**A** and **C**) or nonvisualization (**B** and **D**) of the interface between the nodes (*N*) and aortic lumen (*L*). The misdiagnosis of aortic aneurysm may be made if the interface is not detected (**B** and **D**).

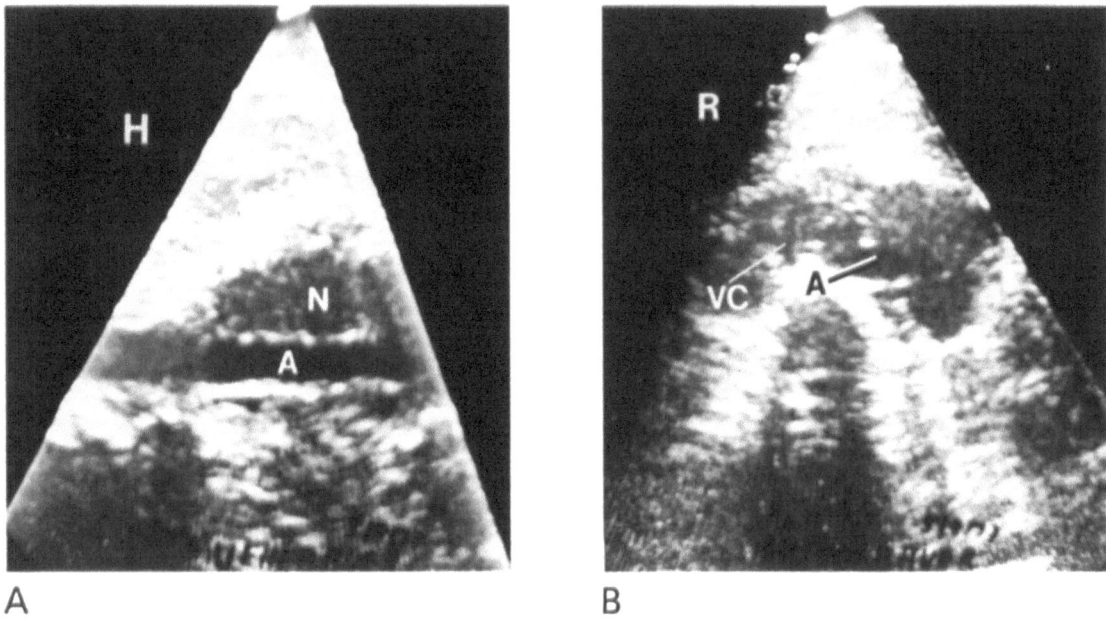

Fig. 8.27. Sagittal (**A**) and transverse (**B**) views of enlarged lymph nodes (*N*) located anterior and lateral but not posterior to the aorta (*A*) and vena cava (*VC*).

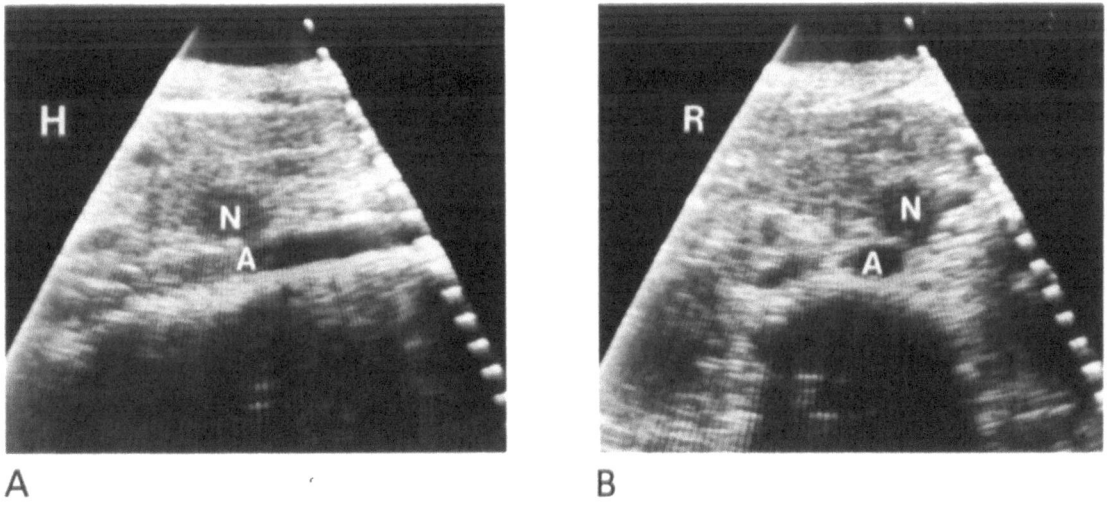

Fig. 8.28. Localized nodal (*N*) enlargement anterolateral to aorta (*A*). Sagittal (**A**) and transverse (**B**) scans.

the central vascular structures. Paravertebral hematoma as a result of a trauma or anticoagulant therapy and paravertebral abscesses can produce a similar picture. It may be very difficult to differentiate a perivascular mantle produced by enlarged lymph nodes from a hematoma or an abscess. Echo levels within enlarged nodes can be extremely low and at times these nodes can demonstrate zones of acoustic enhancement behind them similar to those seen in fluid collections (6).

Fluid- and food-filled small bowel can occasionally mimic a mantle of enlarged nodes anterior to the aorta. The two ways to differentiate bowel from nodal enlargements are by (1) observing peristalsis or change in caliber within the suspected loop of bowel and (2) demonstrating that the suspected bowel loop can change in anteroposterior diameter when greater pressure is applied by the transducer on the anterior abdominal wall (Fig. 3.12A). Solid perivascular masses will show neither of these changes.

Ultrasound Versus Lymphangiography

Although lymphangiography is more sensitive than ultrasound for detecting mildly enlarged paravertebral nodes and for detecting tumor foci within nonenlarged nodes, ultrasound has the advantages of (1) not requiring lymphatic cannulation and injection of contrast agents and (2) being able to visualize nodes that cannot usually be seen with lymphangiography. Such nodes are adjacent to the renal hilum, in the periportal areas, and root of the mesentery which are not routinely filled during pedal lymphangiography, but are appreciated by ultrasound when enlarged. On the other hand, both lymphangiography and computerized tomography scanning have the advantage over ultrasound of being able to more readily visualize enlarged nodes surrounding the iliac arteries since these regions are usually ultrasonically obscured by overlying gas-filled loops of bowel. Only when periiliac nodes become markedly enlarged and indent mar-

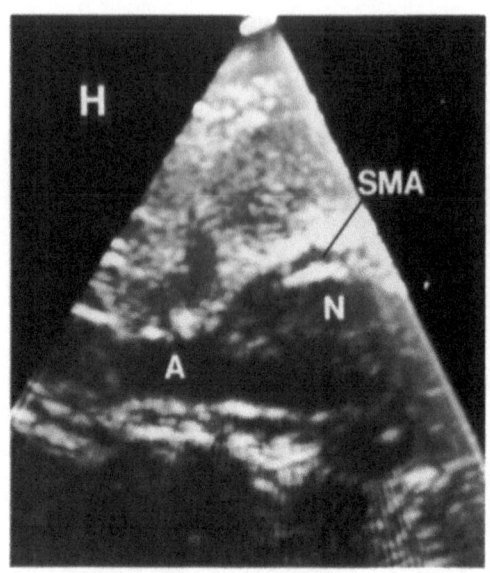

Fig. 8.29. Enlarged lymph nodes (*N*) displacing superior mesenteric artery (*SMA*) anteriorly. Sagittal scan. *A*, aorta.

gins of the bladder or produce a solid mass of tissue extending to the anterior abdominal wall can they be readily appreciated by ultrasound.

Besides being useful as a survey method for initially detecting enlarged perivascular nodes, ultrasound is valuable as a follow-up tool to determine change in nodal size after therapy.

D. Differentiating Enlarged Paravascular Nodes from Aortic Aneurysm

The main ultrasonic distinctions between enlarged nodes and aortic aneurysms relate to the size and shape of the mass and to a lesser extent to the strength of the interface (Fig. 8.30). The mass effect produced by enlarged nodes is usually not simply related to the aorta. It surrounds to a variable degree the vena cava as well, whereas the mass produced by the aneurysm is related only to the aorta. In addition, the outer surfaces of the nodal mass are often lobulated whereas

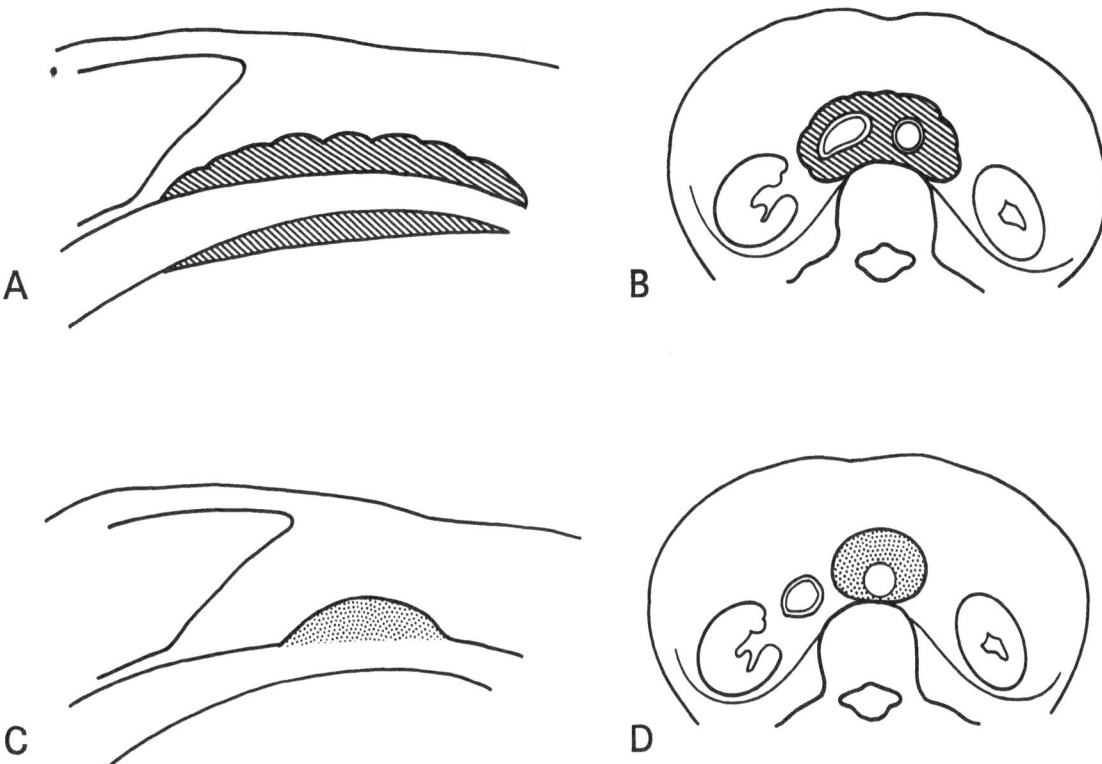

Fig. 8.30. Differentiating enlarged paraaortic lymph nodes from aortic aneurysm. **A** and **B** Enlarged nodes (*shaded*) typically have a lobulated anterior surface, may encase both aorta and vena cava and show a strongly reflective interface with the aorta. **C** and **D** An aortic aneurysm usually has a smooth convex anterior surface, does not involve retroperitoneal structures other than the aorta, and frequently has a weakly reflective interface between clot (*stippled*) and lumen.

those of an aneurysm are smooth. The intensity of the reflections at the interface between the mass and aortic lumen is a less reliable differential sign. In nodal enlargement the interface is often strongly reflective because it is produced by the aortic wall. In an aneurysm containing clot, the interface between the clot and aortic lumen is a weaker one because the acoustic differences between clot and normal liquid blood are slight. However, sometimes an interface between aneurysm and lumen can be strong, presumably because the clot has become organized and the acoustic mismatch between organized clot and blood in lumen is much greater than between soft clot and free blood.

References

1. Willi UV, Teele RL (1979) Hepatic arteries and the parallel-channel sign. J Clin Ultrasound 7:125–127
2. Ralls PW, Quinn MF, Boswell WD, Boger JC, Halls JM (1980) Sonographic anatomy of the hepatic artery. Scientific Exhibit, Space 175, 66th Scientific Assembly and Annual Meeting of the Radiological Society of North America, Dallas, Texas, November 16–21
3. Athey PA, Tamez L (1979) Lateral decubitus position for demonstration of the aortic bifurcation. J Clin Ultrasound 7:154–155
4. Bernardino ME, Libshitz HI, Green B, Goldstein HM (1978) Ultrasonic demonstration of inferior vena caval involvement with

right adrenal gland masses. J Clin Ultrasound 6:167–169

5. Spirt BA, Skolnick ML, Carsky EW, Ticen K (1974) Anterior displacement of the abdominal aorta: a radiographic and sonographic study. Radiology 111:399–403

6. Hillman JB, Haber K (1980) Echographic characteristics of malignant lymph nodes. J Clin Ultrasound 8:213–215

9
Intra- and Extraluminal Fluid

Intraluminal fluid collections are defined for the purposes of this chapter as fluid within bowel since the gallbladder and urinary tract are dealt with in separate chapters. Intraluminal fluid can be seen in both normal and abnormally dilated loops of bowel. Extraluminal fluid refers to fluid external to any hollow viscera, i.e., bowel, gallbladder, urinary bladder. This fluid can either be free within the abdominal cavity, i.e., ascites, or can be loculated in the intra- or extraperitoneal compartment, i.e., hematomas, seromas, abscesses, or lymphoceles. This chapter will discuss applications of real-time ultrasound imaging in the identification and differentiation of intraluminal from extraluminal fluid.

In the normal state fluid collections are present only intraluminally. There is one minor exception: the presence of a few cubic centimeters of extraluminal fluid in the cul-de-sac of some women during the midphase of their menstrual cycles (1). It is, therefore, important during the ultrasound imaging of the abdomen to differentiate intraluminal from extraluminal fluid since extraluminal fluid usually indicates a pathologic state.

1. INTRALUMINAL FLUID

The criteria for determining that the fluid is within bowel are as follows:

1) Detection of peristalsis by observing a change in the configuration of fluid-filled structure or movement of the intraluminal content, or both (Fig. 9.1). Usually the intraluminal fluid is not pure fluid, but a combination of partially digested food mixed with fluid. During peristalsis the particulate material within the fluid moves and demonstrates a changing pattern of echoes.

2) Demonstration of a change in the appearance of the fluid collection by the introduction of fluid or air either orally or rectally, depending upon which region of the intestine is being examined. If the fluid-filled cavity is stomach or duodenum, ingestion of water will produce a sudden change in its appearance because the water entering the bowel churns the intraluminal contents and changes the acoustic echoes (Fig. 9.2). In addition, the swallowed water usually contains gas which produces a varying pattern of acoustic shadows intermixed with fluid. In the pelvis, fluid-filled rectosigmoid can be differentiated from a pathologic retrovesical fluid-filled structure by using a water enema (Fig. 9.3) (2). After preliminary scans of the pelvis are obtained through the full bladder,

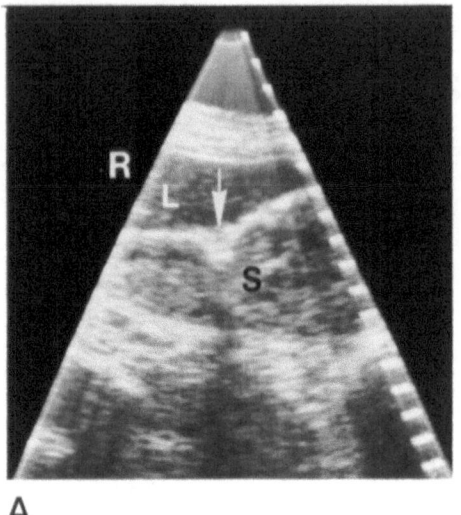 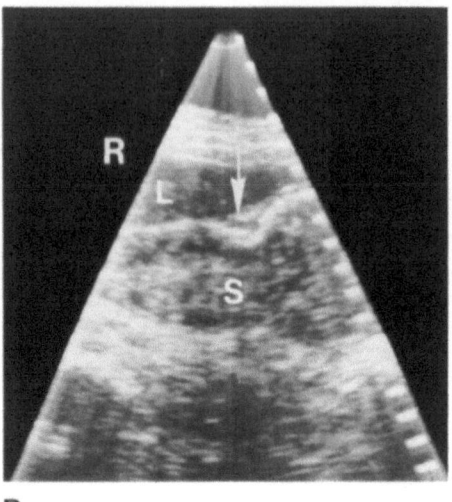

Fig. 9.1. Peristalsis in food-filled stomach (*S*). Note change in shape of anterior wall (*arrow*) between images **A** and **B** taken several seconds apart. Transverse scans. *L,* liver.

a tap water enema is given to the patient while the bladder is still distended. As the enema fluid enters the rectum, the operator scans the pelvis to observe filling of the rectum and sigmoid. The water can be appreciated by observing distention of the bowel and by seeing stool moving within the lumen. In this manner, the mass in question seen on the preenema scans is identified as bowel (because it changes in appearance) or as a mass (because it remains unchanged following the enema). This mass must then be further characterized by size, shape, and echo pattern as a normal organ or pathologic structure. Since only enough water to fill the rectosigmoid is used, the procedure is

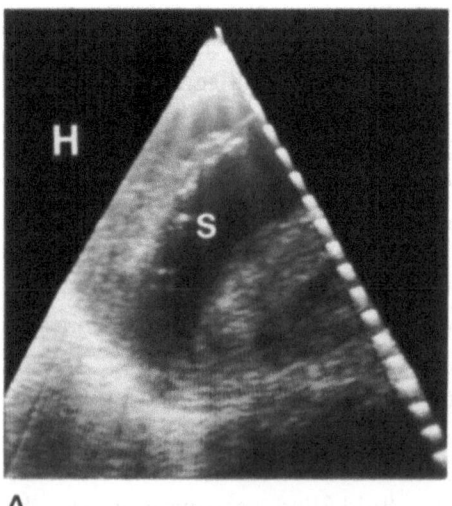 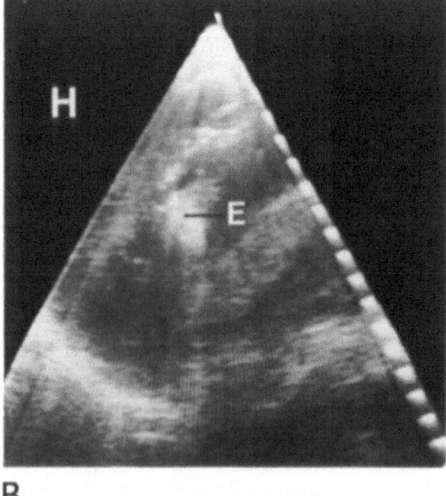

Fig. 9.2. Effect of drinking water. **A** Sagittal view of fluid-filled stomach (*S*) prior to drinking. Stomach is echo free. **B** During drinking. Strong echoes (*E*) within stomach are produced by the entering water mixing with and disturbing the gastric contents.

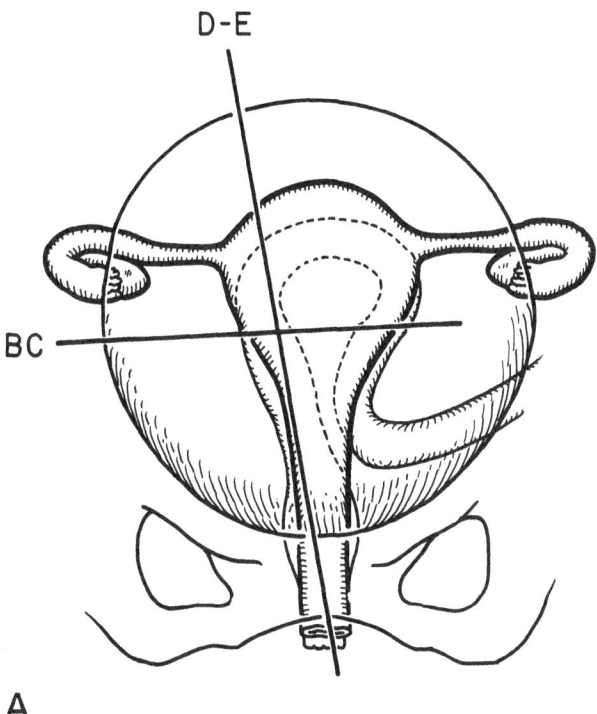

A

Fig. 9.3. Water enema for differentiating rectosigmoid from pelvis mass. **A** Superimposition of bladder and uterus over rectosigmoid. **B** and **C** Transverse scans through uterus before and after water enema. Questionable mass (*M*) on preenema image was shown to be sigmoid (*SIG*) on postenema image. **D** and **E** Sagittal scans through uterus before and after enema to show relationship of rectosigmoid to uterus. Mass not seen on this sagittal preenema image. *R*, rectum; *B*, bladder; *U*, uterus; *O*, ovaries. (Figure continued on page 194)

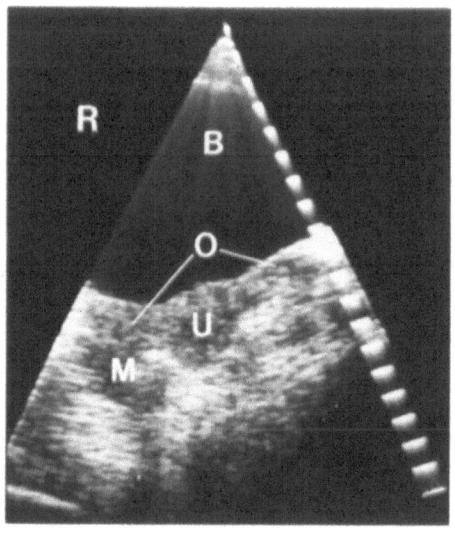

B

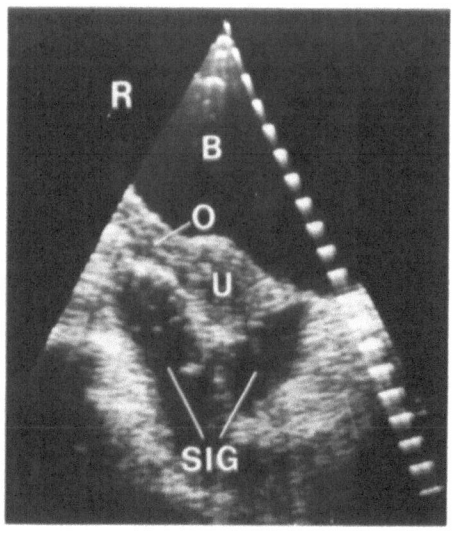

C

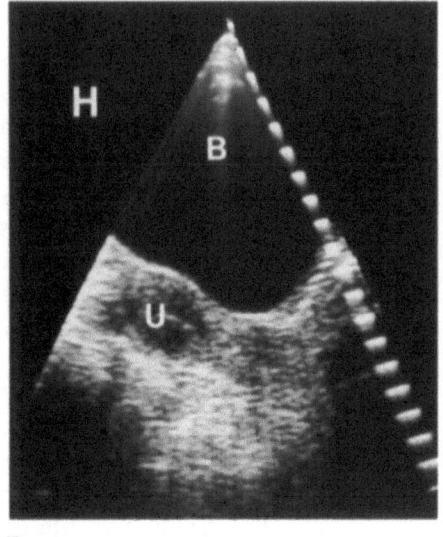

D

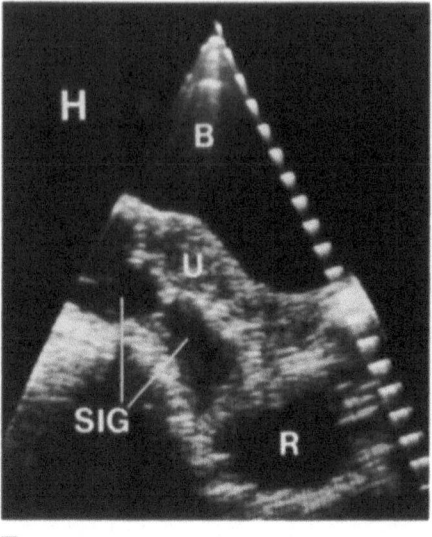

E

Fig. 9.3. (cont.)

well tolerated by the patient. No prior bowel preparation is required. The presence of gas or stool in the colon does not detract from the water enema technique. This technique, however, should not be utilized in any patient in whom an enema is contraindicated.

3) Identification of mucosal folds marginating the fluid-filled structure. Large rugae can be appreciated within the stomach (Fig. 9.4), valvulae conniventes may be seen

in small bowel, and haustral markings noted in colon. However, the internal architecture of the small and large bowel is best appreciated when they are dilated secondary to ileus or obstruction (Fig. 9.5) (3). The gastric antrum, in addition, often has a multi-layered appearance consisting of an inner layer of high level echoes followed by an intermediate layer of low level echoes and an outer layer of high level echoes. These lay-

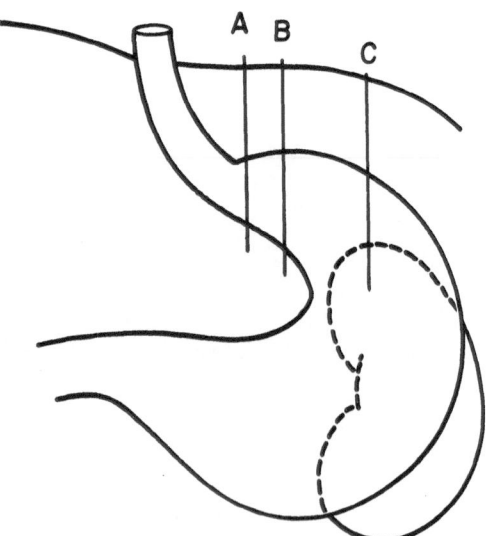

Fig. 9.4. Serial left parasagittal scans through fundus and body of stomach along planes *A, B, C. R,* gastric rugae; *D,* diaphragm; *K,* left kidney.

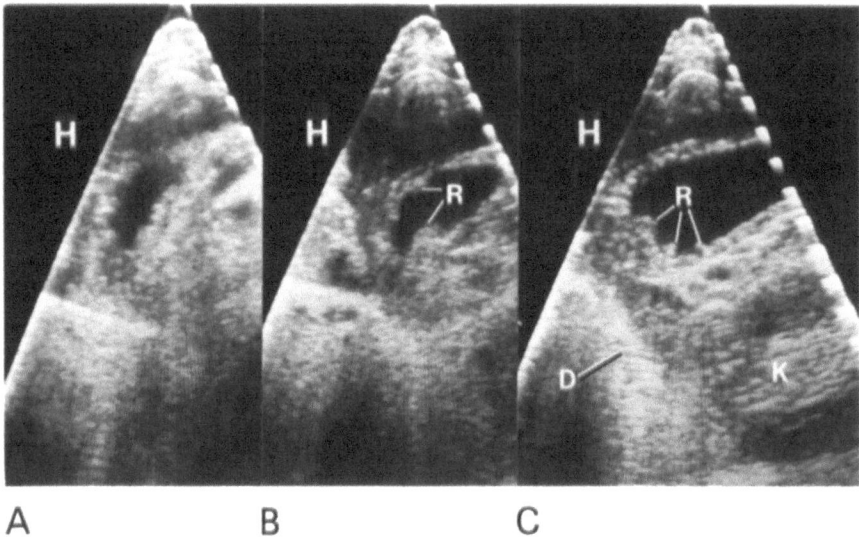

A   B   C

Fig. 9.4. (cont.)

ers presumably represent the mucosa, muscularis, and serosa. In long axis view the stomach appears as a multilayered sandwich, whereas in short axis view the appearance is that of a series of rings of different acoustic intensity representing these three different regions (Fig. 9.6). The pattern is most frequently seen in the antral region.

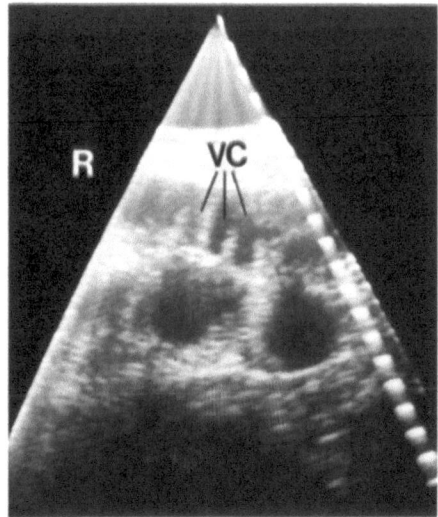

Fig. 9.5. Valvulae conniventes (*VC*) in dilated loop of small intestine. Transverse scan.

2. EXTRALUMINAL FLUID: INTRAPERITONEAL

In our experience the two regions for detecting the smallest quantities of intraabdominal fluid have been (1) between the inferior surface of the liver and right kidney (Morison's pouch) (Fig. 9.7A and B) and (2) in the retrovesical space. As larger amounts of fluid accumulate, the fluid fills the paracolic gutters and partially surrounds the liver, gallbladder, spleen, bowel, and uterus (Figs. 9.8 and 9.9).

Our findings are in accord with the views of Meyers (4) on the movement and accumulation of intraabdominal fluid. Although fluid would be expected to first accumulate in the most dependent part of the peritoneal cavity (retrovesical pouch) because of gravity, fluid may preferentially seek the most dependent part of the right subhepatic space because intraabdominal pressure is reduced in the upper as compared to the lower abdomen as a result of expansive movements of the rib cage during inspiration.

Fine filaments may be seen in the ascitic fluid which connect between solid organs, loops of bowel, mesentery, and peritoneal surfaces. In our experience and in that of

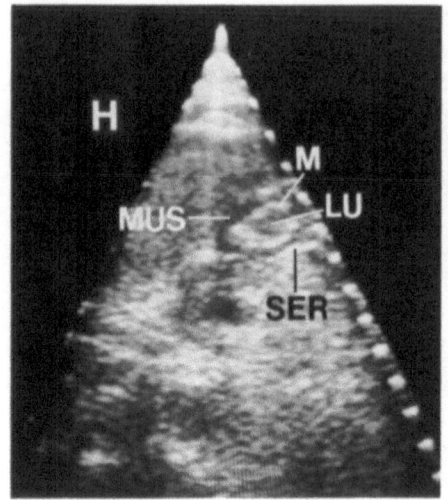

A

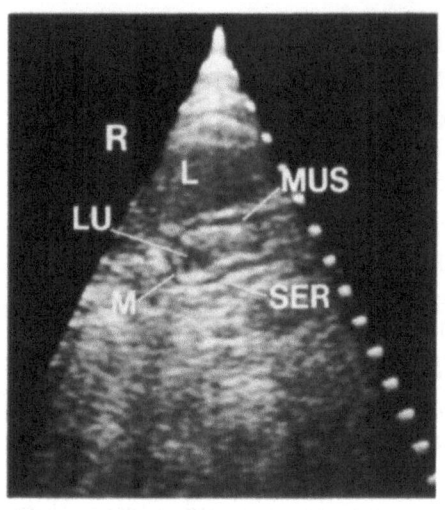

B

Fig. 9.6. Gastric antrum in sagittal (**A**) and transverse (**B**) views. Lumen (*LU*) with minimal contents. *M,* mucosal layer. Low level zone presumed to be muscle layer (*MUS*). Outer strongly reflective layer presumed to be serosa (*SER*). *L,* liver.

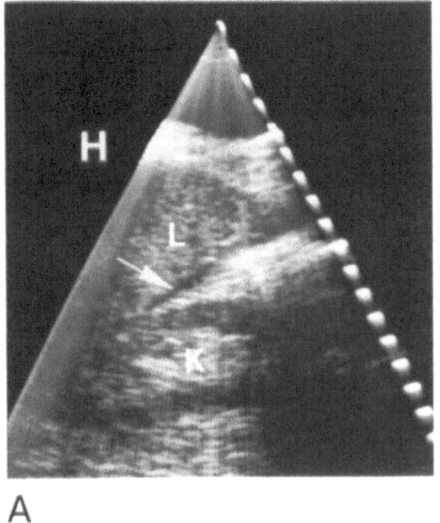

A

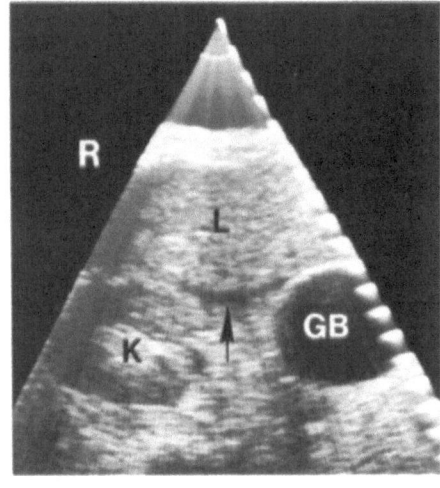

B

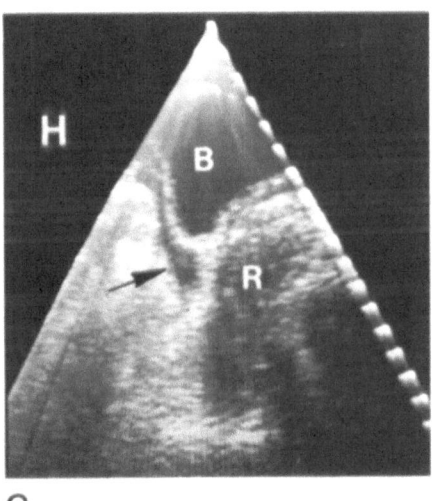

C

Fig. 9.7. Locations for identifying minimal accumulations of ascites (*arrow*) are (1) between liver (*L*) and right kidney (*K*) in sagittal (**A**) and transverse (**B**) scans; and (2) in retrovesical pouch (*arrow*) on sagittal scan (**C**). Fluid and stool are present in distended rectum (*R*) from recent enema. *B,* urinary bladder; *GB,* gallbladder.

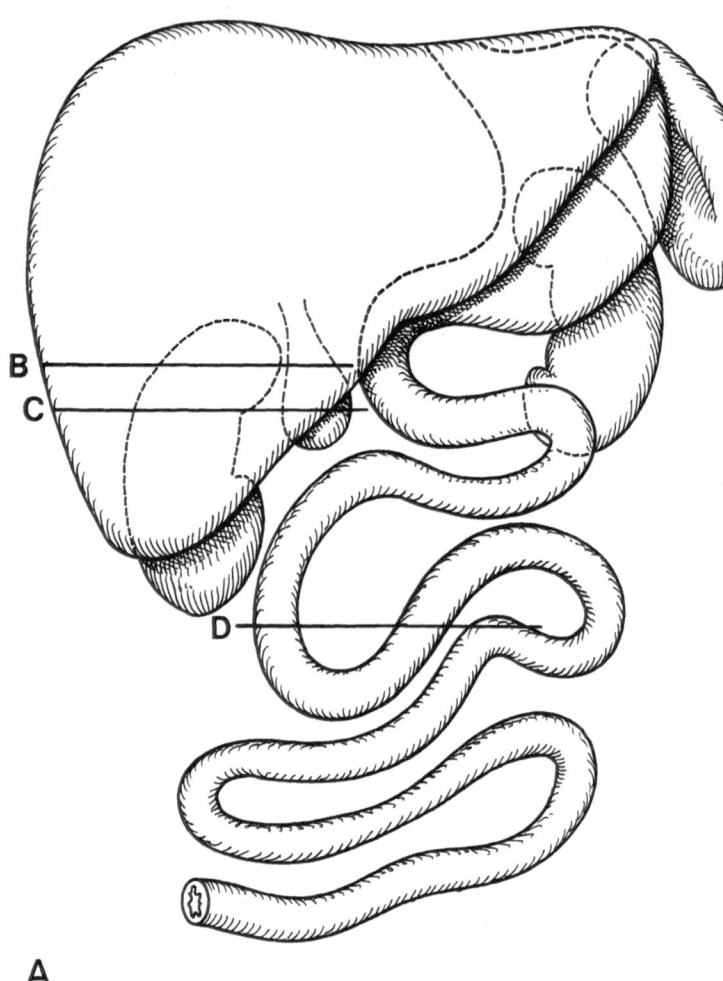

Fig. 9.8. Ascites (*AC*) surrounding intraabdominal organs. Position of images in transverse planes (**B–D**) and sagittal planes (**F-F′–H-H′**) are defined in sketches **A** and **E**. *L*, liver; *GB*, gallbladder; *M*, mesentery; *B*, bowel loop; *K*, right kidney. (Figure continued on pages 199, 200)

A

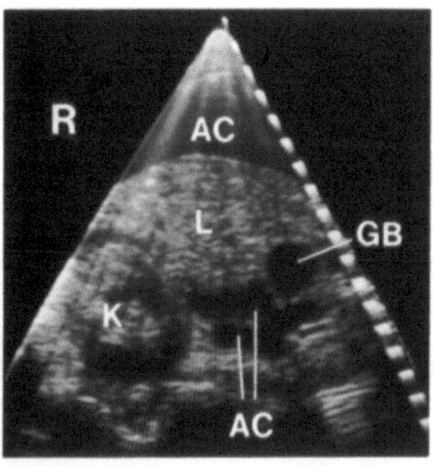

B

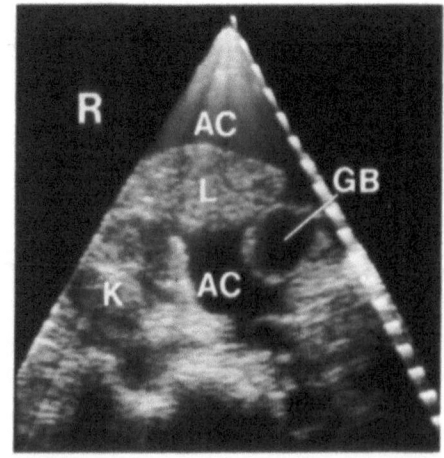

C

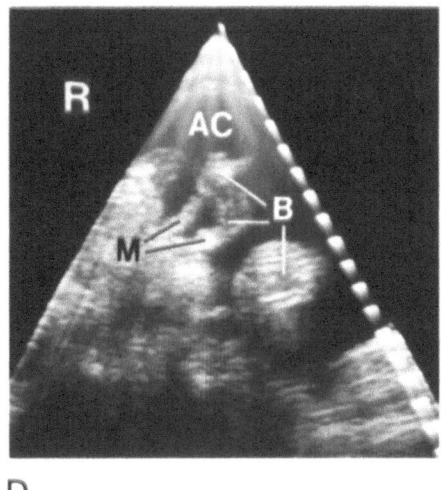

D

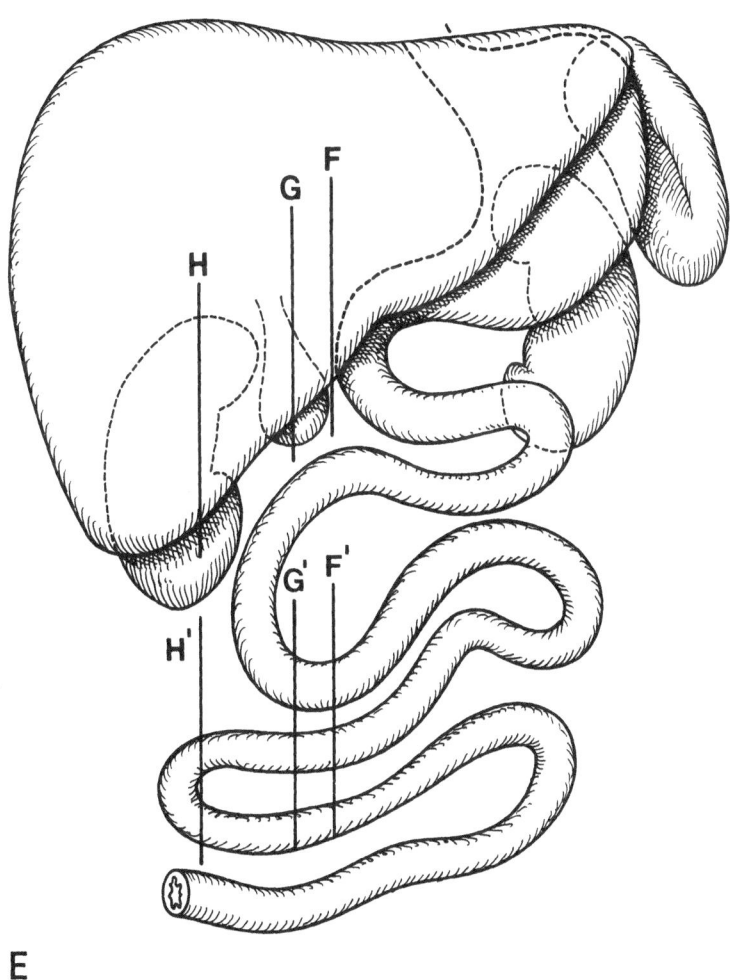

E

Fig. 9.8. (cont.)

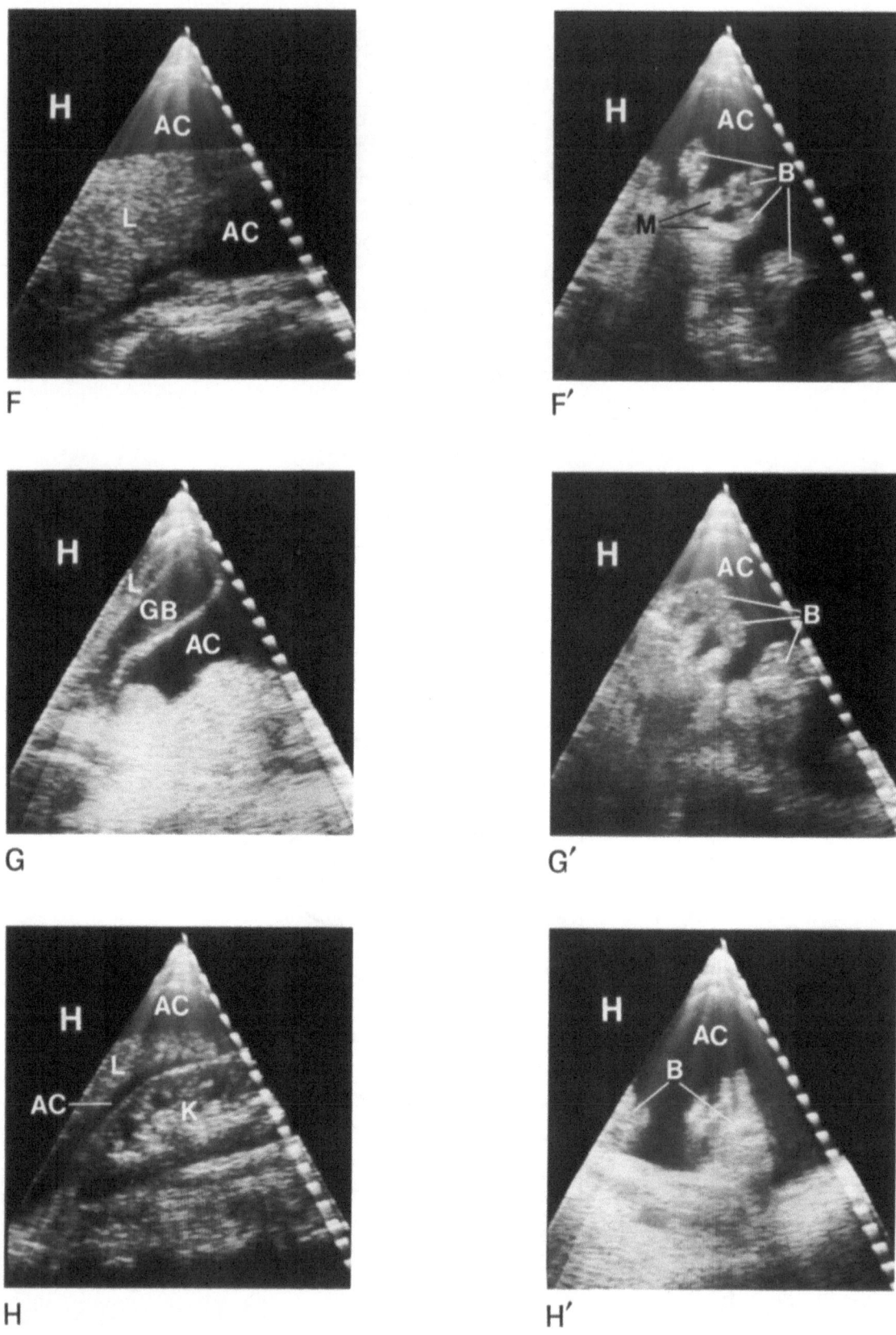

Fig. 9.8. (cont.)

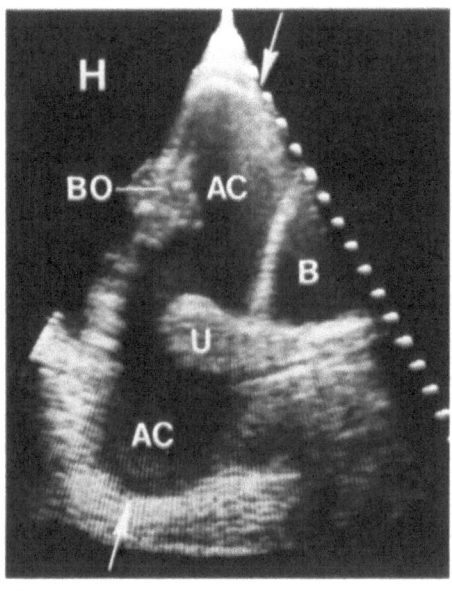
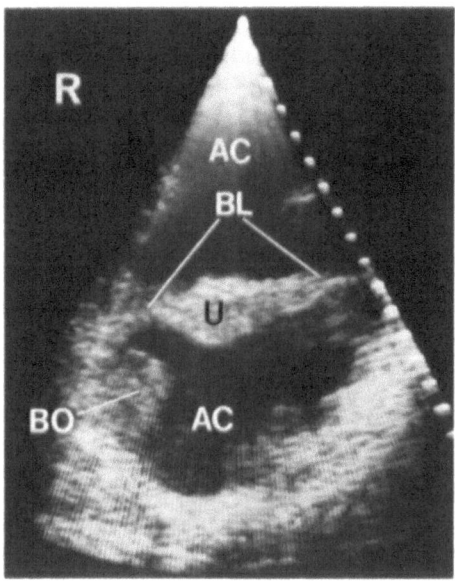

A   B

Fig. 9.9. Ascitic fluid (*AC*) in pelvis outlining uterus (*U*) and broad ligament (*BL*) and delineating superior surface of bladder wall. *B,* bladder cavity; *BO,* collapsed bowel. Sagittal (**A**) and transverse (**B**) scans. *Arrows* indicate plane through sagittal scan at which transverse scan was made.

Edell and Gefter (5), who reported upon 65 cases of proven ascites, both exudative and transudative, such filaments are only seen in peritonitis. These filaments are believed to represent fibrin strands and they may show undulating movements during observation over several seconds (Fig. 9.10). Their motion is probably caused by respiration-

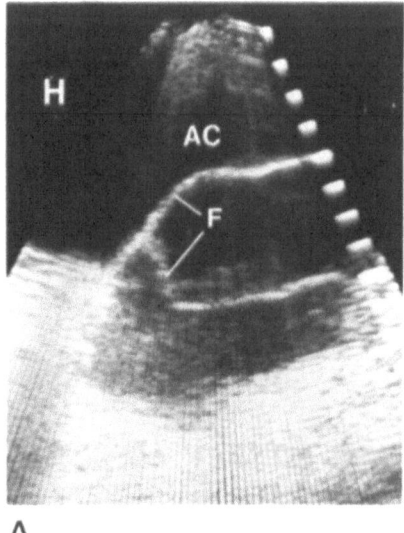
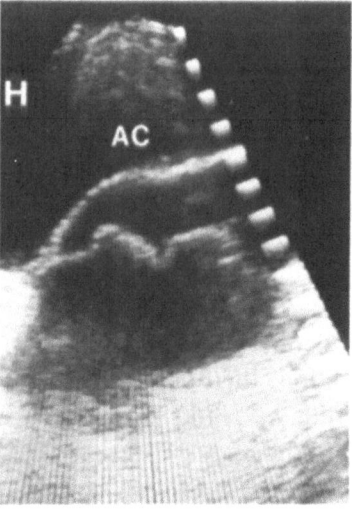

A   B

Fig. 9.10. Filamentous strands (*F*) floating within exudative ascites (*AC*) which rapidly change configuration. Images **A** and **B** are taken a few seconds apart. Patient has bacterial peritonitis.

induced fluid waves within the ascites.

Free intraabdominal fluid may be differentiated from loculated fluid if a shift in the fluid can be demonstrated as the patient is changed from supine to decubitus or erect position. However, this technique does not always prove successful.

In paralytic ileus dilated fluid-filled bowel may be confused with extraluminal fluid if the bowel walls and contents show no change over time and valvulae conniventes or haustral markings are not identified. On occasion an extraluminal fluid collection such as a large abscess can be confused with a loop of fluid-filled bowel because peristalsis of the bowel wall adjacent to the abscess may induce a movement of the particulate material within the abscess.

Sometimes it is difficult to differentiate an extraluminal fluid collection from a normal fluid-filled viscus such as the gallbladder or urinary bladder. To help make this differential diagnosis, it is first important to know whether the gallbladder or urinary bladder is in fact present. A hematoma or collection of bile in the gallbladder bed following cholecystectomy can assume the shape of a normal gallbladder. If the examiner is not aware that the patient had a recent cholecystectomy, this fluid can be confused with the normal gallbladder (6). It is also useful to attempt to change the amount of fluid in the normal urinary bladder or gallbladder by either causing it to empty or to fill so as to distinguish the bladder from a pathologic fluid collection. This technique is especially useful in differentiating the urinary bladder from ascites in the pelvis. The patient should always be examined with a full bladder. If there is a retrovesical fluid collection, then one will see two collections of fluid, i.e., fluid in the bladder and fluid behind the bladder (Fig. 9.9).

If the bladder does not have enough fluid in it to aid in definitive identification, and if it cannot be filled further, one can usually identify a pelvic fluid collection as extravesical by its distinctive shape. The contours of the extraluminal fluid do not form a smooth arcuate margin as does the bladder. Instead the contours have localized concavities where loops of bowel or the uterus project into the fluid (Fig. 9.9A). Sharp angles can be seen in the contours of the fluid when it flows under loops of bowel or in the retrovesical cul-de-sac.

Intraabdominal fluid collections may be multiple rather than singular. In such cases, it is important to distinguish normal fluid-filled structures—intestines, gallbladder, or urinary bladder—from pathologic fluid collections. It is helpful to rescan the patient after voiding or after a brief interval to see if the fluid collection has changed size. However, adynamic loops of fluid-filled bowel may mimic loculated extraluminal fluid collections.

Although ultrasound can usually differentiate an extraluminal from an intraluminal fluid collection, it cannot determine whether the fluid is infected or sterile. In a postoperative patient sunspected of having intraabdominal abscesses, a loculated fluid collection can represent an abscess as well as a hematoma, seroma, or other sterile fluid collection. The differential diagnosis can then be made by using ultrasonic guidance to percutaneously puncture each of the fluid-filled cavities with a fine needle and aspirate a sample of the fluid. This technique is discussed in detail in Chapter 10. At times a loop of paralytic bowel may be mistaken for a pathologic fluid collection and percutaneously punctured. However, since the diameter of the aspirating needle is so fine (22 gauge), the hole through the bowel wall seals itself when the needle is removed.

3. INTRAPERITONEAL ABSCESSES

Patients being examined for suspected intraabdominal abscesses should be studied in a logical manner. If the patient has had recent

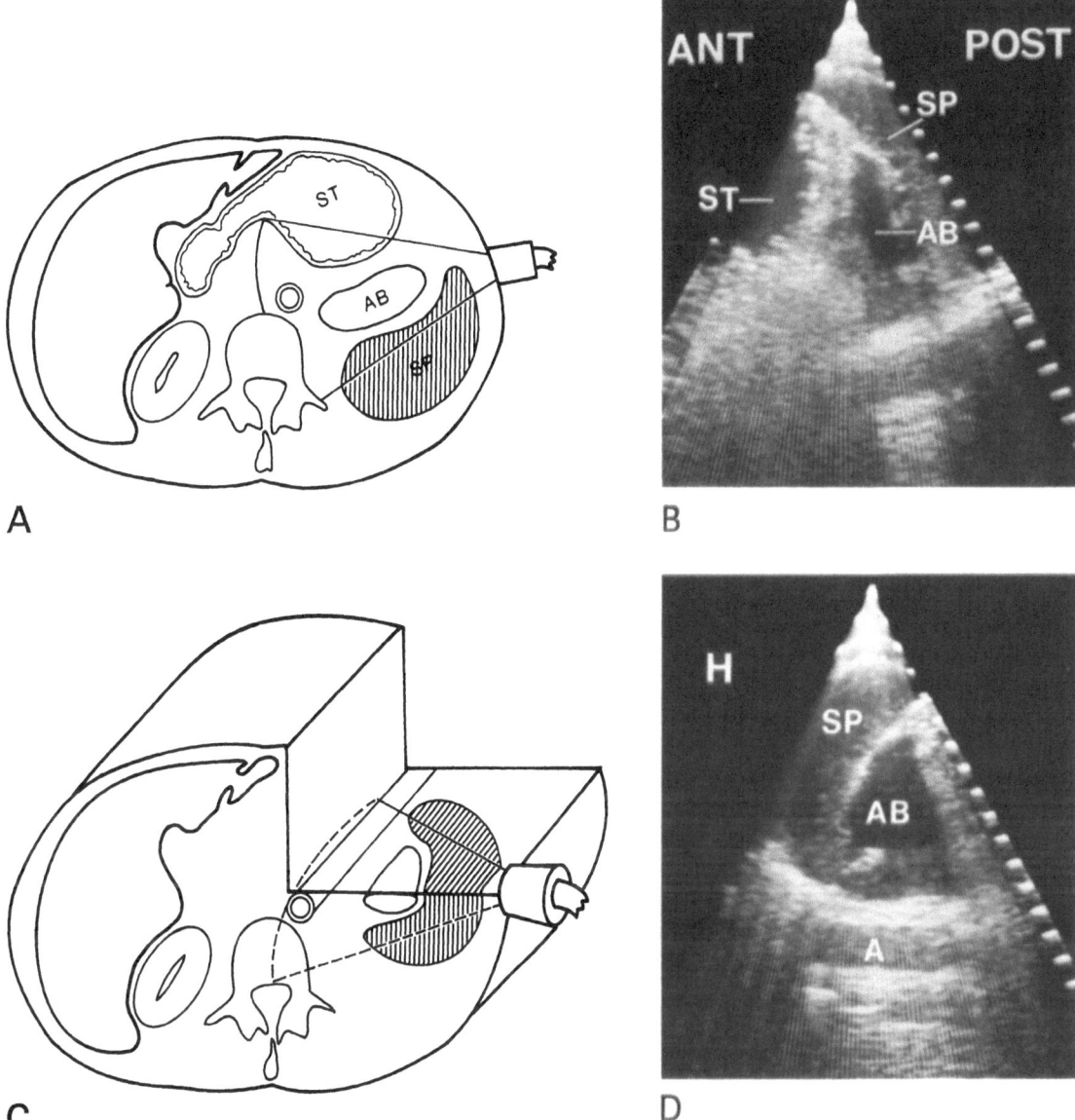

Fig. 9.11. Abscess (*AB*) between spleen (*SP*) and stomach (*ST*) resulting from leak at gastro-enterostomy anastomosis. Images are obtained in transverse (**A** and **B**) and coronal (**C** and **D**) planes by placing the transducer in a lower rib interspace along the mid-axillary line because gas-filled bowel prevents the visualization of abscess when the transducer is placed subcostally or intercostally on the anterior skin surface. *A*, aorta; *ANT*, anterior; *POST*, posterior.

surgery, then the regions around the surgical incision and drainage tubes should be carefully imaged. Next the region overlying the organ(s) that were operated upon should be examined. Lastly, the most common sites for fluid accumulation within the peritoneal cavity should be scanned—the subdiaphragmatic, subhepatic, and subsplenic (Fig. 9.11) spaces, the flanks, and the retrovesical regions. In addition, both lower pleural spaces should be examined because intraabdominal infection can induce pleural effusions which may not be clinically suspected. When examining regions around drainage tubes, the subcutaneous tissues and muscles superficial to the peritoneal cavities should be examined as well as intraperitoneal structures. With some of the sector type of real-time transducers, the first several centimeters of tissue cannot be accurately imaged because this is the area where the sector image converges to a point. With such instrumentation, an acoustic standoff, such as a water bag fabricated by filling a latex glove with water, should be interposed between the transducer and the skin so as to accurately image the superficial structures. A more preferable approach would be the use of a transducer that produces a trapezoid field display or of a linear array that can clearly image near field regions. Otherwise, abscesses and hematomas in the abdominal wall adjacent to the incisions can be missed.

The presence of a large open wound that is secondarily healing does not prevent ultrasonic imaging of tissues directly below the wound. Although it is not advisable to put acoustic gels or oil on the surface of the wound, one can fill the wound cavity with sterile normal saline and then successfully image structures deep to the wound by placing a sterilized transducer gently within the saline. In this manner, the transducer does not press on the wound to cause the patient discomfort. Most transducers can be sterilized either by ethylene oxide gas or cold chemicals. However, one should always first check with the manufacturer of the specific instrument to determine the recommended sterilizing procedures for that instrument.

When the patient presents with surgical dressings covering portions of the abdomen, these dressings should be removed in order to be able to scan as wide an area of the abdomen as possible. If a portion of dressing cannot be removed, or the patient has an ostomy bag that is glued to his skin, then regions deep to these structures can usually be satisfactorily imaged by placing the transducer around the margins of the dressing or bag and angling the beam to the deeper structures lying underneath the bag.

4. INTRA- VERSUS EXTRAPERITONEAL FLUID

The intraperitoneal location of fluid can be differentiated from retroperitoneal location when an intraperitoneal organ can be identified partially or completely surrounded by the fluid. For example, the detection of fluid marginating the liver, surrounding the gallbladder, or in between mobile loops of bowel indicates that this fluid is intraperitoneal. By contrast, fluid can be identified as being retroperitoneal when it is adjacent to organs within the retroperitoneal compartment. We have frequently seen such collections representing hematomas and lymphoceles around renal transplants located within the pelvis (Figs. 4.31 and 4.32).

The shape of the collection may also suggest that the collection is extraperitoneal. For example, extraperitoneal fluid collections in certain locations typically have a distinctive appearance because of the anatomy of the structures surrounding the fluid. A hematoma in the rectus sheath presents as a fusiform echo-free structure bulging into the peritoneal cavity from the under surface of the rectus muscle since the hematoma is confined by the shape of the rectus sheath.

5. PERICARDIAL AND PLEURAL EFFUSIONS

Since the heart and lung bases are frequently seen as part of the routine imaging of the upper abdomen, fluid (often clinically unsuspected) in the pericardial and pleural spaces can be readily detected.

Fluid that is identified in the space bounded by the inferior vena cava, the right atrium, and the right hemidiaphragm can only be fluid in the pericardial space since the inferior vena cava above the diaphragm is completely within the mediastinum (Fig. 9.12) (7). The right pleural space does not form a border with the anterior surface of the inferior vena cava and thus a right pleural effusion cannot be confused with a pericardial effusion in this location. The best plane for detecting a pericardial effusion

around the right atrium is a right parasagittal one through the liver, diaphragm, inferior vena cava, and right atrium (Fig. 9.13). Once fluid is detected, one should determine if the fluid also surrounds the left ventricle by imaging the left side of the heart. For this purpose a left intercostal or subcostal approach is used (Fig. 9.14).

When normal air-filled lung is adjacent to the hemidiaphragm, no echoes are seen above the diaphragm (Fig. 9.15) because the sound is totally reflected at the lung-pleural interface. However, if fluid is present in the pleural space (between the lung and diaphragm), an echo-free space roughly triangular in shape is seen above the hemidiaphragm bounded by the lung superiorly, the parietal pleura anteriorly and posteriorly, and the diaphragm inferiorly (Figs. 9.16 and 9.17). The collapsed lung may be seen as a solid structure projecting into the pleural

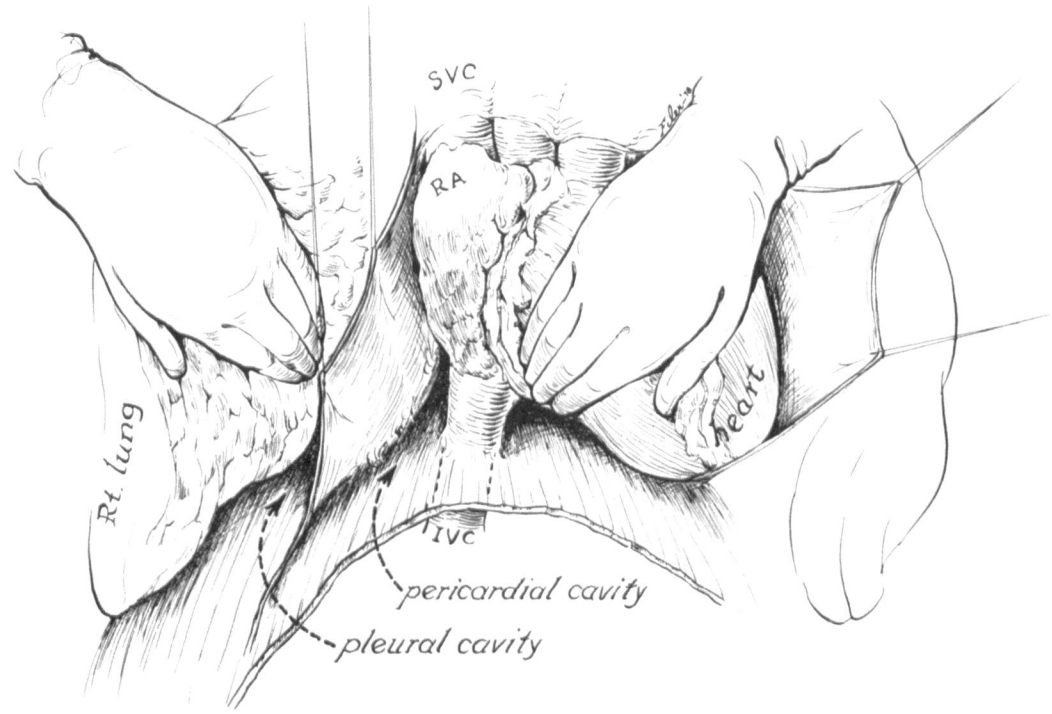

Fig. 9.12. Exposed view of mediastinum demonstrating that inferior vena cava (*IVC*) between right hemidiaphragm and right atrium (*RA*) is completely within the pericardial cavity. *SVC*, superior vena cava. (Reproduced by permission of Clinical Radiology; see ref 7 of this chapter.)

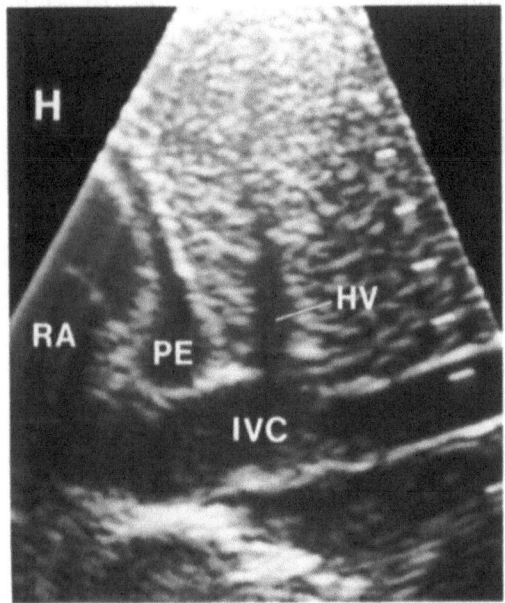

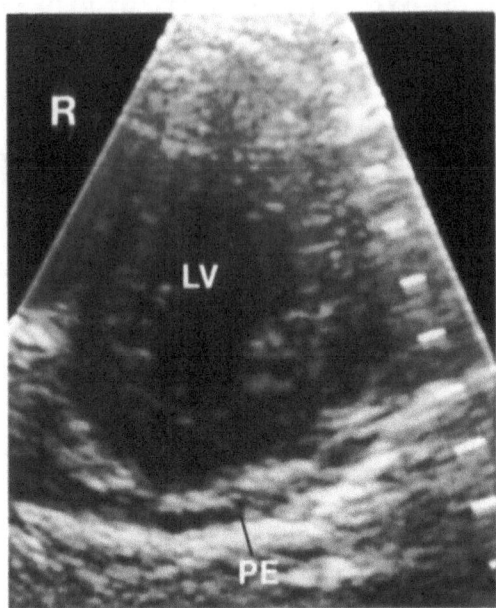

Fig. 9.13. Pericardial effusion (*PE*) between right atrium (*RA*) and diaphragm unexpectedly found during right parasagittal imaging of the superior part of the liver. *IVC*, inferior vena cava; *HV*, hepatic vein.

Fig. 9.14. Same patient as in Fig. 9.13. Pericardial fluid is also posterior to the left ventricle. Transverse scan through a left intercostal space.

fluid (Figs. 9.16C and D and 9.17). During breathing the lung may be seen moving in and out of the fluid. This latter observation is typical for fluid in the pleural space. The presence of an echo-free space separating visceral and parietal pleura can also be caused by coagulated serum or blood in the pleural cavity, and without evidence of lung moving within this space, fluid cannot be differentiated from such echo-free solid material.

Similar scanning planes are used to detect pleural effusions at either lung base. The preferred view is a long axis plane through the lung base, diaphragm, and liver or spleen. In this view fluid above the diaphragm can be more easily distinguished from subdiaphragmatic fluid than in transverse view. On both right and left sides the long axis

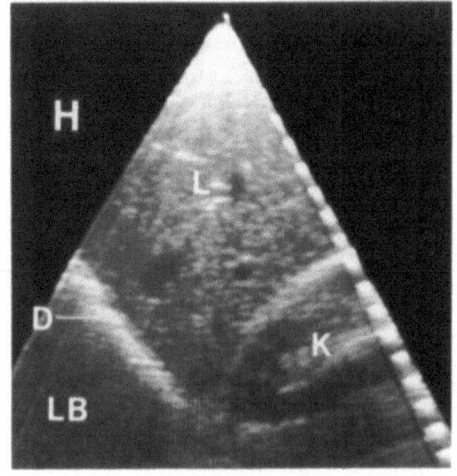

Fig. 9.15. Right parasagittal scan through normal lung base (*LB*), diaphragm (*D*), liver (*L*), and kidney (*K*). Sound does not penetrate through lung because it is air filled.

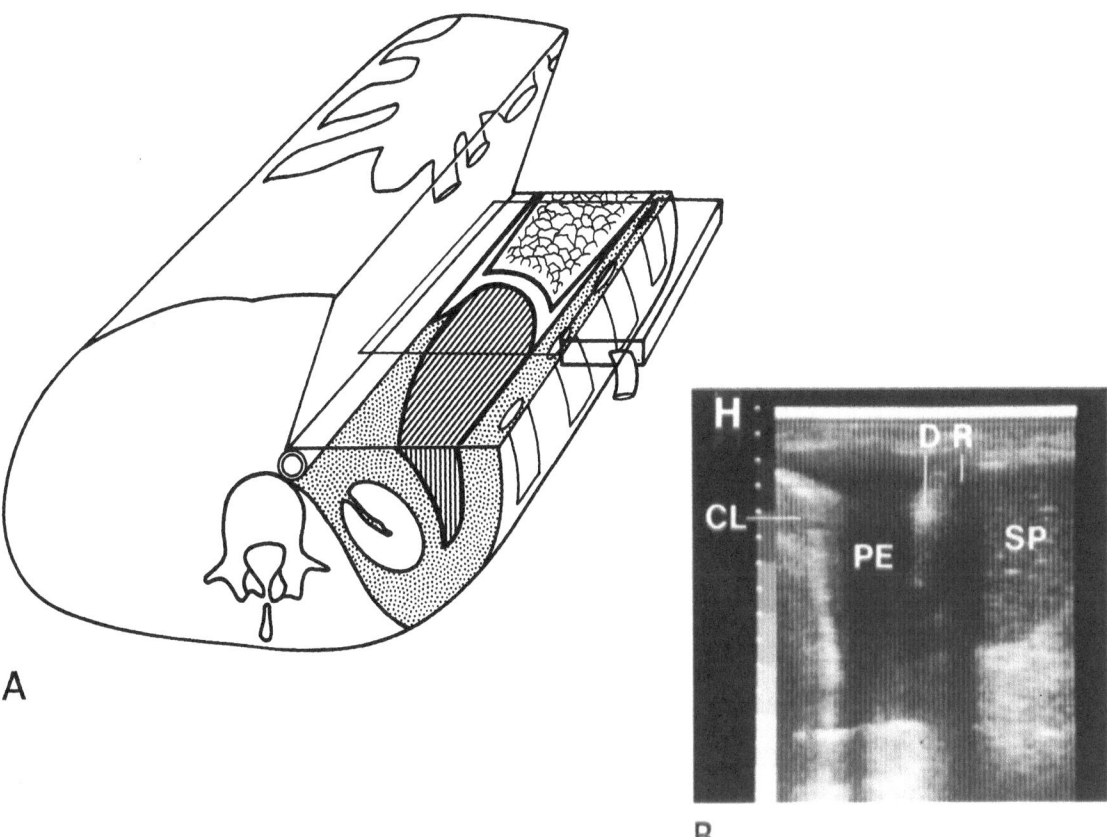

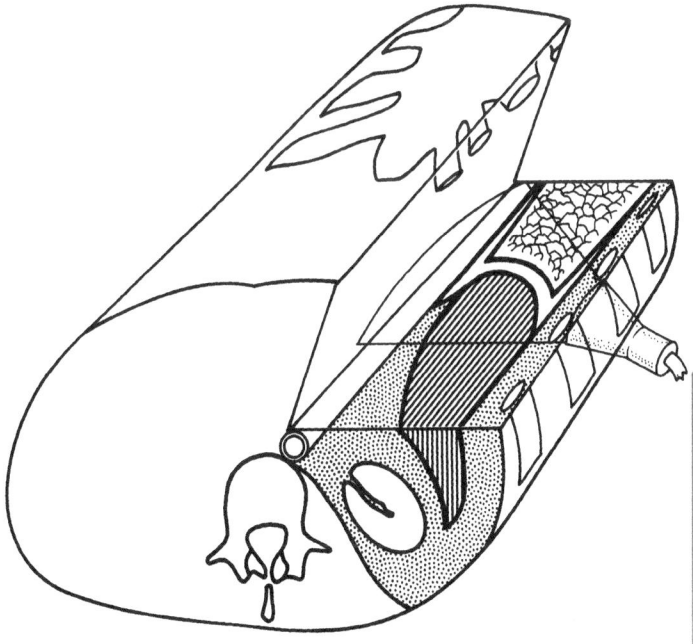

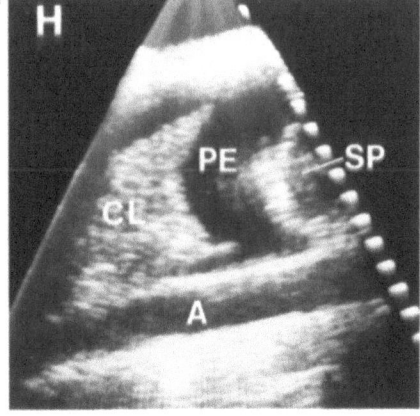

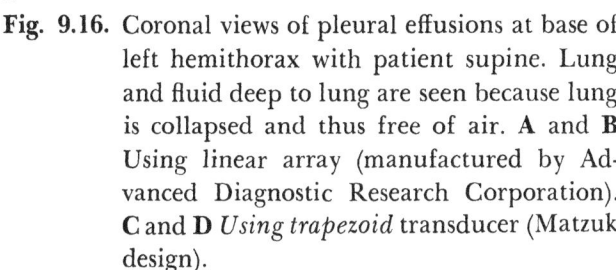

Fig. 9.16. Coronal views of pleural effusions at base of left hemithorax with patient supine. Lung and fluid deep to lung are seen because lung is collapsed and thus free of air. **A** and **B** Using linear array (manufactured by Advanced Diagnostic Research Corporation). **C** and **D** *Using trapezoid* transducer (Matzuk design).

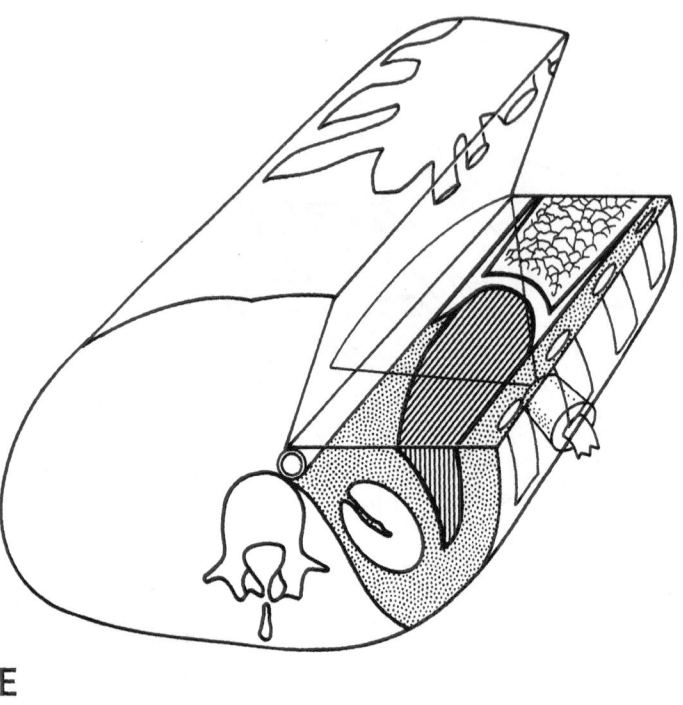

E

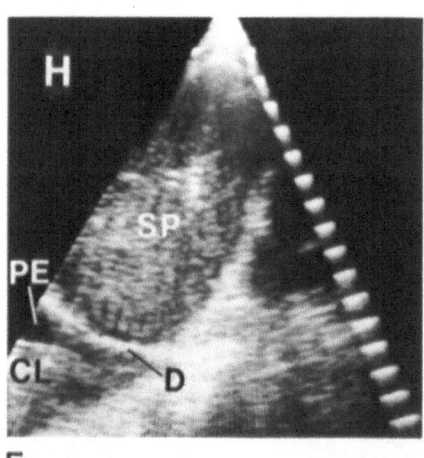

F

Fig. 9.16. (cont.) **E** and **F** Using sector transducer. Since near field is not adequately imaged with this instrument, beam was directed mainly through spleen so as to examine the inferior-medial recess of the pleural space. *PE*, pleural effusion; *CL*, collapsed lung; *SP*, spleen; *D*, diaphragm; *A*, aorta.

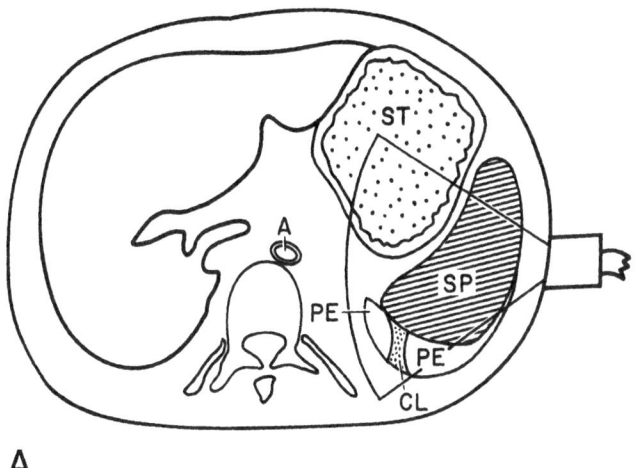

A

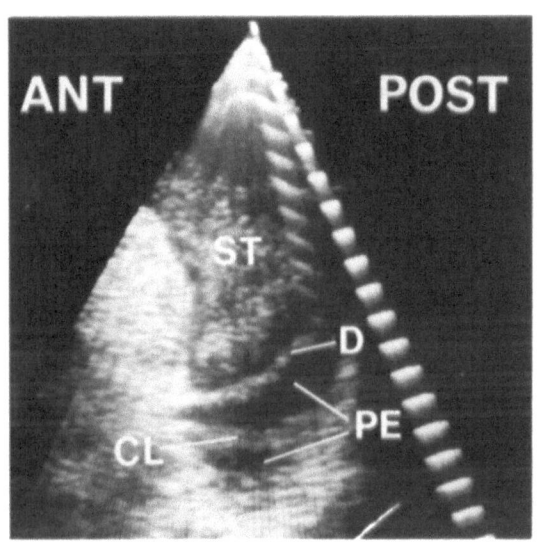

B

Fig. 9.17. A and **B** Transverse views of pleural effusion. Same patient as in Fig. 9.16 E and F. Transducer placed in an intercostal space along midaxillary line and rotated 90° from coronal plane. *ST*, stomach with echoes from ingested food; otherwise same key as in Fig. 9.16. *ANT*, anterior; *POST*, posterior.

plane can be obtained in the coronal section using either a small sector head placed between ribs or a larger format (linear array or trapezoid display) head spanning several ribs (Fig. 9.16B and D). In addition, a sagittal section can often be obtained on the right side by placing a sector format transducer head subcostally and directing the beam superiorly toward the right shoulder (Fig. 9.18). Other shaped heads are usually too large for subcostal approach. On the left side the sagittal scan cannot be obtained because the stomach, which is usually gas filled, is located in the subcostal region and prevents the ultrasound beam from reaching the diaphragm and pleural cavity.

Imaging in the transverse plane is most easily performed with a sector scanner head placed within an intercostal space. Pleural effusions are seen as a crescent-shaped fluid collection below the posterior surface of the liver (Fig. 9.17) or spleen. Large aperture heads (especially linear arrays) may be less effective because the curvature of the flanks can produce incomplete skin contact thereby reducing the width of the image (Fig. 2.16B).

It is important, however, to always confirm via long axis scans that fluid is pleural rather than intraabdominal in location. Ascites located below the liver or spleen can on transverse scans be confused with a pleural effusion (Fig. 9.19), especially if the dia-

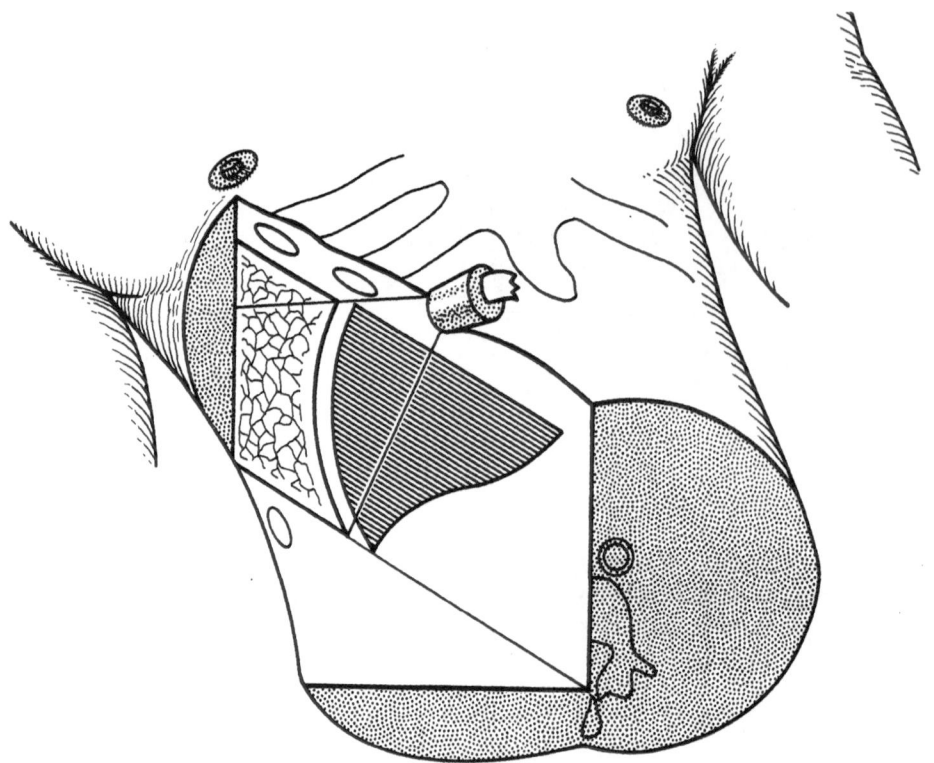

Fig. 9.18. Right subcostal approach to imaging right lower lung (*LU*) and pleural space (*P*) through liver (*L*).

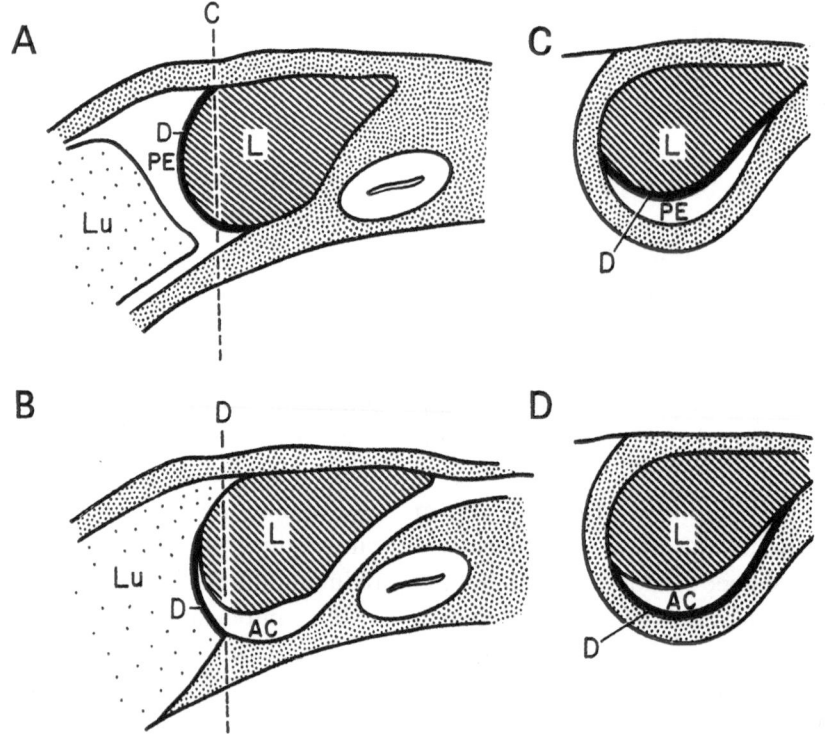

Fig. 9.19. (Legend on page 211.)

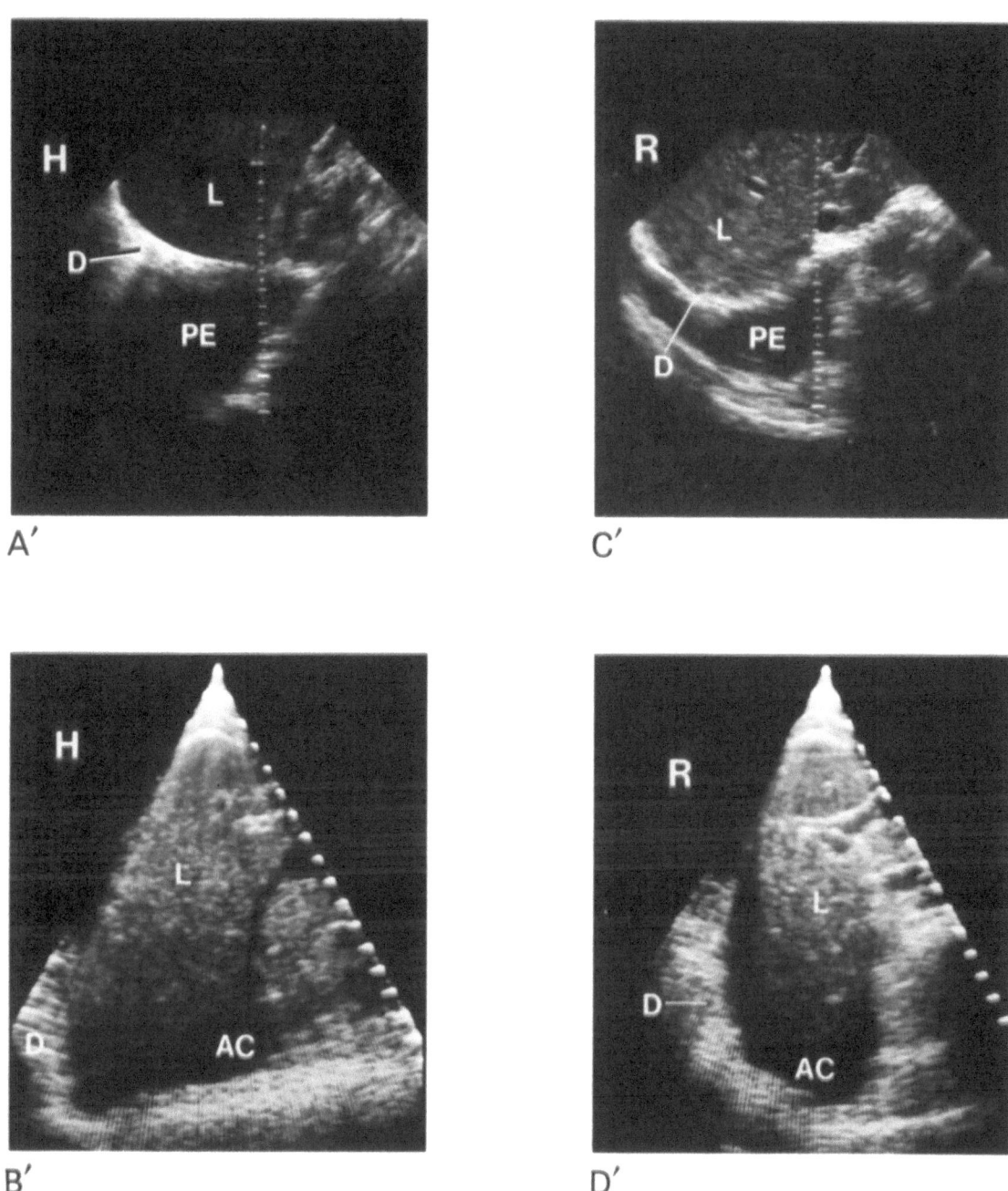

Fig. 9.19. Differentiation of basal pleural effusion (*PE*) from ascitic fluid (*AC*) inferior to liver (*L*) or spleen must be made using images in the sagittal plane. Pleural fluid is above the diaphragm (**A** and **A'**) whereas ascitic fluid is below the diaphragm (*D*) (**B** and **B'**). In transverse planes both pleural effusions (**C** and **C'**) and ascites (**D** and **D'**) have a similar appearance unless the diaphragm is distinctly seen. (Images **A'** and **C'** produced by a Mark III Scanner, manufactured by Advanced Technology Laboratories.)

phragm is not clearly identified and thus one is not sure from the transverse scan on which side of the diaphragm the fluid is located.

References

1. Hall DA, Hann LE, Ferrucci JT, Black EB, Braitman BS, Crowley WF, Nikrui N, Kelley JA (1979) Sonographic morphology of the normal menstrual cycle. Radiology 133: 185–188
2. Rubin C, Kurtz AB, Goldberg BB (1978) Water enema: a new ultrasound technique in defining pelvic anatomy. J Clin Ultrasound 6:28–33
3. Fleischer AC, Dowling AD, Weinstein ML, James AE (1979) Sonographic patterns of distended, fluid-filled bowel. Radiology 133: 681–684
4. Meyers MA (1976) Intraperitoneal spread of infections. In: Dynamic radiology of the abdomen. Springer-Verlag, New York
5. Edell SL, Gefter WB (1979) Ultrasonic differentiation of types of ascitic fluid. Am J Roentgenol 133:111–114
6. Elyaderani MK, Skolnick ML, Weinstein BJ (1979) Ultrasonic detection and aspiration confirmation of intraabdominal collection of fluid. Surg Gynecol Obstet 149:529–533
7. Skolnick ML, Matzuk, T (1979) Ultrasonic detection of pericardial effusions adjacent to the right atrium during routine examination of the upper abdomen. Clin Radiol 30:295–298

10
Invasive Ultrasonography

Although ultrasound is basically considered a noninvasive imaging modality, it is also effective for percutaneously guiding fine needles into deep intraabdominal masses, both solid and cystic, for purposes of sampling their contents. The major applications of this technique are in (1) the aspiration of fluid from cystic masses to characterize the fluid, especially to determine whether it is sterile, infected, or contains malignant cells; and (2) the aspiration of cells from solid masses to determine whether they are benign or malignant. In addition, this technique can guide a needle into an obstructed renal collecting system in order to perform antegrade pyelography so as to determine the cause of the obstructed urinary tract. The needle can then be replaced by a catheter to provide temporary drainage of the obstructed urinary tract until definitive therapy is instituted.

1. ADVANTAGES OF PERCUTANEOUS ASPIRATION

The percutaneous aspiration of intraabdominal masses and fluid collections is not a new technique. It has been used for many years. Prior to the advent of ultrasound, needle guidance has either been done by palpation for superficial masses (1, 2) or x-ray control for deep ones (3). Ultrasonic guidance has several advantages over radiologic localization. The detection of solid or cystic pathologic masses by ultrasound depends upon differences in the acoustic properties of the mass which differentiate it from adjacent normal tissues. Conventional x-ray equipment cannot distinguish most solid and cystic masses from adjacent organs because both the masses and the normal tissues are composed of similar water-density tissue. Only if the mass contains tissue of different x-ray density (gas, fat, calcium) or if the mass deforms an organ that can be selectively enhanced with radiopaque contrast agents can the mass be radiographically appreciated. The precise depth of the mass below the site of skin insertion of the needle cannot be accurately determined radiographically unless biplane x-ray or fluoroscopy is used, whereas this measurement is simple to obtain from the two-dimensional ultrasound scan using the calibrated depth scale on the scanner. The ultrasound cross-sectional images also tell the physician precisely what tissues are situated between the mass and the skin so that he has a better understanding of

213

what organs the sampling needle will pass through on the way to the mass. The patient is exposed to no ionizing radiation during the procedure and no intravenous contrast agents are required to help detect the mass. The time needed to localize the mass by ultrasound is minimal. With certain types of real-time scanners it is even possible to continuously observe the aspiration needle as it is being inserted into the mass.

2. INVASIVE ULTRASONOGRAPHY VERSUS INVASIVE COMPUTED TOMOGRAPHY

Computed radiographic tomography can also be used to percutaneously guide needles into deep intraabdominal masses in a manner similar to that of ultrasonic imaging since with computed tomography (CT) the precise depth of the mass below the skin can be determined, and the needle can be observed in relation to the mass as it is inserted (4). In situations where the mass can be seen both by ultrasound and CT imaging, ultrasound should be the preferred modality because (1) it requires no ionizing radiation or intravenous contrast agents; (2) the time required to localize the mass is usually less; and (3) the cost of the procedure for the patient is considerably less since the initial and operating costs of an ultrasound scanner are much less than that of a CT scanner.

3. SAFETY

The great attractiveness of the fine needle aspirating technique is that the needle, because of its fine caliber, rarely produces significant injury to organs lying between the skin and the mass. Thus, deep masses can be sampled without injury to the intervening tissues even if the needle first has to traverse solid organs, fluid reservoirs, bowel, or blood vessels.

Samples of the mass are obtained by aspiration—by sucking out fluid or cells into the needle—rather than by cutting out a core of tissue. A fine (22 gauge) aspirating needle separates tissue planes as it passes through organs. When the needle is removed, the tissue planes fall back into their former position without leaving a hole. The aspiration needle we use is not a flexible needle of the Chiba variety, but rather the more rigid type used for lumbar punctures since the more flexible needle may deflect away from the mass as it is inserted. By contrast, a conventional biopsy needle, which is usually 14 gauge, is a cutting needle that removes a cylinder of tissue and leaves a hole within the tissue when the needle is removed. If the needle cuts through bowel or a blood vessel, leakage of contents can occur.

Both the literature and our own more limited clinical experience indicate that significant clinical complications such as the spillage of bowel contents from perforation, the development of hematoma or hemorrhage requiring surgery or multiple transfusions, and the spread of abscesses occur infrequently in patients undergoing percutaneous fine needle aspiration procedures (3, 5–9). The spread of tumor along a biopsy needle tract is an exceedingly rare complication. Several large series report no such complications (10, 11), whereas only isolated case reports describe their occurrence(12, 13).

The fine needle aspiration procedure produces minimal discomfort to the patient, often no worse than that caused by the drawing of blood from an antecubital vein or that produced by the intramuscular injection of medication. The procedure, in addition, is quite rapid. The time required for the needle to remain in the patient is only several seconds when a solid mass is being sampled. When a cystic mass is being aspirated, of course, the needle remains in the patient longer, i.e., the time required to remove a 5- to 10-cc sample of fluid. However, once the needle is positioned and the fluid is being aspirated, the needle itself produces almost no discomfort. Pain is mainly produced as the needle is being inserted or removed. Many of our aspiration procedures are performed on out-patients, especially when renal cysts are being sampled.

4. TECHNIQUES

The basic techniques are similar for the aspiration of cystic and solid masses and for the performance of antegrade pyelography and percutaneous nephrostomies. However, minor differences in procedure and instrumentation are used to optimize the examination for the particular purpose.

A. Mass Localization

With most current real-time scanners the needle is *not* under ultrasonic observation during the actual percutaneous insertion. The path and depth of the needle are determined from the initial ultrasound scans and then the aspiration procedure is done using the chosen skin coordinate markers. It is, therefore, necessary that the patient maintain the same phase of respiration for the actual needle insertion as he did for the localizing ultrasound scans.

In order to accurately determine the size and configuration of the mass to be aspirated, two ultrasonic images are obtained in planes perpendicular to each other. From these two views, the site on the skin for the entrance of the puncture needle is chosen. The depth the needle must travel to reach the mass is determined by the centimeter scale that is projected on the images in the line through which the needle will pass (Figs. 10.1 and 10.2). One should lightly touch the transducer to the skin when obtaining an image for measuring the depth of the mass and be careful not to compress the skin with the transducer because compression will shorten

the distance between the skin and the mass. When the aspirating needle is inserted, it may not reach the mass if depth is determined when the skin and subcutaneous tissues are compressed (Fig. 10.3).

Whenever possible, the puncture site is chosen so as to keep the distance between the skin and the mass as short as possible in order to reduce the depth to which the needle has to be inserted. In this way a shorter needle can be used which is easier to guide than a longer one. In addition, it is helpful if the needle can be oriented perpendicular to the horizontal plane in both the transverse and parasagittal scans so as to simplify its insertion into the patient. When the needle is entering in a nonperpendicular angle, the physician must carefully determine the angle of insertion of the needle from the ultrasound image, mark this angle on the patient, and be sure that the needle actually enters at this angle.

To facilitate identifying the site on the skin of needle insertion with a real-time transducer, an instrument that casts an acoustic shadow (needle, tip of hemostat, or paper clip) can be placed between the transducer and skin at the site of needle insertion. The acoustic shadow of this instrument is then cast on the cross-sectional image along the line through which the needle will be inserted (Fig. 10.4).

B. Real-time Biopsy Transducers

Instrumentation is rapidly changing and there are several real-time biopsy transducers that are or soon will be commercially available which will allow the operator to guide and observe the needle as it is being inserted into a solid or cystic mass for the aspiration procedure. In one linear array design (14), the transducer elements are projected out from one side of the case (Fig. 10.5A). A *U*-shaped groove for the biopsy needle is located in the center transducer elements. In another design, the needle shaft goes through the entire thickness of case and

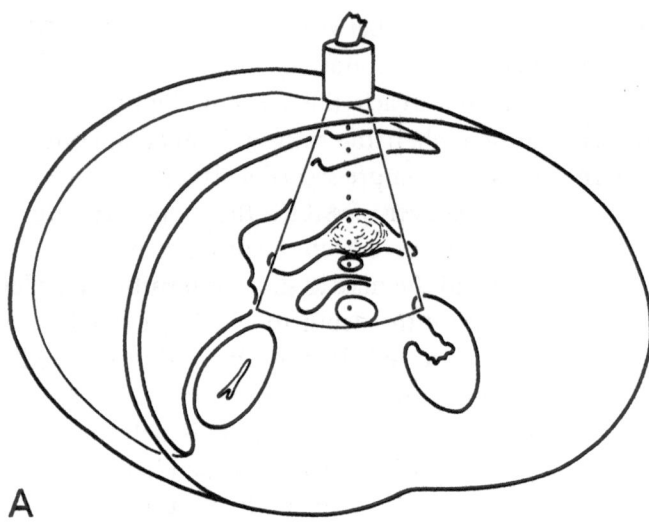

A

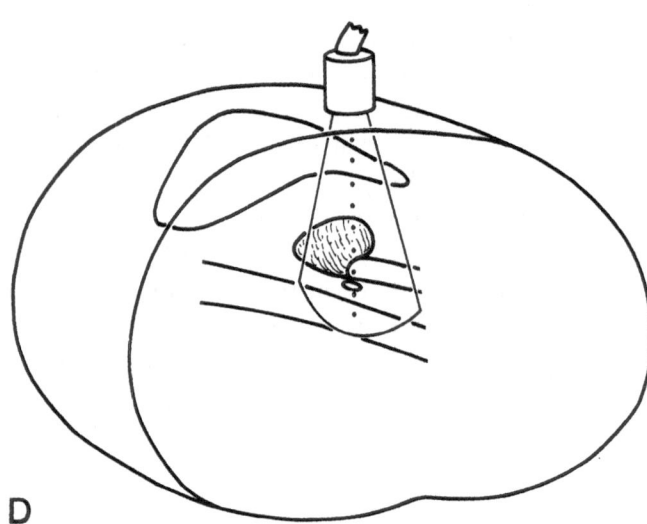

D

Fig. 10.1. Localization of solid mass for aspiration biopsy. Images are obtained in transverse and sagittal planes in order to determine skin site for insertion of aspiration needle. Transverse plane: **A** Sketch relating sector image of pancreatic mass to adjacent structures. Centimeter scale is placed along needle path for accurately determining tumor depth. **B** Ultrasound image of mass. **C** Image of mass with centimeter scale projected through it. Sagittal plane: **D** Sketch relating sector image to ultrasound image of mass (**E**). **F** Image of mass with centimeter scale. *L*, liver; *P*, normal pancreas; *M*, pancreatic mass; *SMA*, superior mesenteric artery; *VC*, vena cava; *A*, aorta.

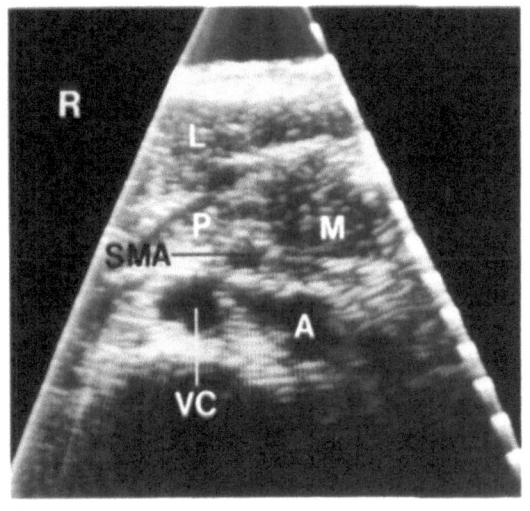

B

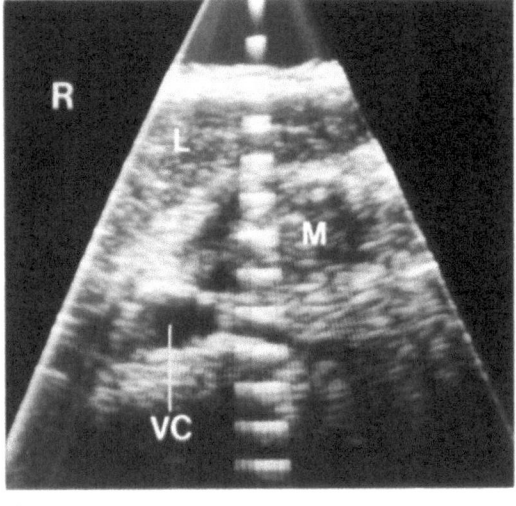

C

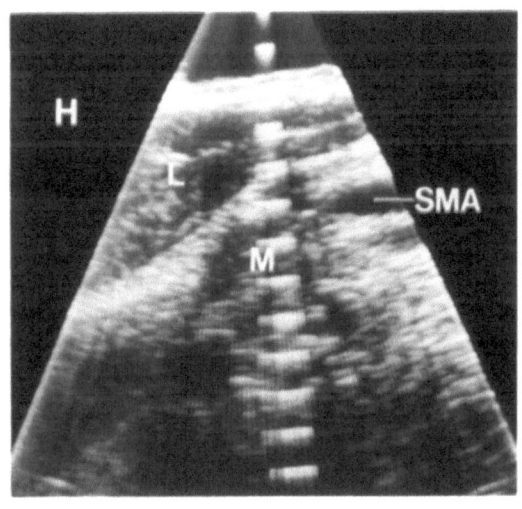

E

F

Fig. 10.1. (cont.)

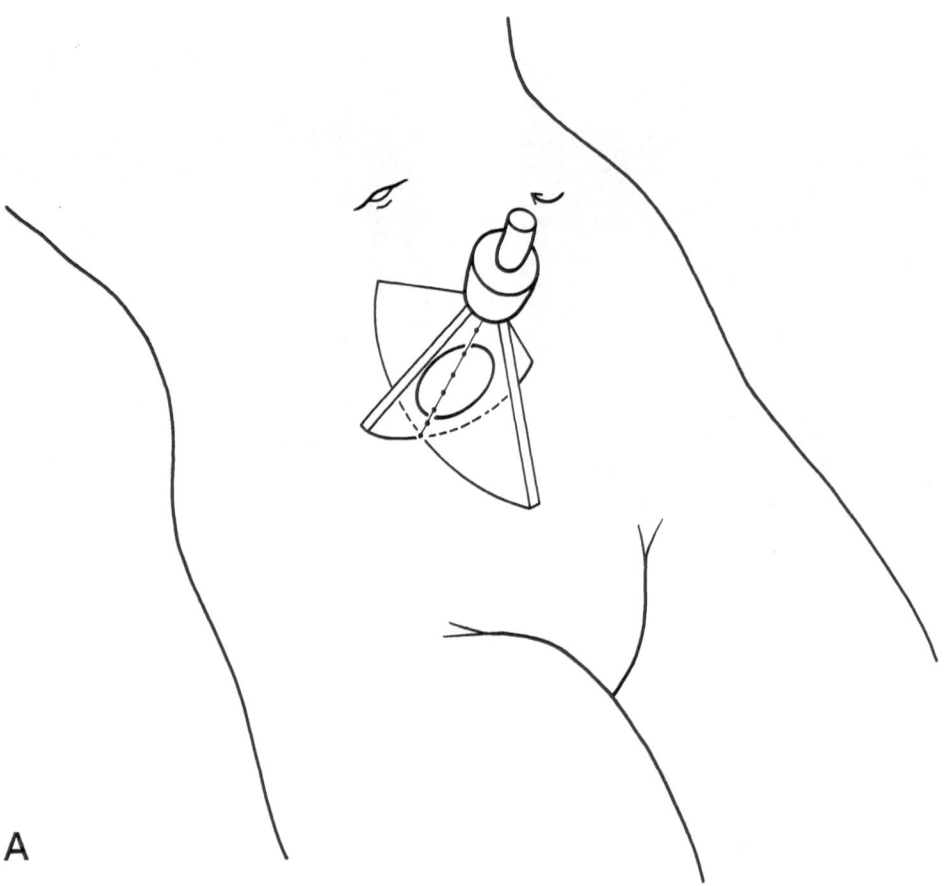

A

Fig. 10.2. Localization of midabdominal abscess (*A*) prior to percutaneous aspiration of 40 cc
of pus. Abscess caused by perforated colonic diverticulum. **A** Transducer placed over
abscess and rotated from transverse to sagittal planes to fully define its size and shape.
Centimeter scale is aligned perpendicular to skin and through center of abscess. Aspiration needle will follow path of centimeter scale. Images are recorded in sagittal
(**B**) and transverse (**C**) planes to confirm position of centimeter scale relative to
abscess.

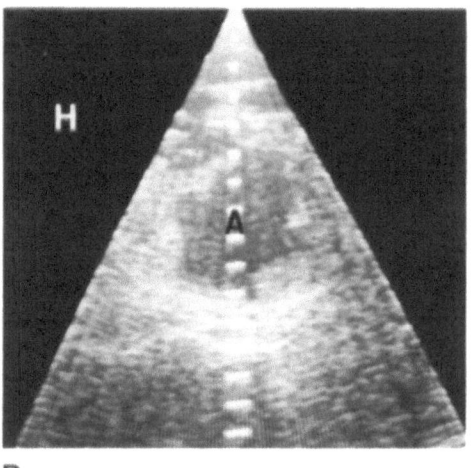

B

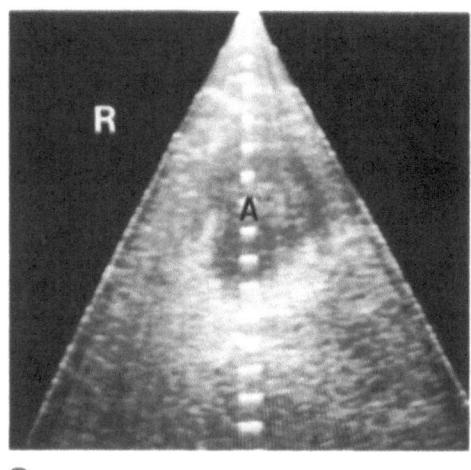

C

Fig. 10.2. (cont.)

transducer elements (15). The transducer is placed on the skin so that the groove is located over the mass along the axis through which the needle is to be inserted into the mass. The needle itself is often not seen because the ultrasound beams are parallel to the needle, but the mass can be continuously observed as it is being sampled. In a sector type of transducer design (16), the needle is inserted off to one side rather than through the center of the transducer system. A protractorlike device is attached to the side of the case so as to guide the needle to intersect the central ray at the depth at which the mass lies (Fig. 10.5B). The angle at which the needle guide should be set is determined by first measuring the depth at which the central ray intersects the mass and then adjusting the needle guide to correspond to this depth. The scale on the needle guide is calibrated in centimeters along the central ray at which the needle will intersect this ray rather than in degrees of an arc.

C. Needle Observation Using Nonbiopsy Transducers

Even without the use of real-time biopsy transducers, in certain instances one can ul-trasonically observe the needle as the aspiration procedure is being performed. The ultrasound beam used to image the mass enters the body from a different direction than does the needle but the beam is broad enough to image most or all of the tissue between the skin and mass through which the needle will pass. Orienting the needle and beam at 90° to each other is often the most convenient method, and it improves needle visualization since the ultrasound beam strikes the needle perpendicularly. The needle might enter from the anterior abdominal wall while the ultrasound beam comes from the flank (Fig. 10.6). For this method to succeed, the anatomic region must be free of gas-filled bowel both in the plane of the ultrasound beam and along the path of the needle so as to image the needle and mass in relation to each other.

5. APPLICATIONS

A. Solid Masses

In the aspiration of solid masses, the purpose of the aspiration procedure is to obtain

A

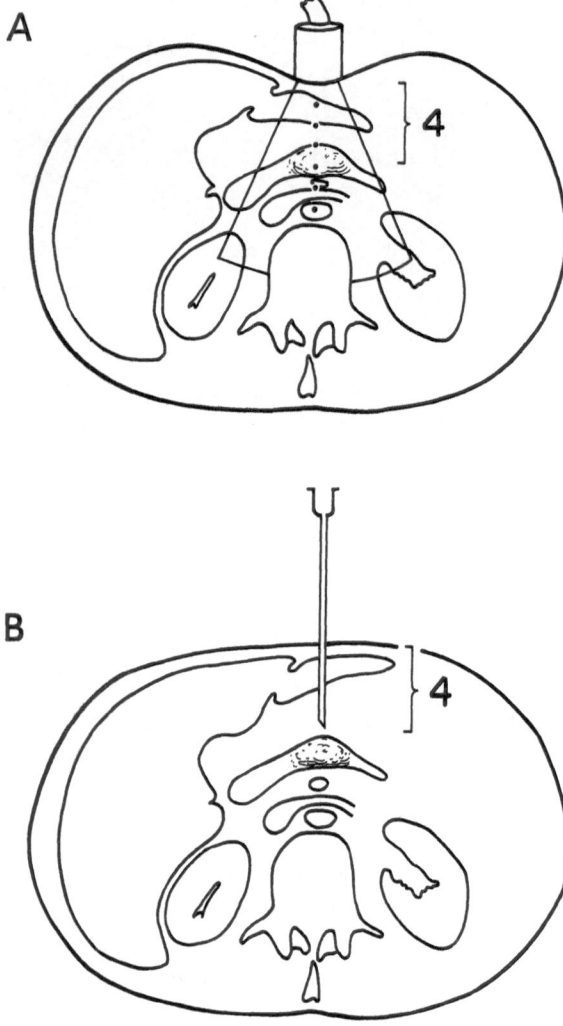

B

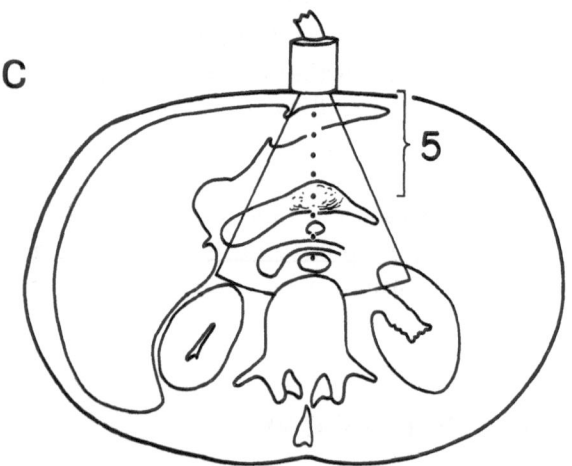

C

Fig. 10.3. An inaccurate measurement of the distance between the skin and the mass to be aspirated can be produced by increased pressure of transducer upon skin. **A** Increased pressure compresses underlying tissues and decreases centimeter distance between skin and mass, thus giving an incorrectly short distance. **B** Needle is inserted to depth determined in Fig. 10.3A. Since needle does not compress tissues as transducer did, tip of needle does not reach mass. **C** Correct method. Transducer just makes contact with skin. Underlying tissues are not compressed and accurate centimeter depth measurement is obtained.

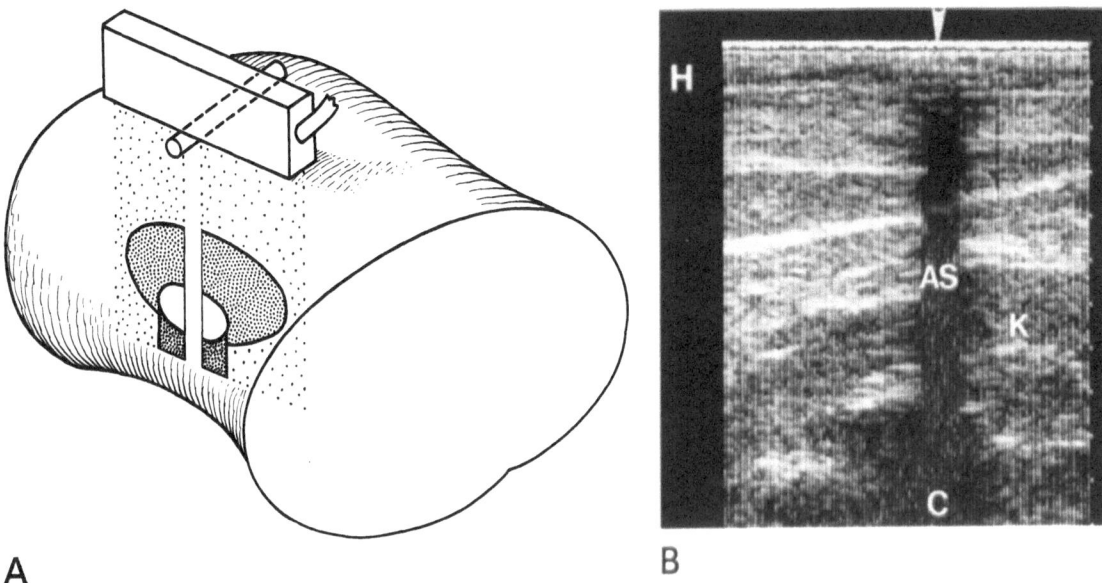

A   **B**

Fig. 10.4. **A** Method for determining the site on the skin at which the aspiration needle should be inserted to puncture an underlying mass. Thin tubular or rod-shaped structure (e.g., opened-up paper clip, hypodermic needle) is placed between the transducer face and skin in such a position that the acoustic shadow which it casts goes through the mass. **B** Application of this technique to localize cyst (*C*) in kidney (*K*). Sagittal scan with patient prone. *Arrowhead,* paper clip on skin; *AS,* acoustic shadow. (Linear array manufactured by Toshiba Corporation, Japan.)

clusters of cells in order to perform a cytologic study of the aspirated material. The determination of whether the tissue is malignant or benign is made on the basis of cytologic rather than histologic criteria.

In order to obtain a satisfactory aspirate, the following technique is used (17). The biopsy needle is attached to a 20-cc disposable plastic syringe. The syringe is inserted in a plastic device called an aspir-gun,[1] which gives the operator one-handed control of the syringe and allows him to rapidly withdraw the plunger of the syringe by squeezing on the hand grip (Fig. 10.7). The other hand is used to help position the needle and stabilize the syringe as the needle is being inserted into the patient. After the skin has been surgically prepared and a small amount of local anesthesia infiltrated, the needle with the syringe and aspir-gun attached is rapidly inserted through the skin to the predeter-

mined depth to pierce the mass (Fig. 10.8). Once the needle has been inserted to its proper depth, the operator squeezes the handle in order to produce maximum suction in the syringe. He then rapidly moves the entire aspiration device up and down several times over approximately a 1-cm excursion in order to fragment bits of tissue and suck cells into the needle. The needle suction is released as soon as fluid or tissue is seen appearing at the hub of the needle, and the device is then completely withdrawn (Fig. 10.9). If the needle is removed from the patient with suction maintained, air will rush into the syringe and the material in the needle will be splattered over the walls of the syringe making its retrieval very difficult. The entire procedure takes several seconds and is performed during suspended respiration.

The syringe and needle are then removed from the aspir-gun and handed to an assistant who smears the contents of the needle on glass slides which are immediately fixed

---

[1] Aspir-gun obtained from Everest Company, Linden, New Jersey, 07036.

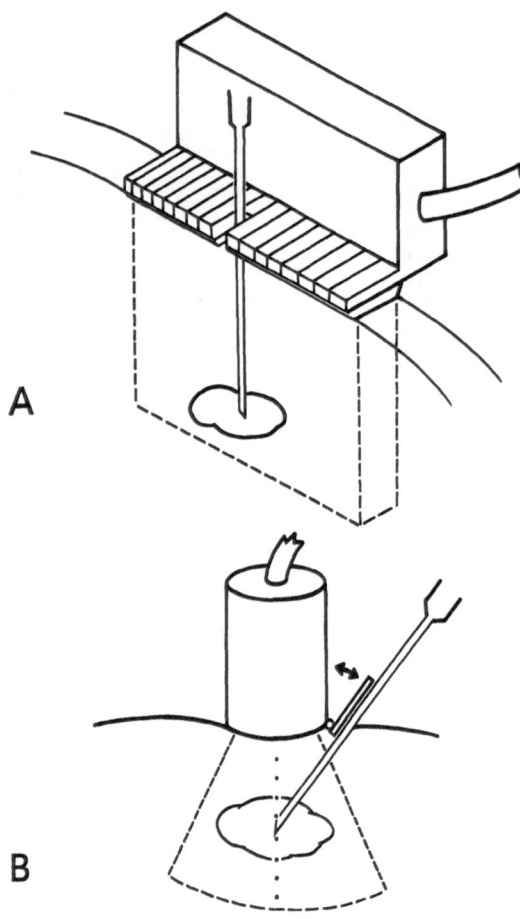

Fig. 10.5. Biopsy transducers. **A** Linear array. Transducer elements are offset to one side of housing. *U*-shaped notch in center of array is positioned above mass and needle is inserted through notch into mass. Because of notch, transducer can be removed from patient without need to remove needle. **B** Sector scanner. Needle is diagonally inserted into mass along needle guide from side of transducer case rather than through center of case as with linear array. Depth along central ray of image at which needle tip intersects mass can be changed by varying angle between needle guide and transducer case.

in 95% alcohol. These slides are subsequently stained using the Papanicolaou technique. The needle and syringe are saved and later washed out with formalin. Any additional cellular material found within the needle or barrel is made into a cell block which is then sectioned and stained using routine histologic rather than cytologic staining procedures. Three to four aspirations are usually performed on a mass. Thus, the pathologist has at his disposal two types of material: the cytologic preparation made from the smeared contents of the needle which can determine whether the cells are benign or malignant, and possible a histologic preparation made from the washings of the syringe and needle which may identify a specific type of tumor.

To improve the accuracy of the aspiration procedure when biopsying a solid mass and

to reduce the number of aspirations performed, the pathologist comes to our ultrasound laboratory during the procedure. His function is to immediately examine a slide made from the aspirated material so as to determine if a diagnostic specimen has been obtained. For this purpose, the slide is stained with hematoxylin and eosin since it is a much faster staining procedure than the Papanicolaou technique. If a diagnostic specimen is obtained on the first attempt, the procedure is terminated. If the sample is not satisfactory, additional biopsies are performed and the specimens are immediately examined. By determining the type of tissue obtained in the specimen, the pathologist can provide information to the physician performing the biopsy so that he may more accurately direct the needle for the next pass if the previous one did not give a satisfactory

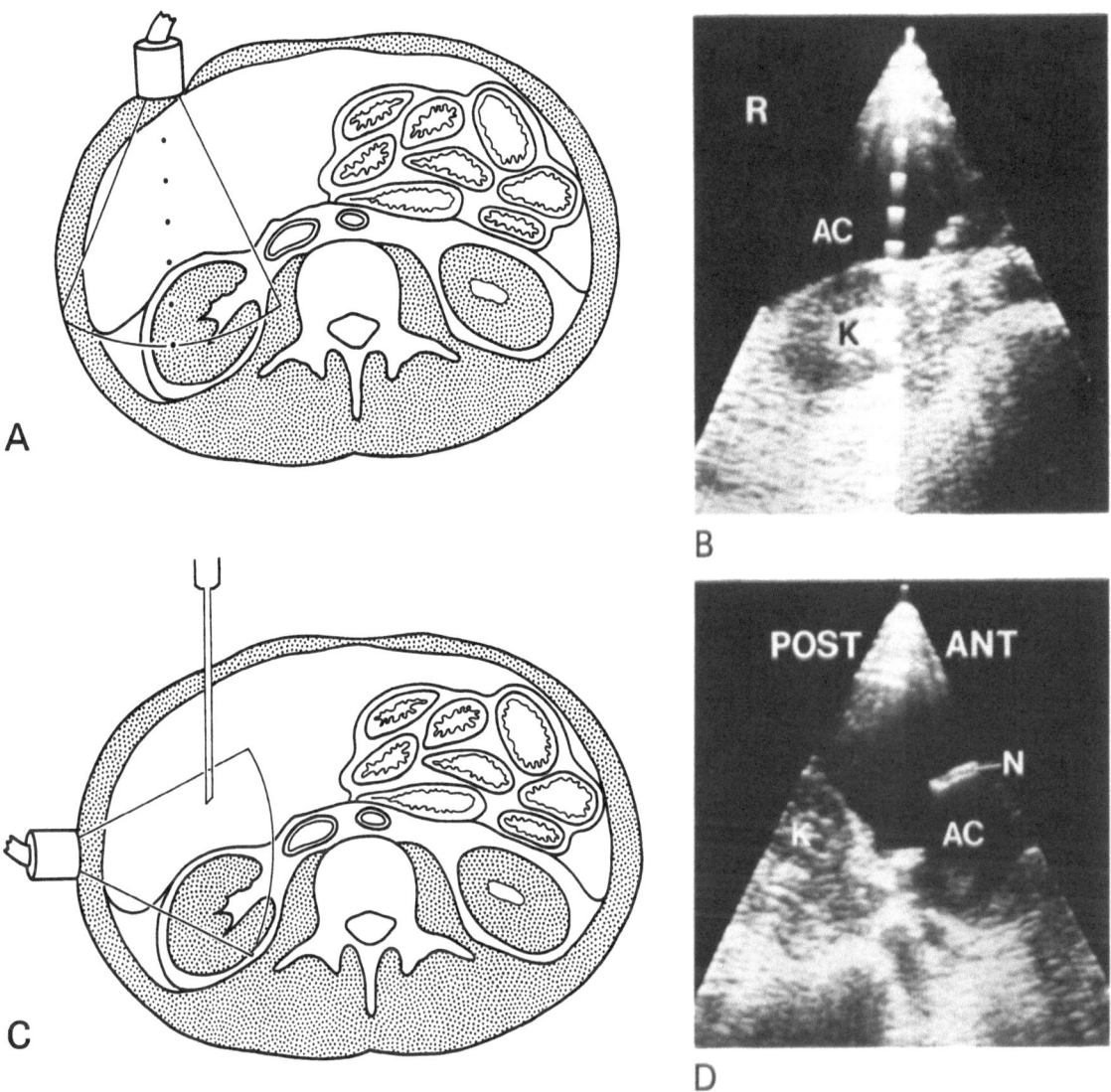

Fig. 10.6. Transducer positioned perpendicular to needle so as to observe insertion of needle. Patient with ascites. **A** and **B** Transducer first positioned over site of needle insertion and path is marked with centimeter scale. **C** and **D** Transducer is then placed on flank with beam positioned to image lower part of needle path. *AC*, ascites; *N*, needle; *K*, right kidney; *ANT*, anterior; *POST*, posterior.

specimen. If no diagnostic material is obtained after four passes, the procedure is ended for that day.

B. Cystic Masses: Nonrenal

The percutaneous puncture of cystic masses is performed, except for some minor changes, in a manner similar to that for solid masses.

The fine needle is usually inserted without a syringe attached to it. Once the needle is at the proper depth, the inner stylet is removed. Frequently fluid will spontaneously flow from the needle if needle placement is correct. A short length of plastic intravenous connecting tubing is attached between the needle and a 10- or 20-cc syringe, and gentle suction is applied to remove a specimen of fluid. If no fluid is obtained,

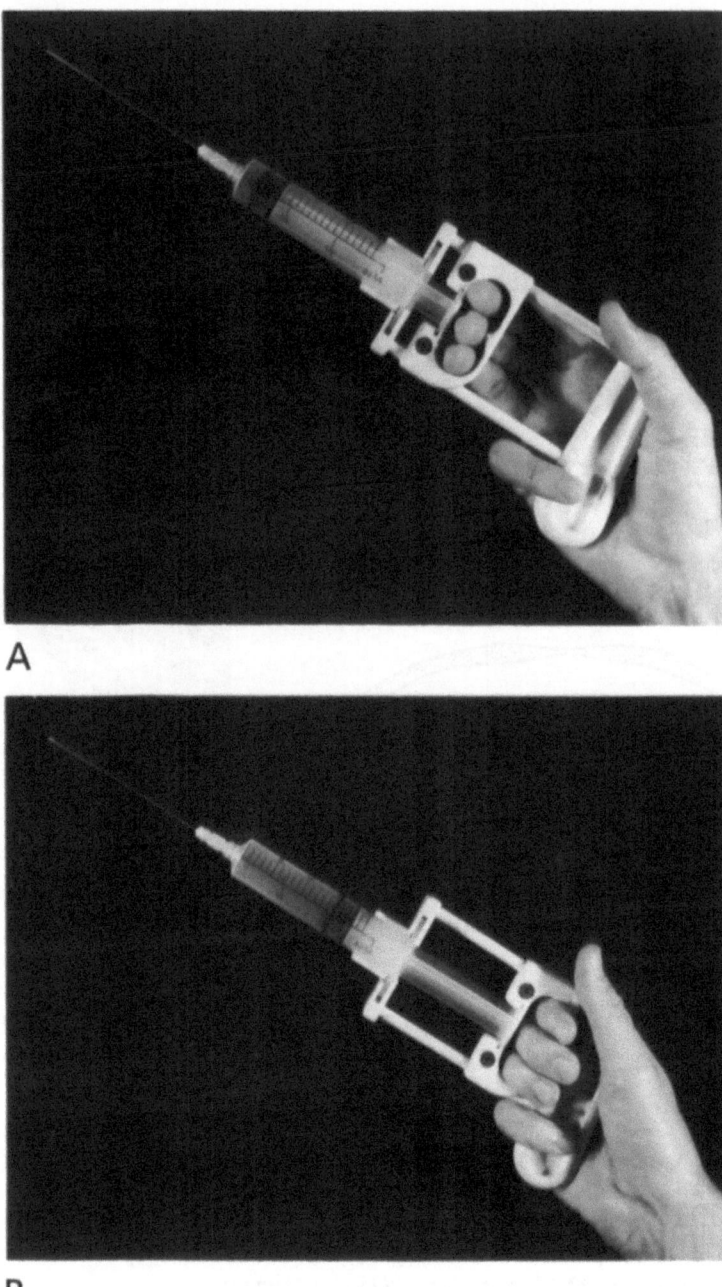

Fig. 10.7. Aspir-gun containing a 20-cc syringe with a 22-gauge spinal needle. **A** Plunger of syringe within barrel. **B** Plunger withdrawn by closing fingers.

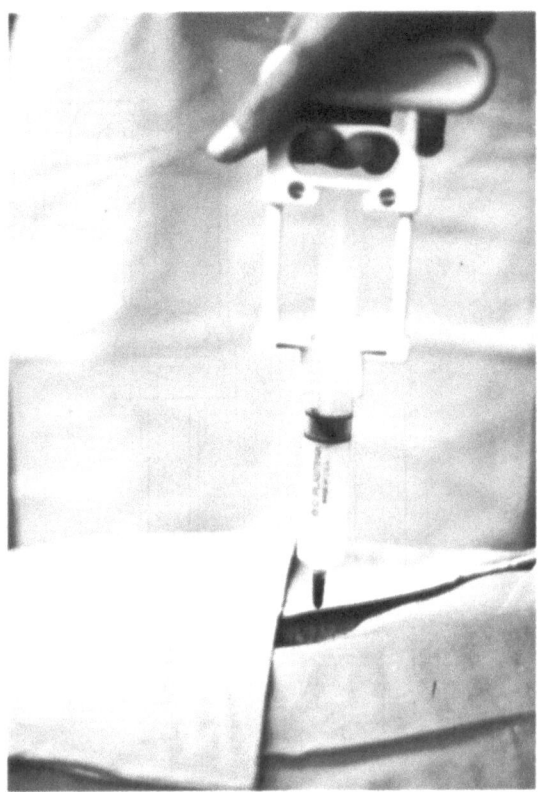

Fig. 10.8. Needle inserted into mass as aspir-gun is controlled with one hand.

the needle should first be slowly advanced to a greater depth with frequent aspirations because there may have been a slight inaccuracy in the depth of the mass if the original measurement had been made with the transducer pressing on the skin and compressing the underlying tissues. After advancing several centimeters, if fluid is still not obtained, the needle should be slowly withdrawn while maintaining suction, hoping to find the fluid at a slightly more superficial level. If the tap is dry, the needle should be reinserted at a slightly different angle.

The connecting tubing allows the needle to move during normal respiration while at the same time permitting the operator to remove fluid. If the syringe were attached to the needle with no intervening plastic tubing and the operator held onto the syringe, the needle could not freely move with breathing. Aspirations could then only be performed during suspended respiration if the needle happened to be in or passing through an organ that moves with respiration. Otherwise, the needle could lacerate the organ through which it traversed as the patient breathed. *Therefore, when the needle is in an organ that moves with respiration, direct needle manipulation should only be done during suspended respiration.*

The main purpose in puncturing a fluid-filled cavity is to obtain a sample of fluid for identification purposes. Occasionally one may desire to completely drain the fluid cavity rather than just to sample it.

Most nonrenal intraabdominal fluid collections are found in patients clinically suspected of having an abscess. In these patients, the percutaneous fine needle aspiration of cystic spaces serves several purposes. An abscess can be detected or excluded. When several intraabdominal fluid collections are ultrasonically detected, each can be percutaneously sampled in order to determine which if any are infected and which are sterile, i.e., seromas, lymphoceles, or urinomas. Occasionally a loop of fluid-filled and adynamic bowel may be confused with a suspected abscess and punctured. However, no harm is done to the bowel from the puncture, and bowel contents can be microscopically differentiated from an abscess. The patient can be spared exploratory surgery if the fluid is sterile or surgically treated if an abscess is detected. The extent of the operative procedure can be reduced because the ultrasound study has located for the surgeon the site of the abscess. This site can be identified by marking the overlying skin. Alternately, the aspiration needle can be left in place and covered with a paper cup to prevent a shift in its position until the patient is in the operating room.

In patients too ill to undergo surgical drainage, the abscess can be drained using a percutaneously inserted catheter although drainage may not be as complete as when operative drainage is instituted.

If the fluid is moderately viscous, it may

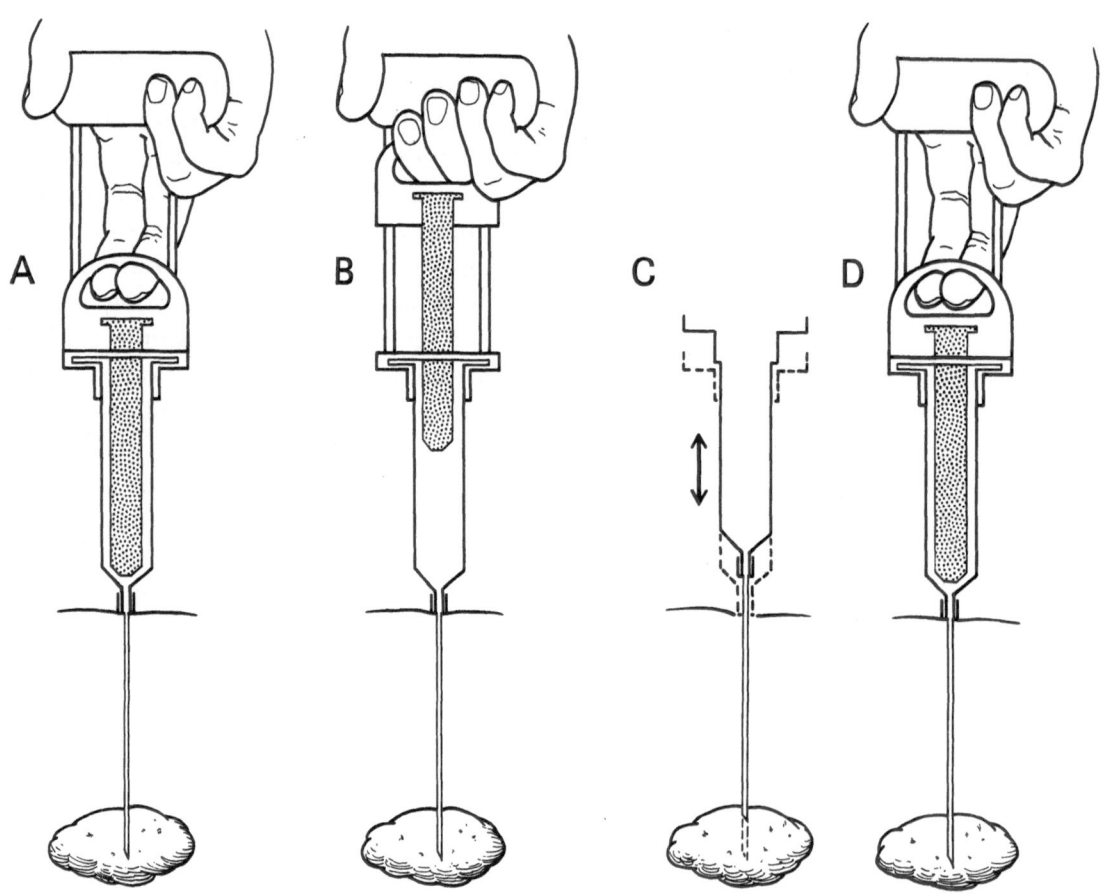

Fig. 10.9. Sequence of manipulating aspir-gun. **A** Needle is inserted into mass with plunger in syringe. **B** Suction produced in syringe by rapidly withdrawing plunger. **C** With suction maintained entire assembly is moved several times in and out of mass through a 1- to 2-cm excursion to dislodge cells and tissue fragments from the mass and suck them into the needle. **D** As soon as tissue or blood appears in the hub of the needle, the suction is released and aspir-gun is removed from the patient.

be difficult to aspirate through a 22-gauge needle. In such situations either a Teflon-sheathed needle of a larger diameter or a larger diameter steel needle can be used.

The Teflon-sheathed needle is a combination of an inner 18- or 20-gauge steel needle with an outer 16- or 18-gauge Teflon sheath that snugly fits around the needle (Fig. 10.10). The steel needle and its Teflon sheath are inserted as one unit to the desired depth. The inner stylet is removed and if fluid is not seen coming through the hollow steel needle, suction is applied using connecting tubing and a syringe to confirm that the tip of the needle is in the fluid space. When fluid is obtained, the steel inner needle is then removed with one hand while holding the hub of the Teflon sheath with the other so as not to withdraw the sheath as well. Fluid contents can be aspirated through the flexible Teflon sheath while permitting the patient to breathe normally (Fig. 10.11). If desired, the hub of the Teflon sheath can be sutured to the skin and a drainage tubing and connecting bag connected to the hub to allow continuous drainage of the fluid.

When one does not plan to keep a per-

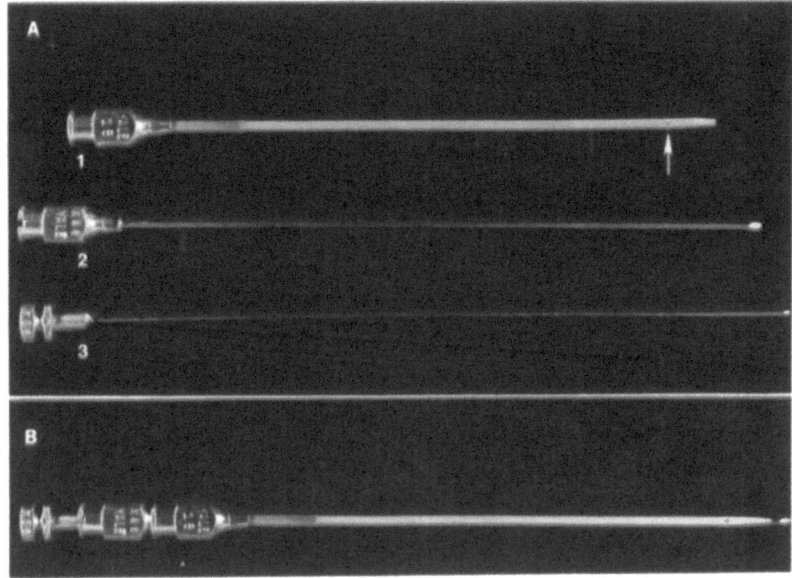

Fig. 10.10. Teflon-sheated needle. **A** Disassembled. *1*, Teflon sheath with side hole *(arrow)*. *2*, steel needle with pointed tip that fits through sheath. *3*, steel stylet that fits within needle. **B** Assembled and ready for insertion into patient.

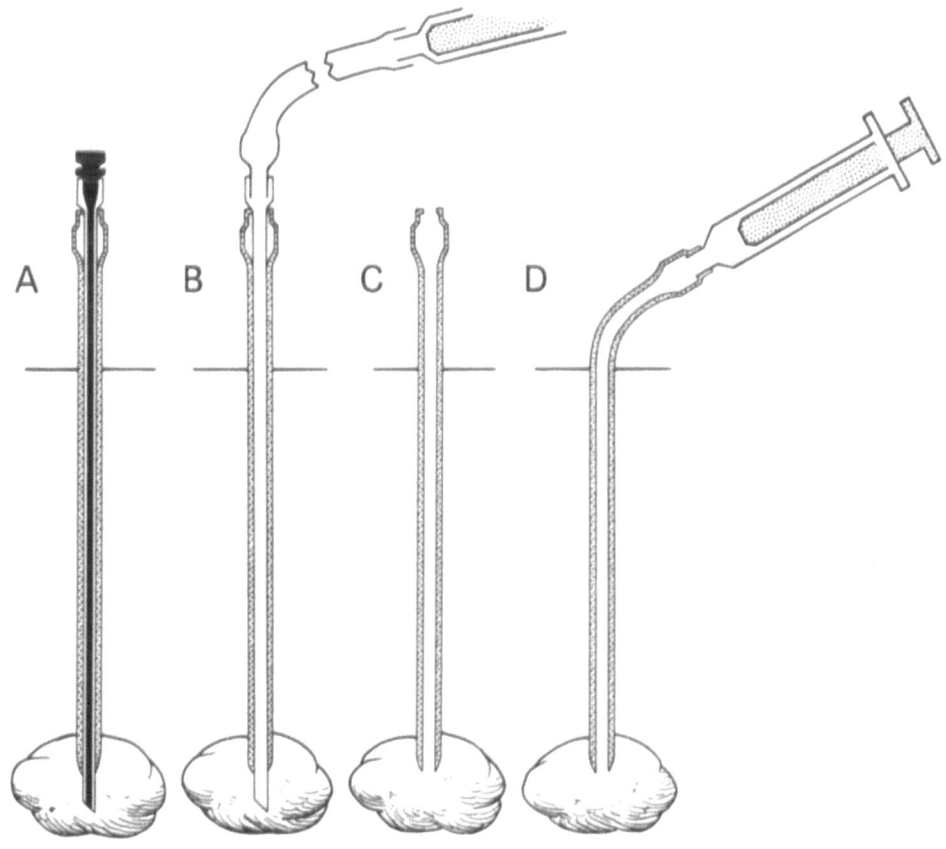

Fig. 10.11. Sequence of insertion of Teflon-sheathed needle into cystic mass. **A** Entire needle assembly (as in Fig. 10.10B) inserted with tip located within fluid. **B** Inner stylet removed. Flexible plastic intravenous tubing is connected between steel needle and syringe. Suction is applied to syringe and sample of fluid is removed. **C** Steel needle is removed. Teflon sheath remains within cystic mass. **D** Syringe is connected directly to Teflon sheath so as to remove additional fluid or insert contrast material.

manent drainage tube in the fluid cavity, then drainage can be performed using an 18- or 19-gauge steel needle in place of the Teflon sheath. After all fluid is aspirated, the needle is removed.

When either the Teflon-sheathed needle or the larger steel needle is used, the operator should be more cautious in its placement than when the 22-gauge needle is used so as to make sure that either of these larger diameter needles does not traverse vital structures on the way to the fluid cavity.

C. Renal Cysts

Puncture of renal cysts, which comprises a major part of our percutaneous puncture procedures, is done in a manner similar to the puncture of other cystic cavities. Since cyst fluid is usually nonviscous, it is easy to aspirate through the 22-gauge needle. We rarely use larger diameter needles because of concern of injuring intrarenal vascular structures. Renal cysts are usually punctured from the flank or back (with the patient in a decubitus or prone position) in order to obtain the shortest route between the cystic mass and the skin. A firm block is placed under the patient to reduce renal motion (Figs. 4.9 and 4.10). The shorter the distance the needle has to travel, the more accurately can one direct the needle into a small cyst. In renal cyst puncture, it is imperative that the patient suspend respiration whenever the needle is being manipulated in order to prevent lacerating the kidney. For this reason, the plastic connecting tubing is always used between syringe and needle when fluid is being drained. When the needle enters the renal cyst, the operator usually feels a change in resistance to the needle and sometimes appreciates the popping sensation as the cyst capsule is pierced. It is usually not necessary to apply initial suction to the needle to see if the tip is in the fluid collection since cyst fluid will spontaneously flow out of the needle, presumably because the fluid is under slight pressure.

The main purpose for puncturing a renal cyst is to demonstrate that the cyst is truly benign. Besides obtaining a sample of fluid for cytologic study, it is also important to demonstrate that the size and configuration of the cyst are the same as the cystic mass demonstrated by intravenous pyelography (IVP) and ultrasonography (Fig. 10.12). One should demonstrate that the margins of the cyst are smooth and contain no irregularities or mass lesions projecting intraluminally from the walls which could represent a rare tumor nodule within a cyst or tumor that has undergone central necrosis.

Usually about 10 to 20 cc of fluid are removed and between 5 and 10 cc of contrast material are instilled. A lesser amount of contrast material is instilled than the amount of cyst fluid that is removed because the radiopaque contrast material is hypertonic and will normally draw extracellular fluid into the cyst cavity. It is not advisable to remove more than 20 cc of fluid for diagnostic purposes because as the cyst decreases in size its wall can become irregular from loss of volume. These irregularities may be confused with tumor nodules.

The roentgenograms obtained following the instillation of contrast material are compared to the IVP in order to determine that the size and configuration of the cyst on the two studies are similar. Occasionally a tumor may be present that has undergone cystic degeneration and the size of the cystic cavity following percutaneous puncture may be smaller than the total mass seen on the IVP. This discrepancy should alert the physician to the presence of a necrotic mass even if the aspirated fluid is free of tumor.

The other reason for insertion of contrast material after the cyst is punctured is to confirm that the structure punctured is the same mass as that seen on the IVP. Occasionally, if the patient has a dilated collecting system as well as a cystic mass, the needle may inadvertently be placed in the collecting system rather than the cyst. Roentgenograms of the contrast-filled punctured mass will prevent this mistake.

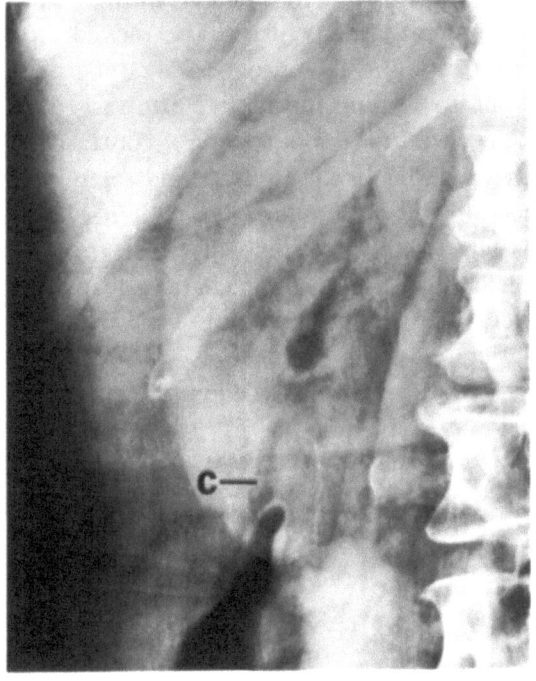

A

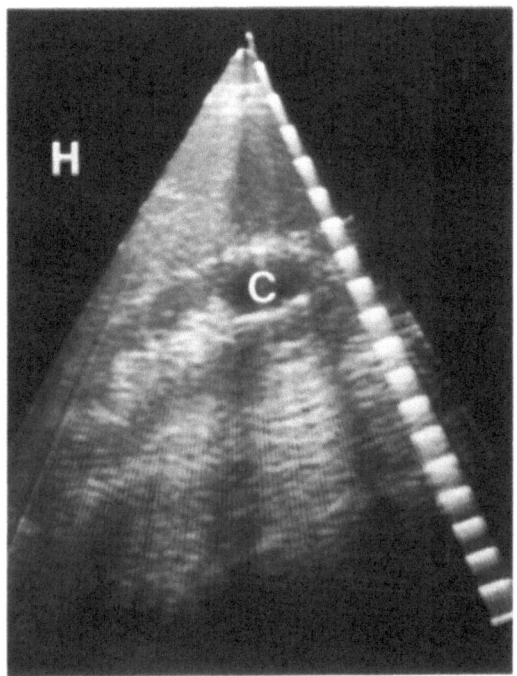

B

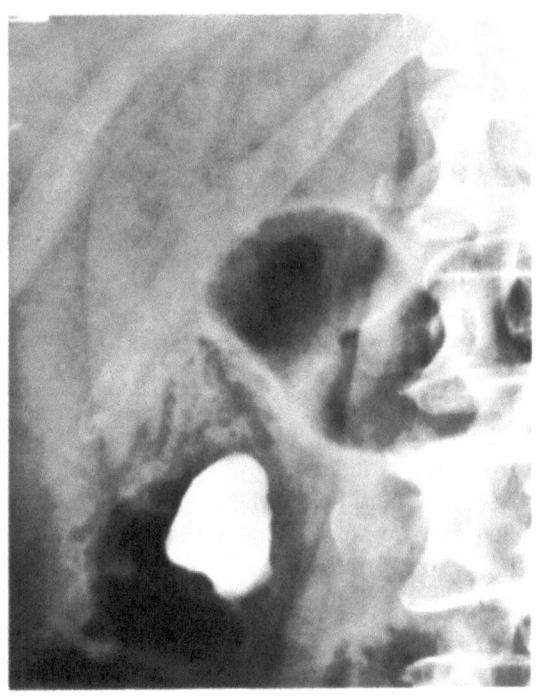

C

Fig. 10.12. Ultrasonically guided percutaneous aspiration of renal cyst. **A** Intravenous pyelogram—0-min nephrogram. Cyst (*C*) with faintly calcified walls is in lower pole. **B** Sagittal scan through lower pole of kidney identifies cyst. **C** Roentgenogram taken after cyst was punctured, 6 cc of fluid removed, and 3 cc of water-soluble contrast material (Renographic 60; Squibb) inserted. Contrast-filled mass has same size and location as cyst identified on IVP, thus confirming that the cystic structure that was punctured was the same as the one seen on the IVP.

Only in patients with a history of pain in the region of the cyst do we attempt to completely drain the cyst. Percutaneous drainage will usually relieve the patient's symptoms for several months to a year. After that time, the fluid usually reaccumulates. The patient may need repeat cyst punctures at yearly intervals. However, repeat cyst punctures are innocuous procedures as compared to open surgical unroofing or resection of the cyst, the surgical alternate choice of treatment.

On rare occasions when the cyst is only 1 or 2 cm in diameter, the cyst may be aspirated dry in the process of obtaining fluid for diagnostic evaluation. Under these circumstances, obviously no contrast material can be instilled. However, we do rescan the area following aspiration to confirm the disappearance of the cyst.

D. Antegrade Pyelography

Antegrade pyelography is a procedure for radiographically visualizing an obstructed renal collecting system proximal to the obstruction. Radiopaque contrast material is instilled by direct percutaneous puncture into the dilated collecting system. The technique for percutaneously directing the needle into the collecting system is the same as that used for the percutaneous puncture of renal cysts.

The purpose of this procedure is twofold: (1) to demonstrate the site of obstruction and (2) to obtain clues as to the possible cause of the obstruction by bacteriologic and cytologic analysis of the aspirated fluid (18, 19). For example, in Fig. 10.13, in which a transitional cell carcinoma obstructed a ureter, a cytologic analysis of the aspirated fluid demonstrated malignant cells and radiographs showed the site of obstruction.

Percutaneous puncture may be performed either with a 22-gauge steel needle or an 18- or 20-gauge Teflon-sheathed needle. The steel needle minimizes risk of injuring the

kidney because of its smaller caliber. Since the patient usually has to be moved from the ultrasound laboratory to a radiographic room to obtain films after contrast is injected, we inject about 10 cc of contrast into the dilated collecting system and remove the needle before moving the patient. If the patient were to be moved with the steel needle in the kidney, the chances of injuring the kidney during the transportation of the patient may be increased.

Advantages of the Teflon sheath are (1)

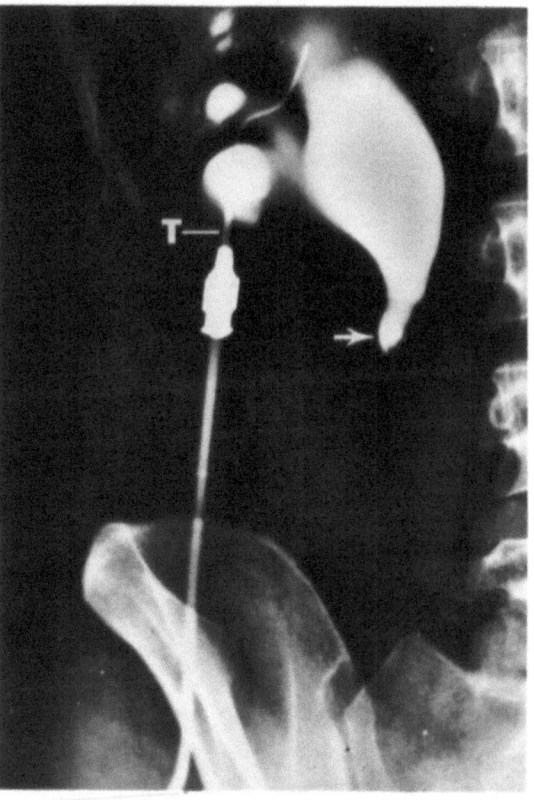

Fig. 10.13. Antegrade pyelogram reveals site and determines cause of obstructed ureter. Teflon catheter (T) was inserted into dilated renal pelvis of nonfunctioning kidney. Contrast material was inserted and obstruction was identified in upper ureter (arrow). Fluid that was removed for cytologic analysis before contrast material was inserted was positive for transitional cell carcinoma.

that it can be left within the patient as he is moved from the ultrasound laboratory to the x-ray room with much less concern about injuring the kidney; (2) that additional contrast material can be inserted into the patient after the initial films are taken if the collecting system has not been well delineated; and (3) that the patient can also be more safely moved into other positions than the original prone position to better direct the contrast material into various parts of the collecting system. We still inject an initial 10 cc of contrast material even when the Teflon catheter is used since this catheter can at times be dislodged as the patient is moved.

However, since the Teflon catheter is of a slightly larger diameter than the steel needle, there is a slight increase in the chance of injuring intrarenal vascular structures

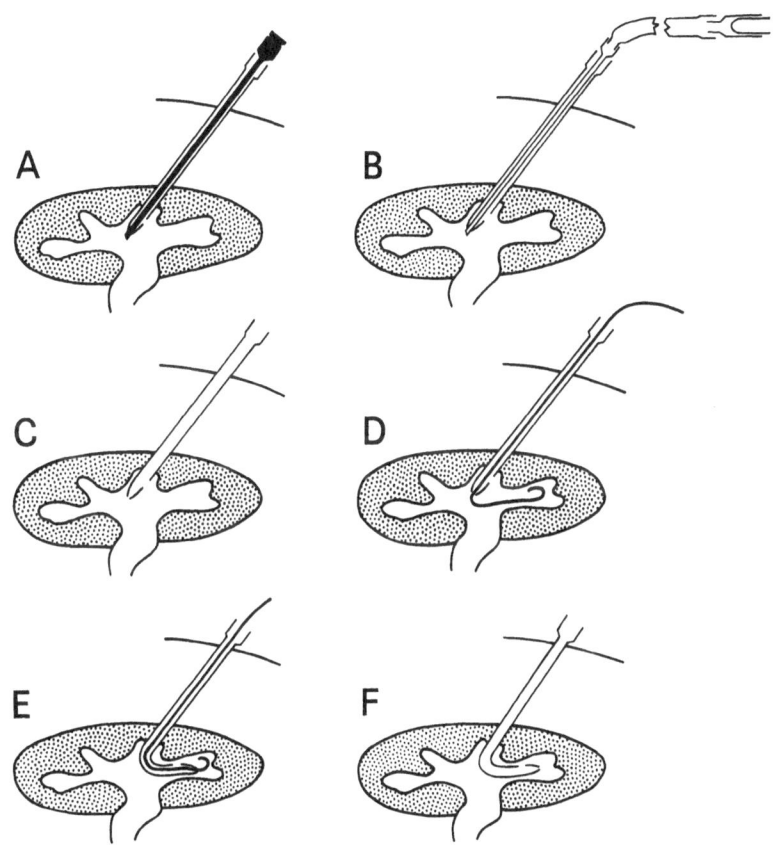

Fig. 10.14. Technique for performing percutaneous nephrostomy using Teflon-sheathed needle assembly. **A** Entire needle assembly has been inserted into dilated renal pelvis or calyx. **B** Stylet has already been removed. Correct position of tip is determined by connecting plastic tubing between needle and syringe and aspirating urine through steel needle. **C** Steel needle has been removed. Teflon sheath with side hole remains. **D** Angiographic guide wire with 3-mm *J*-shaped tip is gently inserted through sheath until it stops. **E** Sheath is advanced over guide wire until sheath can no longer be easily advanced. Sheath should not be forced any further because it may perforate collecting system wall. **F** Guide wire is removed. Suction is applied to sheath to ensure that urine is still obtained and, if so, hub of sheath is sutured to skin to prevent its being pulled out. If no urine is obtained, sheath is slightlyl withdrawn and rechecked until urine flow is established.

during its insertion into the kidney. When the hydronephrosis is gross, then the chance of vascular injury is much less.

If the real-time scanner is readily mobile, an alternate approach would be to perform the entire procedure in a fluoroscopic/radiographic room. Ultrasound would still be used to localize the site and depth of the needle insertion. Once fluid is aspirated, contrast material can be injected under fluoroscopic observation and appropriate roentgenograms taken. Using this approach, the need for transporting the patient from an ultrasound to a fluoroscopic room with a needle projecting from the kidney is eliminated and contrast material is not instilled blindly.

As part of our x-ray filming, we try when possible to obtain an erect view in order to direct the contrast material to the most dependent portion of the collecting system so as to better define the site of obstruction. In addition, prone, supine, and often oblique views are obtained.

E. Percutaneous Nephrostomy

A variation of antegrade pyelography is percutaneous nephrostomy. The main purpose of this procedure is to provide temporary drainage for the obstructed collecting system until institution of definitive therapy for the obstruction. The technique that we use is a modification of that described by Pederson et al. (20). Although it may sound surprising, an 18-gauge Teflon sheath is quite satisfactory for relieving an obstructed collecting system and for allowing an adequate flow of urine so that renal function may return to a more normal state. Since the Teflon catheter may be kept in the collecting system up to several weeks, considerable care is taken to ensure satisfactory placement of the catheter and to prevent its obstruction.

Instead of using the Teflon catheter with a single end hole as we do for antegrade pyelography, one or two side holes are cut in the catheter about 1 to 2 cm from the tip using an angiographic catheter hole cutter (Fig. 10.10). The side holes allow urine to drain into the catheter if the end hole should become plugged by resting against the inner surface of the collecting system.

In order to more deeply position the catheter in the collecting system, we use a short J-shaped guide wire. The guide wire is about 50 cm long and possesses a 3-mm J at one end. The Teflon-sheathed needle assembly is initially placed into the dilated collecting system and the confirmation of correct needle placement is obtained by aspiration of urine through the metal needle. The needle is then removed and the angiographic guide wire is inserted through the sheath until it can no longer easily go any further. The guide wire is held with one hand as the Teflon catheter is advanced with the other hand over the guide wire so as to position the catheter tip deeper within the collecting system. The guide wire is removed and the system is inspected to ensure that an adequate flow of urine still comes out of the catheter (Fig. 10.14).

If this flow is good, the hub of the catheter is sutured to the skin to prevent the catheter from accidentally being pulled out. If flow is poor, a minimal change in the position of the tip (achieved by slightly withdrawing or rotating the sheath) will usually improve flow. Then plastic tubing is used to connect the hub of the catheter to a drainage bag.

The entire procedure is done in our ultrasound laboratory. At the end of the procedure the patient is taken to a radiographic room, radiopaque contrast material is instilled into the kidney via the sheath, and roentgenograms are taken to document the position of the sheath.

However, the procedure could just as easily be done in a fluoroscopic room if the real-time scanner is easily mobile. Then after the catheter and guide wire are inserted into the renal pelvis, final catheter positioning can be done fluoroscopically. When possible, the tip of the sheath should be positioned in the dilated pelvis or proximal ureter so as to reduce its chances of being pulled out of the collecting system during the renal movement that occurs with breathing.

If the urine is infected and viscous, an adequate flow may not be obtainable through the Teflon catheter. In such circumstances, the ultrasonically inserted catheter can be exchanged for a larger catheter under fluoroscopic control. First a guide wire is reinserted through the present catheter and then a series of larger and larger dilators are passed over the guide wire until the tract is wide enough to accept the larger caliber catheter.

References

1. Koss LB (1968) Diagnostic cystology. Lippincott, New York
2. Zajicek J (1974) Monographs in clinical cytology: aspiration biopsy cytology. S. Karger, Basel
3. Tylén U, Arnesjö B, Lindberg LG, Lunderquist A, Akerman M (1976) Percutaneous biopsy of carcinoma of the pancreas guided by angiography. Surg Gynecol Obstet 142: 737–739
4. Haaga JR, Alfridi RJ (1976) Precise biopsy localization by computed tomography. Radiology 118:603–607
5. Hancke S, Holm HH, Koch F (1975) Ultrasonically guided percutaneous fine needle biopsy of the pancreas. Surg Gynecol Obstet 140:361–364
6. Zornoza J, Jonsson K, Wallace S, Lukeman JM (1977) Fine needle aspiration biopsy of retroperitoneal lymph nodes and abdominal masses: an updated report. Radiology 125:87–88
7. Goldstein HM, Zornoza J, Wallace S, Anderson JH, Bree RL, Samuels BI, Lukeman J (1977) Percutaneous fine needle aspiration biopsy of pancreatic and other abdominal masses. Radiology 123:319–322
8. Holm HH, Pedersen JF, Kristensen JK, Rasmussen SN, Hancke S, Jensen F (1975) Ultrasonically guided percutaneous puncture. Radiol Clin North Am 13:493–503
9. Ferrucci JT, Wittenberg J, Mueller P, Simeone JF, Harbin WP, Kirkpatrick RH, Taft PD (1980) Diagnosis of abdominal malignancy by radiologic fine-needle aspiration biopsy. Am J Roentgenol 134:323–330
10. von Schreeb T, Arner O, Skovsted G, Wikstad N (1967) Renal adenocarcinoma. Scand J Urol Nephrol 1:270–276
11. Engzell U, Esposti PL, Rubio C, Sigurdson A, Zajicek J (1971) Investigation on tumour spread in connection with aspiration biopsy. Acta Radiol (Ther) 10:385–398
12. Bush WH, Burnett LL, Gibbons RP (1977) Needle tract seeding of renal cell carcinoma. Am J Roentgenol 129:725–727
13. Ferrucci JT, Wittenberg J, Margolies MN, Carey RW (1979) Malignant seeding of the tract after thin-needle aspiration biopsy. Radiology 130:345–346
14. Goldberg BB, Cole-Beuglet C, Kurtz AB, Rubin CS (1980) Real-time aspiration-biopsy transducer. J Clin Ultrasound 8:107–112
15. Otto R, Deyhle P (1980) Guided puncture under real-time sonographic control. Radiology 134:784–785
16. Saitoh M, Watanabe H, Ohe H, Tanaka S, Itakura Y, Date S (1979) Ultrasonic real-time guidance for percutaneous puncture. J Clin Ultrasound 7:269–272
17. Skolnick ML, Dekker A, Weinstein BJ (1978) Ultrasound guided fine needle aspiration biopsy of abdominal masses. Gastrointest Radiol 3:295–302
18. Weinstein BJ, Skolnick ML (1978) Ultrasonically guided antegrade pyelography. J Urol 120:323–327
19. Sumner TE, Crowe JE, Resnick MI (1978) Ultrasonically guided antegrade pyelography of an obstructed solitary pelvic kidney. J Clin Ultrasound 6:262–263
20. Pedersen JF, Cowan DF, Kristensen JK, Holm HH, Hancke S, Jensen F (1976) Ultrasonically guided percutaneous nephrostomy. Radiology 119:429–431

Index